Preparing Nurses for Disaster Management

Preparing Nurses for Disaster Management

A Global Perspective

JOANNE CHAPERLO LANGAN, PhD, RN, CNE
Professor
TB Valentine School of Nursing
Saint Louis University
Saint Louis, Missouri
United States

ELSEVIER

Elsevier
3251 Riverport Lane
St. Louis, Missouri 63043

PREPARING NURSES FOR DISASTER
MANAGEMENT

ISBN: 978-0-323-77676-9

Notice

Practitioners and researchers must always rely on their own experience and knowledge in evaluating and using any information, methods, compounds or experiments described herein. Because of rapid advances in the medical sciences, in particular, independent verification of diagnoses and drug dosages should be made. To the fullest extent of the law, no responsibility is assumed by Elsevier, authors, editors or contributors for any injury and/or damage to persons or property as a matter of products liability, negligence or otherwise, or from any use or operation of any methods, products, instructions, or ideas contained in the material herein.

Senior Content Strategist: Sandra Clark
Content Development Specialist: Dominque McPherson
Publishing Services Manager: Julie Eddy
Senior Project Manager: Cindy Thoms
Design Direction: Margaret Reid

Printed in The United States of America

Last digit is the print number: 9 8 7 6 5 4 3 2 1

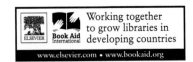

Working together
to grow libraries in
developing countries

www.elsevier.com • www.bookaid.org

I dedicate this book to all who engage in disaster nursing globally, rescue personnel, planning teams, volunteers, and those behind the scenes who work tirelessly to prevent and mitigate the impact of disasters as well as those who assist in recovery. This has been a rewarding journey of teaching and learning.

To my friends who have sustained me throughout this endeavor. To my loving and supportive family:

Husband, Capt. John R. Langan, (USN, Ret.)
Children, John II (wife, Marissa, and
Hadley, Hannah, and Harrison)
Christina (husband, Chad, and Anne
Marie, Nicholas, and Alexis)
Becky (husband, Steve, and Katie, Jack, and Bradley)
LCDR Justin C. Langan, USN (wife, Jen, and
Grace and soon-to-be Baby Langan)

Lavonne M. Adams, PhD, RN, CCRN-K
Associate Professor
Harris College of Nursing & Health Sciences
Texas Christian University
Fort Worth, Texas
United States

Sandy J. Cobb, MSN, FNP-C, RN, REEGT
Graduate Research Assistant
College of Nursing
University of Tennessee Knoxville
Knoxville, Tennessee
United States

Lisa S. Conlon, RN, BSc, MCN, DN
Pre-registration Coordinator
The University of Adelaide
Adelaide, South Australia
Australia

Rhonda K. Cooke, MD
Clinical Pathologist
Laboratory
Missouri Baptist Medical Center
Saint Louis, Missouri
United States

Donna M. Dorsey, RN, MS, FAAN
Regional Disaster Health Service Lead
Disaster Services
American Red Cross Eastern NC Region
Raleigh, North Carolina
United States

Consultant to the Chief Nurse
Office of the Chief Nurse
American Red Cross
Washington, District of Columbia
United States

Jeff F. Evans, RN, BN, MSc, PGCertED, SFHEA
Senior Lecturer, Disaster Healthcare
Faculty of Life Sciences & Education
University of South Wales
Pontypridd
Wales
United Kingdom

Chrystal R. Glinton, BSW
National Emergency Management Agency
(Retired)
Nassau, The Bahamas

Chunlan Guo, PhD
Research Fellow
School of Nursing
The Hong Kong Polytechnic
University
Kowloon
Hong Kong

Karen Hammad, PhD, BN, BN Honours, Graduate Diploma
Associate Director
Torrens Resilience Institute
Daw Park, Adelaide
Australia

Samah Hawsawi, MSN, RN, PhD student
TB Valentine School of Nursing
Saint Louis University
Saint Louis, Missouri
United States

Yoomi Jung, PhD, MSN, BSN
Director
Clinical Nursing Science Department
Korea Armed Forces Nursing
Academy
Daejeon
South Korea

Roberta P. Lavin, PhD, FNP-BC, FAAN
Professor
Nursing
University of New Mexico
Albuquerque, New Mexico
United States

Alice Yuen Loke, RN, PhD, FAAN, FHKAN
Professor, Associate Head of Nursing
The Hong Kong Polytechnic University
Hong Kong
China

Laura Jeanne Mangano, MSN, RN
Graduate Student
School of Nursing
Johns Hopkins
Baltimore, Maryland
United States

Registered Nurse
Neuroscience ICU
VCU Health System
Richmond, Virginia
United States

Xiaorong Mao, PhD, RN
Associate Director
Department of Nursing Research Center
Sichuan Provincial People's Hospital
University of Electronic Science and
    Technology of China
Chengdu, Sichuan
China

Dorcas McLaughlin, PhD, APRN, PMHCNS-BC
Professor
Nursing
Webster University
Saint Louis, Missouri
United States

Charleen C. McNeill, PhD, MSN, RN
Professor
Fran & Earl Ziegler College of Nursing
University of Oklahoma Health Sciences Center
Oklahoma City, Oklahoma
United States

Janice L. Palmer, PhD, RN, CNE
Department Chair and Associate Professor
Nursing
Webster University
Saint Louis, Missouri
United States

Helen Passafiume-Sandkuhl, RN, BSN, MSN, CEN, TNS, CHEP, FAEN
Administrative Director of Nursing
SSM Regional Emergency Medical Services
SSM Saint Louis University Hospital
Adjunct Faculty
TB Valentine School of Nursing
Saint Louis University
Saint Louis, Missouri
United States

Chief Nurse
Missouri Disaster Medical Team
Missouri State Emergency Management
    Agency
Jefferson City, Missouri
United States

Supervisory Nurse
National Disaster Medical Services
Assistant Secretary for Preparedness and
    Response
Washington, District of Columbia
United States

Sallie Shipman, EdD, MSN, RN, CNL, NHDP-BC
Clinical Assistant Professor
College of Nursing
University of Florida
Gainesville, Florida
United States

Jody Spiess, PhD, RN, GCPH
Assistant Professor
Nursing
Webster University
Saint Louis, Missouri
United States

Colleen Kelly Starkloff, RPT
Starkloff Disability Institute
Saint Louis, Missouri
United States

Tener Goodwin Veenema, PhD, MPH, MS, RN, FAAN
Professor
Center for Health Security
Professor
Department of International Health
Johns Hopkins Bloomberg School of Public
    Health
Baltimore, Maryland
United States

FOREWORD

Nursing education for disaster management globally is vital in the second decade of the 21st century. The health threats associated with natural, technological, and human-made disasters are escalating. As I reflect on the situation-at-hand while writing this foreword, it is safe to claim the current global COVID-19 pandemic (ongoing in 2022) has brought into full light the value nursing, public health, communication, and multidisciplinary approaches afford in combatting global health threats. Beyond COVID, nurses globally will continue to be on the frontlines during such disasters. It is my view that we are currently living through a transformative time in our history as a discipline which necessitates us intentionally planning for the future of human and planetary health, drawing upon knowledge of the inextricable interconnectedness of humans, health, and environment. As I reflect on the power nurses have in effecting health especially in the context of crisis and upheaval, including the current pandemic, I am inspired to see a present and future in which nurses in collaboration with other professionals practice with knowledge about the inextricable interconnectedness of humans, health, healing, and the environment. By the transmission and translation of this knowledge, which disaster management nursing is, we can advance the contributions nurses make in advancing the health of the world.

The concepts and strategies presented in this book equip nurses with disaster management knowledge, case examples, experiences, learning activities, toolkits, and specified competencies to respond effectively across a broad range of situations and settings throughout the various stages of disaster management. This book beckons the increasing relevance of disaster management nursing to the world. Its challenge is to present to the largest group of health professionals, nurses and nursing students, a body of knowledge requisite to the fundamental proficiencies to respond effectively. The command to nursing is to provide knowledgeable humanized caring though disaster preparedness, response, and recovery to benefit all humanity. Thus, this book helps the discipline and profession meet a tall order. It is timely, fills a critical need in communicating the evolution of knowledge in disaster management nursing, and reflects well the social contract nurses have with society to protect health, ameliorate suffering, and prevent disease. Disaster management nursing education to prepare nurses globally to respond to human needs emerging in the face of natural, technological, and human-made disasters could not be more important.

Danny G. Willis, DNS, RN, PMHCNS-BC, CNE, HSGAHN, FAAN
Joan Hrubetz Dean and Professor
TB Valentine School of Nursing
Saint Louis University

Each year, hundreds of millions of people across the world are affected by natural and human-made disasters. These events will have a lasting and profound impact on people's health and the communities in which they live. At times, these events will have such an impact that development and progress will be set back for years, even decades leaving individuals and communities vulnerable.

Over the past few years there have been urgent needs to address disasters as a priority area. As such, it has been included as one of the triple billion goals of the World Health Organization to improve the health of billions of people across the world.

Comprehensive progress in this area requires more than the attention of professional responders alone. Each and every one of us has responsibility to protect our homes, communities, and our world. However, nurses have a particular role to play. As the largest providers of health care services in the world, and one of the most trusted professions, the public expects nurses to be there preparing, managing, and responding in times of need.

This book is extremely important and timely. Educators, students, practitioners, and policy makers will find this book a valuable resource of information, ideas, and actions. This book should be used as a reference and resource for all levels of nurses supporting the challenging work that they do and as part of disaster preparedness and practice.

We are living in a time of great complexity with the intersection of a challenging climate in the areas of social, economic, technological, political, and environmental factors. This complex web calls for greater awareness, leadership, social and political acumen, skills, experience, and teamwork. This book, with its collection of expert authors from across the world is a welcome contribution that supports the education and continuing professional development of the nursing profession.

I thank all authors and stakeholders for their contribution and commitment to this valuable resource.

David Stewart, RN, BN, MHN
Adjunct Professor, Queensland University of Technology
Associate Director, International Council of Nurses

PREFACE

It is the belief of every person who contributed to this textbook that every nurse should have the opportunity for basic disaster preparedness education and achieve the related competencies. The *International Council of Nurses Core Competencies in Disaster Nursing, V 2.0* is the foundation of this text. The competencies that every licensed nurse should have in their "tool belt" are listed in this text and applied to the concepts described.

Every nurse needs to be prepared for disasters of all kinds, natural and human-made. We know that disasters will continue to occur, some with little or no warning. Nurses are expected to help victims, rescuers, family members, and friends who have been directly or indirectly affected by mass casualty events. It matters little where nurses live in the world, whether in active practice in acute care, primary care, community-based care or at home in their communities. Nurses are trusted to know what to do and will play key roles in disaster relief. Nurses are obligated to be current in their knowledge base and to provide skilled, competent care.

This textbook will introduce nurses and students to basic disaster nursing concepts and constructs. Some of the contributing authors share their own experiences with disasters and their sequelae. The text begins with basic foundational facts about natural and human-made disasters with a key section on persons with various vulnerabilities and the just treatment of all persons.

Disaster management agencies and organizations are presented in a reader-friendly manner so that all can understand the roles and responsibilities of these essential agencies. With this information, the reader will know where each agency acts in the areas of preparedness, response, and recovery.

Preparedness and Mitigation aspects are treated in the next chapter. If proper time and effort are given to these endeavours, the loss of lives and property can be greatly reduced.

Response efforts including triage and decontamination of survivors are addressed with important assumptions and procedures that must be followed for the greatest good of the greatest number. At times, difficult decisions must be made to distribute scarce resources carefully and ethically.

Recovery efforts are described in a manner that assists communities in reaching some form of normalcy. The Recovery chapter is highly focused on the implications of psychiatric/mental health effects of disasters. The reader will find excellent strategies to assist caregivers in providing comfort to those who have experienced disasters or public health emergencies.

The roles of the general professional licensed nurses and the roles of advanced or specialized nurses follows. Expectations vary for each level of nurses according to the ICN *Core Competencies in Disaster Nursing, V 2.0*. However, nurses need to be made aware of the basic disaster concepts and concepts they are expected to know and apply in their practice settings. A special section is added regarding the responsibilities and difficult decisions encountered by military nurses.

The final chapters describe actual disasters: Natural, Radiation, Chemical, Biologic, or Infectious Disease Outbreaks and Human-Made. Vulnerability Exercises describe methods and toolkits available to assess community risk for disasters. A description of types of Drills follows to help educators and those in service settings to design appropriate drills to fit and test the goals and objectives of readiness efforts.

Most chapters end in Case Study Exercises and "Test Your Knowledge" sections that apply the concepts presented and assist in group discussions and in the evaluation of learning.

I hope this textbook will serve as a resource for those in nursing education and service and provide the impetus toward the achievement of competence in the areas of disaster preparedness, response, and recovery.

Joanne C. Langan, PhD, RN, CNE

ACKNOWLEDGMENTS

I gratefully acknowledge all who have contributed to the creation and completion of this book. I would like to specifically acknowledge:

The SSM St. Clare Emergency Preparedness Team who invited me to serve on their committee, took my advice, and allowed me to share their expertise with my Saint Louis University Emergency Preparedness course students;

Dr. Danny Willis, Professor and Dean, Saint Louis University, TB Valentine School of Nursing, for the support of the Disaster Preparedness course and of this text;

Carol Thomas of Elsevier who put me in touch with the amazing Sandy Clark;

Sandy Clark who ignited the vision for this book and offered sage advice;

The Elsevier team who carefully reviewed and offered excellent edits;

The Society for the Advancement of Disaster Nursing (SADN) colleagues who continue to move forward in preparing nurses to participate in disaster preparedness, response, and recovery Every Nurse a Prepared Nurse is the mission!

Dr. Kristine Gebbie and Mr. David Stewart who invited me to the steering committee and to co-author the *International Council of Nurses Core Competencies in Disaster Nursing, V 2.0*. This work inspired this text and the crucial education of current and future nurses in disaster preparedness on a global level.

CONTENTS

UNIT I: *Overview of Disaster Preparedness   1*

1   Overview of Disaster Preparedness and Considerations for Vulnerable
    Populations   2
    Joanne C. Langan ▪ Colleen Kelly Starkloff

UNIT II: *Stages of Disaster Response   19*

2   Disaster Management Agencies and Organizations, Disaster
    Preparedness and Response Systems, Structures, Logistics,
    and Resources   20
    Sallie Shipman

3   Preparedness and Mitigation   37
    Charleen C. McNeill ▪ Lavonne M. Adams ▪ Rhonda K. Cooke

4   Disaster Response, Triage, and Decontamination   61
    Joanne C. Langan ▪ Rhonda K. Cooke ▪ Helen Passafiume-Sandkuhl

5   Recovery: Promoting Behavioral Health   81
    Dorcas McLaughlin ▪ Jody Spiess ▪ Janice L. Palmer

UNIT III: *Nursing Roles in Disasters and Public Health
           Emergencies   110*

6   Role of the General Professional Nurse   111
    Charleen C. McNeill ▪ Lavonne M. Adams ▪ Lisa S. Conlon ▪ Donna M. Dorsey

7   Role of the Advanced or Specialized Nurse in Public Health,
    Advanced Practice, and Military Service   133
    Alice Yuen Loke ▪ Yoomi Jung ▪ Xiaorong Mao ▪ Chunlan Guo

UNIT IV: *Actual Disasters and Public Health Emergencies   150*

8   Natural Disasters   151
    Joanne C. Langan ▪ Chrystal R. Glinton

9   Preparedness and Response to Radiological Emergencies   171
    Roberta P. Lavin ▪ Laura Mangano ▪ Tener Goodwin Veenema ▪ Sandy J. Cobb

10   Chemical Disasters   194
    Karen Hammad

11   Biological or Infectious Disease Outbreaks   211
    Samah Hawsawi

12   Human-Made Disasters   224
    Joanne C. Langan ▪ Jeff F. Evans

UNIT V: *Anticipating the Future: Brainstorming Exercises*   *237*

13   Anticipating the Future: Hazard Vulnerability Analysis and Resource
     Assessment   238
     Joanne C. Langan

14   Exercises and Drills   248
     Lavonne M. Adams

Appendix A   Core Competencies in Disaster Nursing, Version 2.0   262

Appendix B   Sample List: Readiness Resources and Toolkits   266

Appendix C   Test Answers   270

Index   297

Overview of Disaster Preparedness

Overview of Disaster Preparedness and Considerations for Vulnerable Populations

Joanne C. Langan, PhD, RN, CNE ■ Colleen Kelly Starkloff, RPT

CHAPTER OUTLINE

Introduction   4

Incidence of Natural and Human-Made Disasters: A Global Concern   4

Why Nurses Need to Be Prepared   6

Stages of Disaster Management (Fig. 1.2)   7
Predisaster, Planning, and Mitigation   7
Predisaster and Pre-Impact   8
  Shelter in Place Versus Evacuation of Area   8
Impact and Response   8
Recovery, Reconstruction, and Mitigation   8

Considerations for Vulnerable Populations   10
Independent Living by Persons with Disabilities   10
  Vignette   12

Considerations in Disability Planning and Response   12
  Preparedness Planning   12
  Essential Physical and Communication Needs   12
Issues Faced by Persons with Disabilities During the COVID-19 Pandemic   14
Legal   14

Case in Point   15
Consideration and Planning for Home Evacuation   15
  Questions for Discussion   16

Points to Remember   16

Test Your Knowledge   16

References   17

OBJECTIVES

After reading and studying this chapter, you should be able to:
- Differentiate types of disasters and their impact on the physical, social, economic, and psychological aspects of life.
- List the phases of emergency management and describe the activities associated with each phase.
- Express the value of all nurses having a working knowledge of disaster preparedness, response, and recovery.
- Compare and contrast the competencies of the general professional nurse and the advanced or specialized nurse in at least one of the eight domains in the International Council of Nurses (ICN) *Core Competencies in Disaster Nursing, Version 2.0.*
- Discuss the special considerations for each of three different vulnerable populations in times of disaster preparedness and response.

KEY TERMS

bioterrorism: The use and dissemination of various kinds of microbes or toxins with the intent to intimidate or coerce a government or civilian population to further political or social objectives; humans, animals, and plants are often targets.

chemical terrorism: Attacks meant to cause mass devastation in which terrorist organizations release toxins; chemical attacks meant primarily to terrorize, blackmail, or cause economic damage; a specific attack in a particular product, particularly a food product.

chemical warfare agents: Highly toxic chemicals that can be disseminated as vapors, gases, liquids, or aerosols or adsorbed to dust particles.

disability: A limitation in functional ability resulting from impairment.

disaster: An occurrence, either natural or human-made, that causes human suffering and creates human needs that victims cannot alleviate without assistance.

domestic terrorism: Terrorist acts by individuals or groups within a given country, without foreign direction or involvement.

emergencies: Involve the immediate response to the effects of the event; the immediate community provides assistance or aid because outside sources of aid have not yet arrived or the needs can be satisfied by the immediate community.

human-made disasters: Disaster events, either accidental or deliberate, that are caused by humans; include complex emergencies, technological disasters, and material shortages.

impact stage: A time when the disaster event has occurred and the community experiences the immediate effects; the community is rapidly assessed for damage, types and extent of injuries suffered, and immediate needs.

impairment: Loss of psychological, physiological, or anatomical structure or function.

international terrorism: Terrorist acts directed by foreign groups who transcend national boundaries, affecting people in several countries.

mass casualty event: A situation with a number of casualties that significantly overwhelms available emergency medical services, facilities, and resources.

mitigation: An action taken to prevent or reduce the harmful effects of a disaster on human health or property; involves future-oriented activities to prevent subsequent disasters or to minimize their effects.

natural disasters: Disasters that are caused by nature or emerging diseases.

posttraumatic stress disorder (PTSD): An anxiety disorder that can develop after exposure to a terrifying event or ordeal in which grave physical harm occurred or was threatened.

predisaster stage: Occurs when there is knowledge about an impending disaster; activities include warning, pre-impact mobilization, and evacuation, if appropriate.

radiological and nuclear terrorism: An attack in which a terrorist organization uses a nuclear device to cause mass murder and devastation.

recovery stage: Restoration, reconstitution, and mitigation take place; rebuilding, replacing lost or damaged property, and returning to school and work; when life returns to some semblance of "normal."

response stage: Immediate actions taken to address the needs of those involved in an accident or deliberate act.

terrorism: The systematic use of terror; the deliberate creation and exploitation of fear to bring about political change.

vulnerable: A population or aggregate susceptible to injury, illness, or premature death; those who have special considerations to sustain life including perinatals, neonatals, older persons, persons with disabilities, those with learning and sensory impairments, and the immunocompromised.

Introduction

Disaster preparedness education is imperative for people of varying disciplines, especially in service and health care organizations. This textbook will discuss a variety of actions that nurses should consider in preparing for disasters; responding to disasters; and assisting individuals, families, and communities to return to some degree of normalcy following disaster events. Nurses play key roles in disaster relief whether they are in the emergency department, obstetrics, pediatrics, or general medical surgical units in a hospital, residential facility, ambulartory care, or simply at home in their communities. People throughout the world are sharing an increased awareness of the vulnerability to terrorism. These threats may be bioterrorism, nuclear or chemical weapons, or any number of natural disasters or human-made disasters. This chapter will give an overview of these events and a section to help nurses address special needs of vulnerable populations.

Incidence of Natural and Human-Made Disasters: A Global Concern

Whereas emergencies require a rapid response by appropriate health care and public health officials, disasters typically involve personnel and equipment outside of the community. Most communities are able to respond to and recover from emergencies using their available resources. However, disaster response and recovery require support above and beyond what the community is capable of supplying. This is especially true for mass casualty events when the number of victims overwhelms the available response and health care capacity.

Natural, technological, and human-made disasters occur in every part of the world. Disasters are also classified as either accidental or deliberate. Millions of people are affected by these events through loss of life, property, and basic human needs. In 2018, 394 natural disaster events occurred worldwide. The greatest number of natural disasters that year occurred in Asia. Indonesia experienced the highest number of deaths in the world due to earthquakes and the tsunami in September 2018. In that same year, the United States suffered fatalities from natural disasters in the form of tropical cyclones, wildfires, heat, and drought. Climate change has increased the risk of extreme weather as droughts have become more prevalent and the strength of storms has increased (Fig. 1.1). Elevated levels of water vapor increase storm power and heat in the atmosphere increases ocean surface temperatures, leading to higher wind speeds. As a result, areas that usually are unaffected by the sea become more vulnerable as waves and currents become stronger (Wang, 2019).

It is estimated that worldwide natural disasters in 2018 totaled $160 billion in losses. The costliest natural disaster in 2018 was the Camp Fire in California, which caused $12.5 billion in insured losses. Hurricane Michael in the United States and Cuba resulted in $10 billion in insured losses. Typhoon Jebi in Japan and Taiwan, Hurricane Florence in the United States, and the Woolsey Fire in California caused $9 billion, $5 billion, and $4 billion in losses, respectively (Insurance Information Institute, 2019a, 2019b).

Human-made disasters in 2016 resulted in $8 billion in losses. These catastrophes included fires; explosions; and maritime, aviation, and rail disasters in attrition to terrorism and social unrest. A nuclear power plant generator failure in France and a floating storage and offloading vessel accident in Ghana were the worst human-made disasters in 2016. The deadliest human-made disasters in 2016 were multiple migrant boats capsizing and a church roof collapse in Nigeria, which caused 160 deaths. However, the September 11, 2001, terrorist attack in the United States was the costliest human-made disaster in history (Insurance Information Institute, 2019a, 2019b). Some of these human-made disasters were accidental and others were deliberate acts, such as domestic and international terrorism, intending to inflict great harm and terror in populations. Terrorists use a great number of devices and agents, including biological agents (bioterrorism,

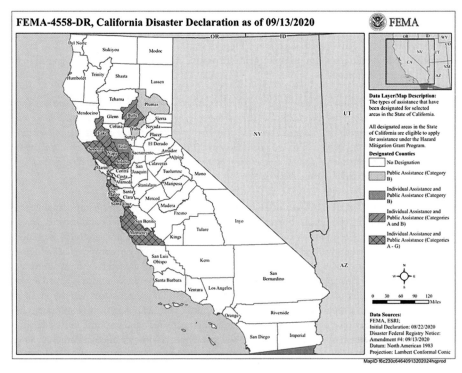

Fig. 1.1 Map of California showing disaster declarations due to wildfires.

agroterrorism), chemical warfare agents (chemical terrorism), and radiological dispersion bombs (radiological and nuclear terrorism).

The international community has developed a universal legal framework against terrorism. The Terrorism Prevention Branch (TPB) of the United Nations Office on Drugs and Crime (UNODC) has been instrumental in providing counterterrorism technical assistance to United Nations member states (UNODC, 2019). All types of disasters have the potential to threaten international peace and security. Caring for populations of people who are affected by these events is truly a global concern.

Top priorities for all who work in disaster preparedness and response are providing relief and shelter to those who have been displaced from their homes and businesses and addressing their health needs. Another priority is the need for information that will guide those who will make critical decisions to help those in need. Disaster preparedness education is imperative for people of varying disciplines. Through collaborative efforts, we can make a difference now and in the future (Khanna, 2017). We have learned that disaster preparedness and response includes the staging of equipment and the appropriate personnel to operate the equipment. Health care professionals, faculty, administrators, students, and volunteers all work together to provide the best services for those in need.

Although all persons in service and health care organizations are essential in their roles in disaster preparedness and response, the primary focus of this text is the preparation of nurses. Nurses are key to disaster relief regardless of their service site, from acute care to community-based care centers to at-home care in their communities.

Why Nurses Need to Be Prepared

In recent years, nurses have experienced many types of war in their own communities. This brings the realization that all nurses, not just emergency department (ED) or military nurses, need to be trained in disaster competencies.

Nurses, as the largest group of committed health personnel, often working in difficult situations with limited resources, play vital roles when disasters strike, serving as first responders, triage officers and care providers, coordinators of care and services, providers of information or education, and counselors. However, health systems and health care delivery in disaster situations are only successful when nurses have the fundamental disaster competencies or abilities to rapidly and effectively respond. (International Council of Nurses, 2019, p. 3)

The ICN (2019) *Core Competencies in Disaster Nursing, Version 2.0* includes eight domains: preparedness and planning, communication, incident management systems, safety and security, assessment, intervention, recovery, and law and ethics. Each domain lists competencies for both the general professional nurse and the advanced or specialized nurse. The first category of competencies addresses expectations for all nurses who have completed a basic nursing curriculum and have been authorized to practice nursing by the regulatory body of their country. This level of expectations is aimed at staff nurses in acute care, clinics, and public health facilities as well as all nurse educators. On the advanced level, nurses who are in a supervisory capacity, who lead nurses within an organization's disaster plan, or who represent nurses on a planning committee and all preparedness and response nurse educators are expected to be competent in a higher level of skills and duties. More detailed information about expectations for both Level I and Level II nurses is presented in other chapters.

In addition to the updated ICN (2019) *Core Competencies in Disaster Nursing, Version 2.0* (see Appendix A), a number of nursing organizations and accreditation bodies are endorsing nurse competencies in disaster nursing. For example, the American Association of Colleges of Nursing (AACN) lists disaster-related content within its published essentials for baccalaureate, master's, and doctoral education (AACN, 2006, 2008, 2011). Additional documents that address disaster preparedness as essential competencies for nurses include those by the World Health Organization (WHO), public health nursing competencies for surge events, and emergency preparedness and response core competencies for perinatal and neonatal nurses (Langan et al., 2017). All nurses, whether students, retired, or working in acute care, long-term care, ambulatory care, or at home in their communities, need to be alert and well informed regarding actions to take to be safe and to preserve life. Nurses are trusted to know the correct, appropriate, and priority steps to take in disasters and public health emergencies and to be able to communicate those actions to others.

If registered nurses are retired or simply not working as licensed nurses but wish to become involved if needed for disaster response and recovery, a number of organizations welcome their assistance. For example, the Red Cross has multiple roles that nurses can engage in to help populations across the globe. The Emergency System for Advance Registration of Volunteer Health Professionals (ESAR-VHP) is another type of volunteer agency. Nurses are invited to preregister on these organizations' websites to verify their licensure status and availability for volunteer service. Volunteer agencies such as these also need to know whether the individual is available to serve, how much predeployment notice is necessary, and the amount of time the volunteer is able to be away from their job and home (Missouri Show-Me Response, n.d.). As the largest segment of the health care workforce (Carlson, 2019), nurses are needed to deliver health care in times of peace, war, disasters, and public health emergencies. To fully understand what might be expected of nurses during disaster preparedness, response, and recovery, it is important that nurses become familiar with the phases of disaster management and the associated activities at each phase or stage.

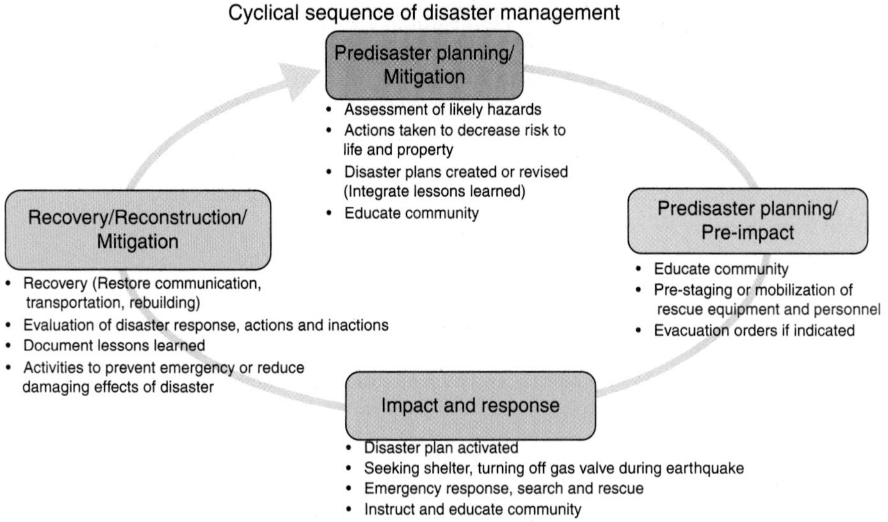

Cyclical sequence of disaster management

Predisaster planning/ Mitigation
- Assessment of likely hazards
- Actions taken to decrease risk to life and property
- Disaster plans created or revised (Integrate lessons learned)
- Educate community

Predisaster planning/ Pre-impact
- Educate community
- Pre-staging or mobilization of rescue equipment and personnel
- Evacuation orders if indicated

Recovery/Reconstruction/ Mitigation
- Recovery (Restore communication, transportation, rebuilding)
- Evaluation of disaster response, actions and inactions
- Document lessons learned
- Activities to prevent emergency or reduce damaging effects of disaster

Impact and response
- Disaster plan activated
- Seeking shelter, turning off gas valve during earthquake
- Emergency response, search and rescue
- Instruct and educate community

Fig. 1.2 The cyclical sequence of disaster management. (Courtesy Joanne C. Langan.)

Stages of Disaster Management (Fig. 1.2)

PREDISASTER, PLANNING, AND MITIGATION

Nurses are integral in all stages of disaster management. To perform well in each phase of disaster management, nurses must understand the work to be accomplished at each stage and what nurses can do to support the effort. Nurses are expected to work within the disaster management system of their own communities; they are not asked to create their own plans of action for community members. At the predisaster stage, much assessment and planning is happening. Communities conduct hazard vulnerability analyses to consider the most likely threats to the community and assess their capabilities for each of the threats. They then use this information to plan, prepare, and implement mitigation activities to prevent or reduce the harmful effects on human life or property. For example, buildings may be reinforced, highway overpasses may be rebuilt, and communication backup systems may be placed. In addition, the predisaster phase calls for a great deal of education for professionals and the public to prepare them for probable and possible disasters and public health emergencies.

Preparedness activities include plans and preparations to help response and rescue operations through collaborative efforts among disaster management agencies and organizations, ultimately to save lives. An important concept is the inclusion of community members and representatives of those potentially affected by the disaster to be present during the creation of the plan. This inclusive, collaborative effort ensures a more thorough plan and buy-in of the plan's directives. Educating the public in disaster readiness includes stocking up of food, water, first aid supplies, medicines, important documents, and comfort items that are necessary for various age groups and family members. This is also a time to conduct public service announcements (PSAs) regarding appropriate times to evacuate the residence, school, or work environment or to shelter in place. If there is a noxious agent in the atmosphere, citizens would be advised to shelter in place. If a building is on fire, not safe, unstable, or deemed unsuitable in any way, its inhabitants must choose the safest evacuation route and alternate care site or shelter. An example of a PSA is the Centers for Disease Control and Prevention (CDC) list of recommendations for public safety behaviors during the COVID-19 pandemic (Box 1.1).

BOX 1.1 ■ Steps to Reduce Your Risk of Getting COVID-19

Practice everyday preventive actions to help reduce your risk of getting sick and remind everyone in your home to do the same. These actions are especially important for older adults and people who have severe chronic medical conditions.

■ Wear a mask when you interact with others.

■ Avoid close contact with people who are sick; keep space between yourself and others.

■ Stay home when you are sick, except to get medical care.

■ Cover your coughs and sneezes with a tissue and throw the tissue in the trash.

■ Avoid touching your eyes, nose and mouth with unwashed hands.

■ Wash your hands often with soap and water for at least 20 seconds, especially after blowing your nose, coughing, or sneezing; going to the bathroom; and before eating or preparing food.

■ If soap and water are not readily available, use an alcohol-based hand sanitizer with at least 60% alcohol. Always wash hands with soap and water if hands are visibly dirty.

■ Clean and disinfect frequently touched surfaces and objects (e.g., tables, countertops, light switches, doorknobs, and cabinet handles).

From Centers for Disease Control and Prevention. (2021). *Steps to reduce your risk*. https://www.cdc.gov/coronavirus/2019-ncov/need-extra-precautions/older-adults.html

---

PREDISASTER AND PRE-IMPACT

Shelter in Place Versus Evacuation of Area

The pre-impact stage is a time when a disaster is imminent but has not yet occurred. It is considered the warning or threat stage. Communities are warned of the impending disaster when there is time to predict the time of impact, pre-staging or mobilization of rescue equipment and personnel are activated, and persons are evacuated if appropriate. Shelters are opened and manned, and emergency supply kits are taken with citizens as they seek safer locations. Citizens are given instructions through PSAs as to whether to shelter in place or evacuate to safer areas or shelters (Box 1.2).

IMPACT AND RESPONSE

At this stage the disaster has occurred and the community is experiencing the effects of the event. Citizens go to the aid of those who need assistance, and agencies outside of the affected area are deployed to assist in search and recovery efforts. Response efforts are started by the local agencies until outside assistance can arrive. Emergency work is often done during the continued impact of the disaster, depending on the scope and degree of damage incurred. Many agencies often set up instruction and recovery aid centers in shelters or prominent areas of the community to assist citizens toward recovery (Fig. 1.3).

RECOVERY, RECONSTRUCTION, AND MITIGATION

Recovery is the stage in which disaster survivors seek to find a new kind of normalcy. Those who are able to rebuild their homes or restore some kind of routine through work, school, and recreation are those who can see an end to the devastation many have experienced. Recovery includes securing financial assistance to help pay for home repairs and replacement of some essential items. However, some survivors are forced to relocate, as their primary residence may be in an area that is

---

BOX 1.2 ■ Emergency Training and Information

General training for all employees should address:
- Individual roles and responsibilities
- Information about threats, hazards and protective actions
- Notification, warning and communications procedures
- Means for locating family members in an emergency
- Emergency response procedures
- Evacuation, shelter and accountability procedures
- Location and use of common emergency equipment
- Emergency shutdown procedures

From: https://www.fema.gov/pdf/library/bizindst.pdf
Emergency Management Guide for Business and Industry A Step-by-Step Approach to Emergency Planning, Response and Recovery for Companies of All Sizes FEMA 141/October 1993 Retrieved Sept. 13, 2021.

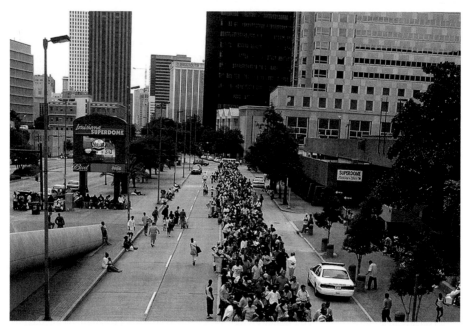

Fig. 1.3 A line to enter a shelter in New Orleans after Hurricane Katrina.

deemed uninhabitable after the disaster event. As expected, the toll on human life and the psyche can be devastating. Post-traumatic stress disorder (PTSD) is common among rescue personnel, health care providers, and disaster survivors. Part of disaster recovery may be postdisaster debriefings or psychiatric or mental health sessions with professionals. This type of support is discussed extensively in a later chapter.

Evaluation and lessons learned from the disaster or public health emergency that just occurred will inform disaster management personnel and planners of what to modify in their disaster preparedness plans. Mitigation work will continue after a disaster, and officials will know what actions need to be taken to prevent or lessen the impact of future disasters. An extensive discussion of disaster preparedness for vulnerable populations follows. All of the stages of disaster preparedness and response are critical to prepare and mitigate the suffering and loss of individuals, families, and communities regardless of a person's ability or inability to help themselves.

Considerations for Vulnerable Populations

The preparedness phase is critical for vulnerable populations, those who have special considerations to sustain life. Those who are susceptible to injury, illness, or premature death often include perinatals; neonatals; older persons; persons with disabilities; those with learning, sensory, and communication impairments; and the immunocompromised; these are all examples of persons who need special consideration in times of disaster. Some individuals have personal or social conditions that make them unusually susceptible, resulting in a decreased ability to cope with traumatic situations. The vulnerability may cause them to be more dependent on assistance from others. Plans must be made for each of these persons to be cared for appropriately in the event of a disaster. For example, persons with special needs may have their names and locations registered with rescue personnel. In this way, if a disaster or public health emergency occurs in that geographical area, rescue personnel are alerted to the appropriate rescue equipment that may be necessary to evacuate or treat individuals safely.

Approximately 1 billion people (15% of the global population) live with some form of disability. This number is expected to double to 2 billion by 2050. It is estimated that 2% to 4% of these individuals experience significant difficulties in functioning. Many of these people require assistive technologies such as low-vision devices, wheelchairs, or hearing aids. Low- and middle-income countries have higher rates of disability than high-income countries, and the impact of disability on people in poorer areas is compounded by issues of accessibility and lack of health care services. Indigenous persons, internally displaced or stateless persons, refugees, migrants, and prisoners with disabilities also face particular challenges in accessing services. In recent years, the understanding of disability has moved away from a physical or medical perspective to one that takes into account a person's physical, social, and political context.

Today, disability is understood to arise from the interaction between a person's health condition or impairment and the multitude of influencing factors in their environment. Great strides have been made to make the world more accessible for people living with a disability; however, much more work is required to meet their needs (WHO, 2020). Sixty-one million adults in the United States live with a disability (CDC, 2019). Although some older adults may experience some type of debilitation or degree of infirmity, most senior citizens do not consider themselves disabled even though their loss of hearing, sight, cognition, limbs, mental health, or mobility puts them in the category of "people with disabilities."

Given the enormous number of people whose needs for support escalate dramatically and instantly in a disaster, it makes sense for nurses to understand the subject of disability from a holistic perspective. Nurses play key roles in acute, long-term, and ambulatory care settings as well as in education, administration, and policy arenas. When a person with a disability is affected by a disaster, they are likely to interact with nurses very soon after a disaster strikes. With education and active drills prior to disasters, nurses' actions become instinctive and effective. Generally speaking, nurses have the training to manage the health care traumas experienced by persons with disabilities, but nurses need further education to understand the intricacies of persons learning to live with specific disabilities and the sequelae of these life-changing events.

INDEPENDENT LIVING BY PERSONS WITH DISABILITIES

Worldwide, an ever-increasing number of people with disabilities are living independently, in their own homes and in communities of their choice. The independent living movement in the United States has defined people with disabilities as "independent" when they are able to make decisions about their own lives and make choices that influence their lives based on access to a reasonable framework of options. This includes hiring, training, and managing people who can provide personal assistance (bathing, dressing, transferring, personal hygiene assistance, housekeeping, shopping, etc.). This new definition of independence does not require a person to do everything for themselves in order to live independently, which is in contrast to how senior communities define independent living. Living independently in the community is possible now because of changes brought about by Section 504 of the Rehabilitation Act of 1973 and the subsequent Americans with Disabilities Act (ADA) of 1990. Curb cuts; lifts on buses; and access to public buildings and spaces, schools and universities, government spaces, airplanes, and more allow persons with disabilities to live and move freely in communities. Housing access lags behind, but people with disabilities make modifications in their homes that are personal to their needs. The internet, technology, and better rehabilitation have leveled the playing field for persons with disabilities to live and work in their communities, which is bring-ing about a change in attitude toward people with disabilities and their capacity to live full, productive, and independent lives. For example, an individual who is quadriplegic due to a car accident would be considered to be living independently if they live in a home, apartment, or condominium in a neighborhood of their choice and have either a spouse or a personal assistant (attendant, caregiver) living with them or available to them on a schedule that they determine. Because this individual decides who to hire, provides training for the personal assistant (PA) in activities of daily living, and arranges to pay the PA (through Medicaid, personal income, or another source) that individual has taken control over their life and is considered to be living independently.

All persons with disabilities who live independently create their own environment and system of supports that make their independence possible. What is independent for one person who is deaf, is blind, has a spinal cord injury, or has some other significant disability may differ from that of another person with the same disability, in terms of choices, living arrangements, and types of job situations. Therefore, in times of disaster, these individuals cannot necessarily recreate their specific environment in a public shelter, hotel, or family or friend's home.

When disaster strikes there is often little or no warning available to the public. For people with disabilities worldwide, preparations to protect, rescue, and save their lives are not well enough established in advance and, therefore, many lives are lost. When an advisory is issued to leave the area, where will disabled people go? People living in their own homes or those in nursing homes have nowhere to go. Visions of seniors sitting in their wheelchairs in 3 feet of water in a nursing home in New Orleans after Hurricane Katrina still haunt many who watched the news about this disaster on television.

Persons with disabilities require, at bare minimum, accessible entrances, bathrooms, and bed-rooms. People on ventilators, with diabetes, are blind or deaf, and children with significant dis-abilities such as cerebral palsy, forms of muscular dystrophy, or Down syndrome all have very specific needs for medications, personal assistance, technology, electricity, communication, and more. These are the people who first responders encounter in their homes or institutions in disaster situations.

When cities set up emergency shelters in large public spaces, such as convention centers, there are likely accessible public restrooms. However, transfer devices, medications, technology, people who understand and are skilled in assisting people with significant disabilities, and so on are often nonexistent in such emergency shelters. Persons with disabilities often end up at hospitals. Where will they go upon discharge?

The following vignette relates the true-to-life experience of a man with a disability and his wife and their unfortunate encounters as a result of the health care providers' assumptions.

Vignette

Colleen Kelly Starkloff, a physical therapist (PT) by training, who married Max Starkloff in 1975, learned so much about living with disability that she ended her career as a PT after 3 years of practice and got involved in the emerging independent living/disability rights movement in the United States. Colleen remarked that her husband, quadriplegic at C3, C4, and C5 resulting from a car accident was continually considered remarkable by nurses and doctors whenever he went to a hospital for health care. They were surprised that he was married; had children; had a full-time job; and was a local, national, and international disability rights leader. Upon discharge, nurses were surprised that he would return home to his family rather than to a nursing home.

A nurse's attitude toward a person living with disability is critical to that person's health outcome, in and out of the hospital. Often a nurse is the first person someone with a disability will meet in a hospital or clinical setting. First impressions matter. If nurses greet a person with disabilities with lowered expectations for their health care outcomes and their capacity to live a normal life, this has a negative impact on that person, often for quite a long time. Conversely, if a nurse is positive toward someone with a disability, expecting them to live a normal life in their community, shored up by the supports needed to do so, such as accessibility and personal assistance, the impact can be tremendously uplifting for that person and their family. A nurse can offer great hope for the future to someone with a disability.

Colleen saw this firsthand once when her husband was rushed to the ED. The ED doctor knew that Max needed intubation and asked if there was a Do Not Resuscitate (DNR) order before she would attempt intubation to protect his airway. The Starkloffs were very offended. This happened on the hospital floor as well. Max lived to age 73 and died of the flu, not from complications related to his spinal cord injury. Max Starkloff and millions of Americans with disabilities live lives worth living. This encouragement can begin with that first interaction with a nurse in a wide variety of settings.

CONSIDERATIONS IN DISABILITY PLANNING AND RESPONSE

Preparedness Planning

The best preparation is to have people who are able to evacuate to a safer environment do so. However, first responders and health care professionals must be prepared to rescue and treat people with disabilities who have no place to go and who are likely to be heavily represented at mass care areas (Fig. 1.4). Preparing for disaster responses must include factors that affect people with disabilities. It is imperative to have people with disabilities on disaster preparedness teams. Disaster preparedness guides are available to assist with disability preparedness planning (Kailes, 2020).

Kailes (2020) emphasizes the importance of making emergency shelter programs accessible, which includes the physical, equipment, programmatic, and effective communication access required by the ADA.

Essential Physical and Communication Needs

Physical access in shelters: Accessible entrances (level or slightly sloping ramps), wide doorways (at least 32 inches wide), accessible restrooms, and portable shower units.

Signage: Clear directional signage with text; accessibility logo and arrow showing locations of accessible parking, entrances, and restrooms.

Communication access: Televised public announcements must include sign language interpreters and open captions; access to sources of communication for use by the public to contact family or support services such as computers, cell phones, and charging stations.

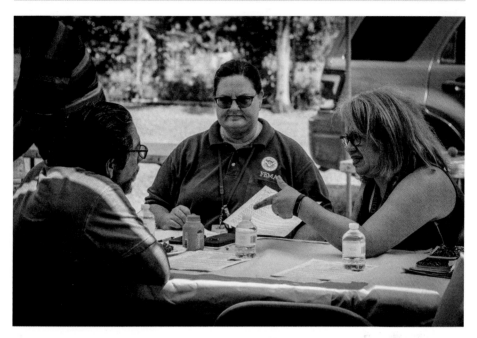

Fig. 1.4   Federal Emergency Management Agency (FEMA) disability integration staff.

Transportation: Identification and location of people who require transportation assistance and have vehicles with lifts available for emergency evacuation or rescue as soon as rescuers begin searching for people who need this assistance. In the case of flooding, boats that will accommodate people in wheelchairs should be available.

Personal assistance: Having continued access to personal assistance through a family member, friend, paid attendant, or nurse can mean the difference between life and death. PAs must be welcomed in hospitals, clinics, and shelters and provided with personal protective equipment (PPE) and medical care supplies in order to ensure their safety and ability to continue to provide personal assistance to persons with disabilities. They also can help with communication and cooperation by persons affected by disaster, displacement, and subsequent worry. Nurses also can teach persons with disabilities and their attendants about new ways to better care for themselves. This continuation of personal assistance support can prevent institutionalization. For persons with disabilities who have worked hard to create an independent lifestyle in the community of their choosing, having to live in a nursing home is unacceptable.

Loss of electricity: For those who must have electricity to operate their durable medical equipment (DME)—ventilators, suction machines, wheelchairs, scooters, computers, cell phones, nebulizers, power transfer devices, electric beds, refrigerators to keep medications safe, and so many more supports in their daily lives—loss of electricity is dangerous and life-threatening. It is life-saving to have a generator in their home, but most persons with disabilities cannot afford to buy and install a home backup generator.

Communication: Individuals who are deaf or hard of hearing are particularly dependent on sign language interpreters during disasters, to be aware of impending disasters, and guidance on what to do once a disaster occurs. Sign language interpreter certifications for health care settings should be RID (Registry of Interpreters for the Deaf) Advanced, RID Master, BEI (Board for Evaluation of Interpreters) Advanced, or BEI Master. In disasters where such

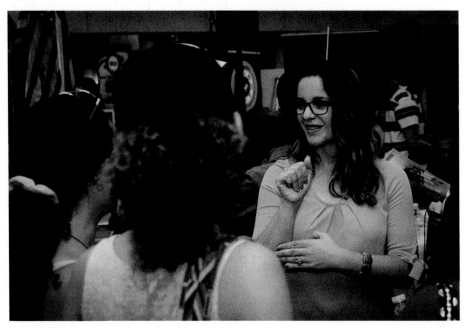

Fig. 1.5   An American Sign Language interpreter.

qualified interpreters are not available to nurses, a family member or friend should be welcomed to help with communication. Telehealth can be used in disasters, but sign language interpreters who work for relay companies are not trained to handle health care communication and should be used only when there is no other option (Fig. 1.5).

Personal protective equipment (PPE): Access to PPE is essential for all people to protect themselves and others from disease spread. The disability community quickly realized during the COVID-19 pandemic that PAs need to be classified as "essential workers" who should be provided with PPE.

ISSUES FACED BY PERSONS WITH DISABILITIES DURING THE COVID-19 PANDEMIC

Persons with disabilities were losing their PAs during the COVID-19 pandemic for several reasons; PAs had contracted the virus; they had children to care for at home during school closures; they did not have access to PPE, causing them to feel unsafe working in their clients' homes. Persons with disabilities did not feel safe having PAs who also worked for other clients in their homes, regardless of access to PPE. In addition, PAs did not feel safe working for persons who did not have access to PPE for themselves or their PAs. Nursing homes quarantined their residents. People living in nursing homes died after exposure to COVID-19, brought into the nursing home by staff who did not have PPE (Fig. 1.6).

LEGAL

Persons with disabilities worry that crisis standards of care will cause them to "go to the end of line" for health care during disasters. Several statements reiterating disability rights in disasters have been

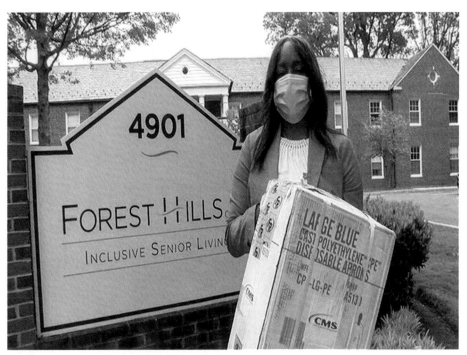

Fig. 1.6 A nursing home employee with personal protective equipment (PPE).

issued by the US Department of Health and Human Services (HHS) regarding the same rights to treatment, visitors, communication, and supports during situations such as pandemics. The HHS Office for Civil Rights in Action (2020) clarified protections provided to persons with disabilities to receive equal access to health care under Section 504 of the Rehabilitation Act of 1973 and the subsequent ADA of 1990. On April 14, 2020, the Healthcare Resilience Task Force (2020; composed of HHS, the Federal Emergency Management Agency [FEMA], and the Army Corps of Engineers) issued documents titled *Crisis Standards of Care* and *Civil Rights Laws*. Both of these documents assert that disabled people have the same right as anyone else to health care in disaster situations and to deny care is illegal and discriminatory. (See additional resources in Appendix B.)

In summary, all persons must be considered during each phase of disaster preparedness, response, and recovery. The gravity of this work and the intense time commitment needed to achieve a dynamic disaster preparedness plan are acknowledged. However, the effort will contribute to multitudes of persons saved from harm or death and the protection of property for individuals, families, communities, tribes, and populations around the world.

Case in Point

CONSIDERATION AND PLANNING FOR HOME EVACUATION

Ms. L. lives in a low-lying area that is less than half a mile from the river. Her house is not on stilts. She is a young, single mother with an infant. She also cares for her mother who has multiple health comorbidities and is on oxygen and has difficulty walking. It has been raining for 7 days straight, and Ms. L. has heard that the river has breached the levee 10 miles upstream.

Questions for Discussion

1. What should Ms. L.'s immediate plan include?
2. If she decides to evacuate her home, what should Ms. L consider taking with her?
3. What items should be taken for the care of the infant?
4. What items should be taken for the care of her mother?

Points to Remember

- Natural disasters are events caused by nature or emerging diseases and include floods, tornadoes, earthquakes, volcanoes, tsunamis, hurricanes, mudslides, avalanches, epidemics, and famine.
- Human-made disasters are complex emergencies, technological disasters, material shortages, and other disasters not caused by natural means and either accidental or deliberate.
- Each country, geographical location, city, town, or village needs to assess the most likely disasters or public health emergencies that might occur. This assessment informs the disaster management planners in steps to take to mitigate or prevent damage to human lives or property.
- Nurses in all practice settings or at home in their communities are trusted to know what to do in emergency situations. Nurses are essential at every step of disaster preparedness, response, and recovery cycle.
- Persons with disabilities, regardless of their disability, have the right to be treated equally as those without disabilities; to deny care based on disability is discriminatory and illegal.
- Disability and other "special considerations" experts must be included in local disaster planning efforts.
- Access to communication supports, personal assistance, and accessibility is a must.
- A nurse's attitude toward persons with disabilities living independent lives is critical to persons with diabilities' independence and health outcomes.

Test Your Knowledge

1. Which of the following is an example of an accidental disaster?
   a. A car loaded with bombs that steers into a bus loaded with passengers
   b. A fuel tanker that runs aground due to poor visibility in a storm
   c. Anthrax spores that are disseminated to a large population through the mail
   d. A toxic agent that is discovered in a jar of baby food
2. The final stage of recovery after a disaster, which involves future-oriented activities to prevent subsequent disasters or to minimize their effects is called:
   a. Reconstruction
   b. Recovery
   c. Mitigation
   d. Reconstitution
3. The types of activities that occur during the pre-disaster or pre-impact stage include: *(Choose all that apply.)*
   a. Rescue equipment is pre-staged
   b. Citizens are evacuated to safe areas
   c. Rescue and recovery teams are mobilized
   d. Public service announcements are made to instruct communities on appropriate safety actions

4. After a disaster event, which of the following actions should take place? *(Choose all that apply.)*
   a. Review actions taken that were most helpful
   b. Review actions taken that were of little use
   c. Transfer the persons who made errors to a different department
   d. Modify the disaster plan to include lessons learned

5. Mitigation includes which of the following activities? *(Choose all that apply.)*
   a. Reinforcing existing structures
   b. Building new structures to withstand the forces of a disaster
   c. Recruiting and preparing volunteers to assist in disaster prevention, preparedness, and relief efforts
   d. Extensive education for health care providers in multiple settings about types of injuries that might occur in future disasters

6. Key activities that occur during the preparedness stage include: *(Choose all that apply.)*
   a. Plans and preparations made to save lives and help with response and rescue operations
   b. Evacuation plans that include routes, shelters, and alternate care sites
   c. Stocking food and water
   d. Mobilizing rescue units and equipment

7. Responding safely in an emergency includes: *(Choose all that apply.)*
   a. Actions taken to save lives and prevent further immediate damage
   b. Putting preparedness plans into action
   c. Seeking shelter
   d. Turning off gas valves in an earthquake

8. Recovery from an emergency or disaster situation takes time. Some of the activities during the recovery stage include: *(Choose all that apply.)*
   a. Actions taken to return to normal
   b. Return to one's home to inspect the damage
   c. Getting financial assistance to pay for home repairs
   d. Making one's home safer than it was prior to the disaster

9. Which of the following persons would be considered vulnerable and need special consideration by nurses in a disaster situation? *(Choose all that apply.)*
   a. Near-term pregnant woman
   b. Person who is sight impaired
   c. Person who is hearing impaired
   d. Person who does not understand the primary language where the disaster is occurring

10. An example of a deliberate human-made disaster is:
    a. A multiple-car pileup on the highway during a snowstorm
    b. A technological block in services due to a rodent entering a power generator
    c. Multiple deaths after patrons ate anthrax-contaminated food from a restaurant salad bar
    d. A storm surge that floods a community

References

American Association of Colleges of Nursing. (2006). *The essentials of the doctoral education for advanced nursing practice.* https://www.aacnnursing.org/Portals/42/Publications/DNPEssentials.pdf.

American Association of Colleges of Nursing. (2008). *The essentials of baccalaureate education for professional nursing practice.* https://www.aacnnursing.org/Portals/42/Publications/BaccEssentials08.pdf.

American Association of Colleges of Nursing. (2011). *The essentials of master's education in nursing.* https://www.aacnnursing.org/Portals/42/Publications/MastersEssentials11.pdf.

Carlson K. *2020 is the year of the nurse: Is your organization preparing?.* : MultiBriefs: Exclusive; 2019. http://exclusive.multibriefs.com/content/2020-is-the-year-of-the-nurse-is-your-organization-preparing/medical-allied-healthcare.

Centers for Disease Control and Prevention. (2019). *Disability and health promotion.* https://www.cdc.gov/ncbddd/disabilityandhealth/infographic-disability-impacts-all.html#:~:text=61%20million%20adults%20in%20the,is%20highest%20in%20the%20South.

Healthcare Resilience Task Force. (2020). *Crisis standards of care and civil rights laws.* https://files.asprtracie.hhs.gov/documents/crisis-standards-of-care-and-civil-rights-laws-covid-19.pdf.

Insurance Information Institute. (2019a). *Facts + statistics: Global catastrophes.* https://www.iii.org/fact-statistic/facts-statistics-global-catastrophes#Natural%20andMan-made%20Disasters.

Insurance Information Institute. (2019b). *Facts + statistics: Man-made disasters.* https://www.iii.org/fact-statistic/facts-statistics-man-made-disasters.

International Council of Nurses. (2019). *Core competencies in disaster nursing, version 2.0.*

Kailes JI. *COVID-19 challenges in college reopening plans for students with disabilities.* : The Partnership for Inclusive Disaster Strategies; 2020. https://disasterstrategies.org/blog-post/covid-19-challenges-in-college-reopening-plans-for-students-with-disabilities/.

Khanna G. *Pulling together in a time of need.* : Agency for Healthcare Research and Quality; 2017. https://www.ahrq.gov/news/blog/ahrqviews/pulling-together.html.

Langan JC, Lavin R, Wolgast KA, Veenema TG. Education for developing and sustaining a health care workforce for disaster readiness. *Nursing Administration Quarterly.* 2017;41(2):118–127.

Missouri Show-Me Response. (n.d.) FAQ. https://www.showmeresponse.org/faq.php.

United Nations Office on Drugs and Crime. (2019). *Terrorism prevention.* https://www.unodc.org/unodc/en/terrorism/index.html.

US Department of Health and Human Services Office for Civil Rights in Action. (2020, March 28). *Bulletin: Civil rights, HIPAA, and the coronavirus disease 2019 (COVID-19).* https://www.hhs.gov/sites/default/files/ocr-bulletin-3-28-20.pdf.

Wang T. *Annual number of natural disaster events globally from 2000–2018.* : Statista; 2019. https://www.statista.com/statistics/510959/number-of-natural-disasters-events-globally/.

World Health Organization. (2020). *Disability.* https://www.who.int/health-topics/disability#tab=tab_1.

Stages of Disaster Response

Disaster Management Agencies and Organizations, Disaster Preparedness and Response Systems, Structures, Logistics, and Resources

Sallie Shipman, EdD, MSN, RN, CNL, NHDP-BC, CNE

CHAPTER OUTLINE

Introduction	22	Resources and Logistics	31
Emergency Preparedness		Personal and Family Preparedness	31
Organizations and Frameworks	23	Communication—Incident	
Global/Regional Level	23	Management Systems	32
National/Regional Level	24	Exercises and Lessons Learned	32
Community/Local/State Level	28	Case in Point	33
Principles of Health Care Emergency		Formation of a Rural Hospital Health	
Preparedness and Disaster		Care Coalition	33
Management	29	Questions for Discussion	33
Emergency Preparedness Steps for		Points to Remember	33
Health Care Systems Planning	29	Test Your Knowledge	33
Threat Assessment and Risk Management	29	References	35
All-Hazards and Mass Casualty Incidents	30		
Operational Readiness	31		

OBJECTIVES

After reading and studying this chapter, you should be able to:

- Define emergency preparedness and disaster management organizations on the community, national, and global levels.
- Identify emergency planning frameworks to assist with health care planning.
- Discuss the steps needed for health care system emergency preparedness planning.
- Explain the importance of threat assessment and risk management.
- Define a mass casualty incident.

- Appreciate the benefits of an all-hazards approach to planning.
- Recognize health care system challenges regarding resources and logistics.
- Describe the importance of personal and family preparedness.
- Explain the importance of the National Incident Management System.
- Define the importance of exercises and lessons learned in emergency preparedness.

KEY TERMS

all-hazards: Assuring that the emergency response can address any type of situation that can affect society and the health of people, including both natural (e.g., hurricanes, tornados, earthquakes) and human-made (e.g., terrorist attacks, mass shootings, cybersecurity breach) events.

emergency: An event or threat that produces or has the potential to produce a range of consequences that require urgent, coordinated action.

emergency preparedness: The knowledge, capacities, and organizational systems developed by governments, response and recovery organizations, communities, and individuals to anticipate, respond to, and recover from the impacts of likely, imminent, emerging, or current emergencies.

emergency response plan (ERP), standard operating procedure (SOP), or emergency operations plan (EOP): A document describing how an agency or organization will manage its response to emergencies. An ERP describes the objectives, policies, and concept of operations (CONOPS) for the response, as well as the structure, authorities, and responsibilities to make that response systematic, coordinated, and effective.

health care coalition: A group that supports a collaboration between and among health care agencies and assists the community during planning, response, and recovery.

mass casualty incident (MCI): An event that overwhelms the local health care system with a number of casualties that vastly exceeds the local resources and capabilities in a short period of time.

national disaster management agency (NDMA): The equivalent bodies at subnational and local levels often designated as responsible for coordinating preparedness and response to many types of emergencies, including those caused by natural and technological hazards.

plan: A document designed to identify, at various levels, responsibility for a range of activities aimed at meeting specific objectives and implementing accompanying strategies and tactics.

public health event: Any event that may have negative consequences for human health, including events that have not yet led to disease in humans but have the potential to cause human disease through exposure to infected or contaminated food, water, animals, manufactured products, or environments.

risk: The potential for an unwanted outcome resulting from an incident or caused by systemic degradation, as determined by its likelihood, associated consequences, and vulnerability to those consequences.

risk assessment: The process of identification of risks that could occur along with prioritization of those risks based on the needs and capability of the community.

risk communication: How the agency communicates with people in the community so that they can make informed decisions to address their potential emergency risk.

risk management: Coordinated activities to direct and control risk in order to minimize potential harm. These activities include risk assessments; implementing risk treatment or response measures; and evaluation, monitoring, and review.

Introduction

On January 30, 2020, the World Health Organization (WHO) declared a Public Health Emergency of International Concern for COVID-19, a novel coronavirus, which led to the largest public health emergency response of our lifetime (WHO, 2020a). The unbelievable magnitude and scale of this event affected millions of people across the globe, but we must remember that this disaster started with patient number one in a local community in Wuhan, China. A view from the local perspective highlights the essential point that "the most effective disaster response and recovery efforts are locally developed and executed, state/tribal/territorially managed, and federally supported" (White House Office of Intergovernmental Affairs, 2018, p. 2) and each level of the preparedness planning and response should support the local community (WHO, 2017a, 2017b) where the people "live, learn, work, and play" (Riley, 2010).

The COVID-19 response also highlighted the importance of resources, logistical supply chains, and the structures that provide the foundation of our health care system. Shortages of personal protective equipment (PPE), ventilators, and medications created many challenges for those working on the front lines of this public health emergency (Ranney, Griffeth, & Jha, 2020) (Fig. 2.1). Nurses found themselves thrust into this public health emergency response, caring for patients with COVID-19 in hospitals and clinics, demonstrating unquestionably the importance of health care workers, and the role they play in emergency preparedness planning and response. Emergency preparedness is "the knowledge, capacities and organizational systems developed by governments, response and recovery organizations, communities, and individuals to effectively anticipate, respond to, and recover from the impacts of likely, imminent, emerging, or current emergencies" (WHO, 2017a, p. 14).

This chapter outlines the emergency systems currently in practice; however, as in every emergency response, there will be many lessons learned from the challenges of COVID-19, leading to an improved response for future generations (WHO, 2017a, 2017b). This discussion will guide

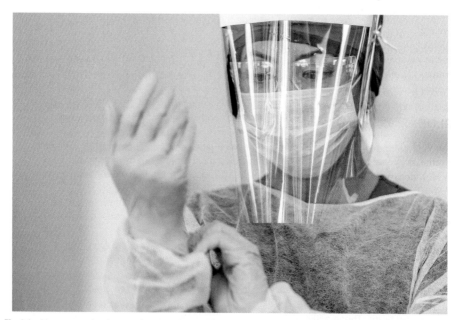

Fig. 2.1 Nurses wearing layers of personal protective equipment and clothing designed to protect from injury or infection. (iStock.com/FatCamera)

the reader to a more thorough understanding of the way in which health is integrated into the overall emergency response. We begin with the agencies and organizations that coordinate planning efforts and provide frameworks. Next, we examine the principles of health care emergency preparedness and disaster management by discussing the emergency preparedness steps for health care systems planning. The structure of the chapter is based on a variation of the WHO (2017a) levels of organization terminology: Global/Regional Level (global and regional countries), National/Regional Level (national and regional governments), and Community/Local/State Level (state and local governments, volunteers, hospitals, clinics, and other agencies on the front line of the response in the community). For the purposes of this discussion, the terms *emergency preparedness* and *disaster management* are used interchangeably.

Emergency Preparedness Organizations and Frameworks

Global and national frameworks guide emergency planners through the process of emergency preparedness planning (Federal Emergency Management Agency [FEMA], 2019; WHO, 2017a, 2017b, 2019). The COVID-19 pandemic demonstrated an unprecedented global response, highlighting the need for emergency preparedness on all levels. Most disaster responses begin in a local community, involve people, and require a coordinated effort where agencies work together to address the emergency. As nurses, we understand that when people are involved, there will be health concerns. The WHO (2017b p.4) defines a public health event as "any event that may have negative consequences for human health." The community is very complex and includes many stakeholder groups, including individuals, families, households, volunteers, nonprofit agencies, private sector, nongovernmental organizations, academia, law enforcement, fire services, emergency medical services, state and local health departments and emergency management agencies, clinics, hospitals, and other agencies who serve on the front lines of the response (FEMA, 2015, 2016b; WHO, 2017a, 2019). In addition, many times the capacity of a disaster exceeds what the local community can handle, causing the needs to progress up the levels of response (WHO, 2017a, 2017b). For instance, the COVID-19 pandemic started with patient number one in Wuhan, China, at a local hospital, then progressed through local, state, and national government levels of response, then to the global level of response of the WHO declaring a Public Health Emergency of International Concern (WHO, 2020b).

GLOBAL/REGIONAL LEVEL

The WHO was enacted on April 7, 1948, and is divided into six regional offices: Africa, Americas, Southeast Asia, Europe, Eastern Mediterranean, and Western Pacific (WHO, 2020a). Several WHO documents aid with global, regional, national, and community emergency planning. *A Strategic Framework for Emergency Preparedness* provides guidance for member regional offices and countries (WHO, 2017a) (Fig. 2.2). This document outlines the role of the WHO in responding to public health events and emergencies:

1. Undertake a timely, independent and rigorous risk assessment and situation analysis.
2. Deploy sufficient expert staff and material resources early in the event/emergency to ensure an effective assessment and operational response.
3. Establish a clear management structure for the response in-country, based on the Incident Management System.
4. Establish coordination with partners to facilitate collective response and effective in-country operations.
5. Develop an evidence-based health sector response strategy, plan, and appeal.

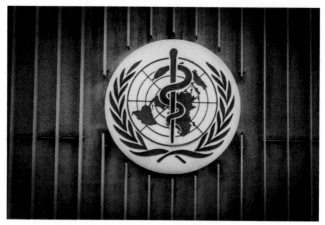

Fig. 2.2 World Health Organization symbol. (iStock.com/Ekaterina79)

6. Ensure that adapted disease surveillance, early warning, and response systems are in place.
7. Provide up-to-date information on the health situation and health sector performance.
8. Coordinate the health sector response to ensure appropriate coverage and quality of essential health services.
9. Promote and monitor the application of technical standards and best practices.
10. Provide relevant technical expertise to affected Member States and all relevant stakeholders. (WHO, 2017b, pp. 10–11)

Health Emergency and Disaster Risk Management Framework (EDRM) helps planning agencies develop a comprehensive emergency planning approach. The Health EDRM components and functions for emergency planning efforts are (1) policies, strategies, and legislation; (2) planning and coordination (national, subnational, local); (3) human resources; (4) financial resources; (5) information and knowledge management; (6) risk communications; (7) health care infrastructure and logistics; (8) health and related services (before, during, and after emergencies including routine, emergency, and surge services); (9) community capacities for health; and (10) monitoring and evaluation (WHO, 2019).

Emergency Response Framework (ERF) provides guidance to WHO staff on how to grade and respond to public health events (WHO, 2017b). The criteria the WHO uses for assessing needs impact and operational environment include the scale and scope of the event along with the capacity of the affected country (WHO, 2017b). The WHO grades each public health emergency event on a scale from ungraded to three (3). The grading depends on scale, urgency (of mounting or scaling up the response), complexity, capacity, and reputation risk (WHO, 2017b; Table 2.1). It is important to note that the Centers for Disease Control and Prevention (CDC) and 49 global health security countries are working together to decrease health security risks and to build capacities in the event of outbreaks and pandemics (Cassell et al., 2017). The following sections address the plans and efforts on national, regional, and local or community levels.

NATIONAL/REGIONAL LEVEL

National and state plans must be built to support the community response. The (WHO, 2017a) outlines the following strategic objectives for the national level:
1. Operational readiness to respond to emergencies;
2. Resilient health system;

TABLE 2.1 ■ **World Health Organization (WHO) Levels for Graded Emergencies**

	A public health event or emergency that is being monitored by WHO but that does not require a WHO operational response.
	A single country emergency requiring a limited response by WHO, but that still exceeds the usual country-level cooperation that the WHO Country Office (WCO) has with the Member State. Most of the WHO response can be managed with in-country assets. Organizational and/or external support required by the WCO is limited. The provision of support to the WCO is coordinated by an Emergency Coordinator in the Regional Office.
	A single country or multiple country emergency, requiring a moderate response by WHO. The level of response required by WHO always exceeds the capacity of the WCO. Organizational and/or external support required by the WCO is moderate. The provision of support to the WCO is coordinated by an Emergency Coordinator in the Regional Office. An Emergency Officer is also appointed at headquarters to assist with the coordination of Organization-wide support.
	A single country or multiple country emergency, requiring a major/maximal WHO response. Organizational and/or external support required by the WCO is major and requires the mobilization of Organization-wide assets. The provision of support to the WCO is coordinated by an Emergency Coordinator in the Regional Office(s). An Emergency Officer is also appointed at headquarters, to assist with coordination of Organization-wide inputs. On occasion, the WHE Executive Director and the Regional Director may agree to have the Emergency Coordinator based in headquarters. For events or emergencies involving multiple regions, an Incident Management Support Team at headquarters will coordinate the response across the regions.

From World Health Organization. (2017). *Emergency response framework* (2nd ed., p. 28). https://www.who.int/hac/about/erf/en/

3. One Health at the human-animal-environment interface; and

4. A whole-of-government, whole-of-society approach. (p. ix)

Each nation or country is required to develop emergency preparedness strategies to address disaster management (WHO, 2019). "The national disaster management agency (NDMA) and/or the equivalent bodies at subnational and local levels are often designated as responsible for coordinating preparedness and response to many types of emergencies, including those caused by natural and technological hazards" (WHO, 2017a, p. 5). Many agencies plan and respond on the national-level emergency preparedness efforts. For the purpose of this discussion, we focus on the health components of the United States' national response.

The Federal Emergency Management Agency (FEMA) is a part of the US Department of Homeland Security (DHS) and the NDMA coordinating agency for the United States' overall emergency preparedness response. During times of emergency, the president declares an emergency under the authority of the Robert T. Stafford Disaster Relief and Emergency Assistance Act, as amended, and Related Authorities, which gives FEMA the authority to coordinate national emergency efforts. FEMA has ten regional offices, which provides the agency with the flexibility to scale the response up or down depending on need (FEMA, 2019).

BOX 2.1 ■ National Preparedness System—Five Mission Areas

Prevention: The capabilities necessary to avoid, prevent, or stop a threatened or actual act of terrorism. Within the context of national preparedness, the term "prevention" refers to preventing imminent threats.

Protection: The capabilities necessary to secure the homeland against acts of terrorism and manmade or natural disasters.

Mitigation: The capabilities necessary to reduce loss of life and property by lessening the impact of disasters.

Response: The capabilities necessary to save lives, protect property and the environment, and meet basic human needs after an incident has occurred.

Recovery: The capabilities necessary to assist communities affected by an incident to recover effectively.

From Federal Emergency Management Agency. (2016). *National mitigation framework* (2nd ed., p. 1). https://www.fema.gov/media-library-data/1466014166147-11a14dee807e1ebc67cd9b74c6c64bb3/National_Mitigation_Framework2nd.pdf

---

The National Preparedness System organizes the United States' emergency preparedness efforts into five mission areas—prevention, protection, mitigation, response, and recovery—with the National Preparedness Goal of providing "A secure and resilient nation with the capabilities required across the whole community to prevent, protect against, mitigate, respond to, and recover from the threats and hazards that pose the greatest risk" (FEMA, 2019, p. 5). FEMA's National Planning Frameworks provide emergency planners with guidance for all mission areas to help state and local communities plan for all stages of emergency preparedness (Box 2.1).

FEMA's *National Response Framework* is organized into 15 Emergency Support Functions (ESFs) annexes that provide structure for private and public entities' emergency response. Table 2.2 contains a list of the ESFs and provides an example of how health and medical entities could be supported during an emergency response.

The nursing role best fits into ESF #6 and ESF #8. ESF #6 is mass care, emergency assistance, temporary housing, and human services, which is where mass care shelters are coordinated. ESF #8 is public health and medical services, which includes hospitals, clinics, and all entities involved in the health component of the emergency response (FEMA, 2019). The ESF #8 response includes:

- Assessment of public health/medical needs
- Health surveillance
- Medical surge
- Health/medical/veterinary equipment and supplies
- Patient movement
- Patient care
- Safety and security of drugs, biologics, and medical devices
- Blood and tissues
- Food safety and defense
- Agriculture safety and security
- All-hazards public health and medical consultation, technical assistance, and support
- Behavioral health care
- Public health and medical information
- Vector control
- Guidance on potable water/wastewater and solid waste disposal
- Mass fatality management, victim identification, and mitigating health hazards from contaminated remains
- Veterinary medical support (FEMA, 2016a, p. 2)

TABLE 2.2 ■ **Example Actions an Emergency Support Function (ESF) May Take to Support Stabilizing the Health and Medical Lifeline During Incident Response Operations**

ESF	Example Supporting Actions or Capabilities
ESF #1 Transportation	Coordinate the opening of roads and manage aviation airspace for access to health and medical facilities or services.
ESF #2 Communications	Provide and enable contingency communications required at health and medical facilities.
ESF #3 Public Works & Engineering	Install generators and provide other temporary emergency power sources for health and medical facilities.
ESF #4 Firefighting	Coordinate federal firefighting activities and support resource requests for public health and medical facilities and teams.
ESF #5 Information & Planning	Develop coordinated interagency crisis action plans addressing health and medical issues.
ESF #6 Mass Care, Emergency Assistance, Temporary Housing & Human Assistance	Integrate voluntary agency and other partner support, including other federal agencies and the private sector to resource health and medical services and supplies.
ESF #7 Logistics	Provide logistics support for moving meals, water, or other commodities.
ESF #8 Public Health & Medical Services	Provide health and medical support to communities and coordinate across capabilities of partner agencies.
ESF #9 Search & Rescue	Conduct initial health and medical needs assessments.
ESF #10 Oil & Hazardous Materials Response	Monitor air quality near health and medical facilities in close proximity to the incident area.
ESF #11 Agriculture & Natural Resources	Coordinate with health and medical entities to address incidents of zoonotic disease.
ESF #12 Energy	Coordinate power restoration efforts for health and medical facilities or power-dependent medical populations.
ESF #13 Public Safety & Security	Provide public safety needed security at health and medical facilities or mobile teams delivering services.
ESF #14 Cross-Sector Business and Infrastructure	Be informed of and assess cascading impacts of health or medical infrastructure or service disruptions, and deconflict or prioritize cross-sector requirements.
ESF #15 External Affairs	Conduct public messaging on the status of available health and medical services or public health risks.

From Federal Emergency Management Agency. (2019). *National response framework* (4th ed., pp. 21–22). https://www.fema.gov/media-library-data/1582825590194-2f000855d442fc3c9f18547d1468990d/NRF_FINALApproved_508_2011028v1040.pdf

The lead agency for ESF #8 is the US Department of Health and Human Services (HHS) (FEMA, 2016a). HHS has many offices and agencies that are involved in preparedness efforts, but the main ones that coordinate emergency preparedness efforts are the Office of the Assistant Secretary for Preparedness and Response (ASPR) and the CDC. On the national level, there are many frameworks and tools to help with the steps of the planning process. Technical assistance is provided to health care emergency planners by the Technical Resources, Assistance Center, and Information Exchange (TRACIE), or ASPR TRACIE.

The Centers for Medicare and Medicaid Services (CMS) (governmental) and The Joint Commission (TJC) (private) are the main national agencies that regulate health care facilities' emergency planning efforts and require:

- Emergency operations plans
- Policies and procedures
- Communication plans
- Training and testing
- Integrated health care systems

The CMS outlines health care emergency requirements for agencies that receive federal funding in Medicare and Medicaid programs; Regulatory Provisions to Promote Program Efficiency, Transparency, and Burden Reduction; Fire Safety Requirements for Certain Dialysis Facilities; Hospital and Critical Access Hospital (CAH) Changes to Promote Innovation, Flexibility, and Improvement in Patient Care (CMS, 2019). The TJC's Emergency Management (EM) chapter outlines what is required for health care agencies seeking accreditation (TJC, 2019).

State and local governments can request federal emergency medical supplies and pharmaceutical assistance from the Strategic National Stockpile (SNS) and CHEMPACK, both of which are managed by the CDC. Other national agencies that assist in the ESF #8 response are the US Public Health Service (USPHS) Commissioned Corps, National Disaster Medical System (NDMS), and Federal Medical Stations (FMS) (ASPR, 2019).

COMMUNITY/LOCAL/STATE LEVEL

All levels of emergency preparedness should support the local community level (FEMA, 2019; White House Office of Intergovernmental Affairs, 2018; WHO, 2017a, 2017b). The local and community preparedness planning is a complex process with many stakeholders (FEMA, 2015, 2016b; WHO, 2017a, 2019). The ESFs and planning issues are the same as at the state and county levels, and governmental plans have the same format as the national FEMA plan (FEMA, 2019). Local, regional or area, and state health departments are the lead agencies for the area or district ESF #8 efforts for the state or region, with the goal of supporting health care facilities. The CMS (2019) identifies the following as health care facilities:

- Ambulatory surgical centers
- Home health agencies
- Hospices and hospitals
- Federally qualified health centers
- Rural health clinics
- Critical access hospitals

A health care coalition is a group that supports a collaboration between and among health care agencies and assists the community during planning, response, and recovery. The HHS provides emergency planners with topic collections to assist health care coalitions with administrative issues, models and functions, and response operations (including mutual aid) (ASPR, 2020). A comprehensive document created for the HHS is *Medical Surge Capacity and Capability: The Healthcare Coalition in Emergency Response and Recovery* (Barbera & Macintyre, 2009). This document is a great resource to those communities who wish to create a health care coalition to enhance recovery efforts and to build resilience among their populations.

The focus of local efforts is to create a resilient environment in which the community is self-sufficient and efforts are sustainable during an all-hazards event. Health care planners need to understand that emergency preparedness "is fostered not only by government, but also by individual, organization, and business actions" (FEMA, 2016b, p. 2); therefore, it is essential to solicit wide community support throughout the process. The Community Preparedness Toolkit provides steps to overall community planning: (1) partner identification, (2) team building,

(3) goal setting, (4) community service, and (5) celebrating success (Ready.gov, 2021). FEMA's Individual and Community Preparedness Division provides information to assist communities through the emergency preparedness process. Volunteer agencies and volunteers are also a tremendous resource for the local community, with their understanding of the importance of coordination and training prior to an emergency response. Some communities have local chapters of the National Voluntary Organizations Active in Disaster (VOAD), American Red Cross, and Medical Reserve Corps, which can help provide communities with trained volunteer assistance.

Principles of Health Care Emergency Preparedness and Disaster Management

Emergency situations can occur without warning (e.g., active shooter) or have a slow arrival (e.g., hurricane with several preparation days before landfall) (WHO, 2017b). The WHO (2017a) defines principles for health care emergency preparedness as (1) "safeguarding, maintaining and restoring the health and well-being of communities"; (2) understanding that "communities are critical"; (3) sustaining "political commitment, partnerships, and funding"; (4) realizing that the cost is worth the investment; (5) appreciating that "health systems and emergency preparedness reinforce one another, and along with other systems contribute to the resilience of communities and countries"; (6) using an "all-hazards approach"; (7) using risk management in all planning and response phases; and (8) valuing that a "whole-of-society approach is critical."

EMERGENCY PREPAREDNESS STEPS FOR HEALTH CARE SYSTEMS PLANNING

All levels from the local community to the global level must participate in the emergency planning process and develop a plan for the needs of their agency. The WHO defines a plan as "a document designed to identify, at various levels, responsibility for a range of activities aimed at meeting specific objectives and at implementing accompanying strategies and tactics" (WHO, 2017a, p. 14). Many terms can be used by an agency or organization to identify a plan, *such as emergency response plan (ERP)*, *standard operating procedure (SOP)*, or *emergency operations plan (EOP)*. Regardless of the terminology used to identify the plan, the emergency planning process working directly with key stakeholders and all levels of personnel to identify the why, what, when, who, and how of a potential emergency response is key to any agency or organization (FEMA, 2016b). Emergency preparedness plans must coordinate within all levels and agencies so that duplication of efforts is minimized (Fig. 2.3). Broad stakeholder consensus should be a priority in the planning process (WHO, 2017a).

Threat Assessment and Risk Management

The first steps in developing an EOP are identifying potential threats the community could face and prioritizing. Each community's list of concerns will differ depending on what threats they face in a specific region (FEMA, 2018; WHO, 2017a). FEMA defines risk as "the potential for an unwanted outcome resulting from an incident or caused by systemic degradation, as determined by its likelihood, associated consequences, and vulnerability to those consequences" (FEMA, 2016b, p. 6). Threat and risk assessment is the process of identifying emergency situations that could occur along with prioritizing those risks based on the needs and capability of the community (WHO, 2017a). A coastal community would need to plan for a hurricane, whereas a community located close to a fault line would need to plan for a potential earthquake. Identifying risk is just the beginning; the agency must then use risk management measures by continuing to "emphasize prevention measures to avoid hazards and reduce vulnerability" (WHO, 2017a, p. 3).

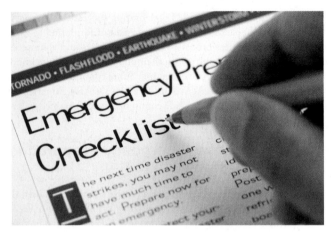

Fig. 2.3 Emergency Preparedness Checklist. (iStock.com\zimmytws)

All-Hazards and Mass Casualty Incidents

An "all-hazards" approach means assuring that the emergency response can address any type of situation that may affect society and the health of people, including both natural (e.g., hurricanes, tornados, earthquakes) and human-made (e.g., terrorist attacks, mass shootings, cybersecurity breach) events (FEMA, 2016b, 2019; WHO, 2017a, 2017b, 2019). Annually, approximately 190 million people are affected directly by emergency events (WHO, 2019). Natural and human-made emergency events also have a significant financial impact, costing an average of $300 billion annually (WHO, 2019). All-hazards planning efforts are not directed to a certain type of emergency event but focus on the structures that support the emergency response and include the ability to scale up or down depending on the need (FEMA, 2019). The response to a small tornado in a town with few casualties might or might not require activation at the state level, whereas a pandemic affecting millions of people would require all levels to respond. The overall emergency response should be seamless and include basic principles for emergency preparedness, with each preceding level supporting the successive level regardless of how many levels are involved (FEMA, 2016b, 2019; WHO, 2017a, 2017b).

Mass casualty (WHO, 2019) or a mass casualty incident (MCI) is "an event that overwhelms the local healthcare system, with number of casualties that vastly exceeds the local resources and capabilities in a short period of time" (Ben-Ishay et al., 2016, p. 1). For example, one person treated in a local emergency department (ED) with pneumonia-like illness is an everyday occurrence, but when clusters of patients demonstrating the same symptoms overwhelm the capacity of the organization's response, the event then progresses to an MCI. In addition, the threshold for an MCI would be much lower in a rural hospital with limited resources than in an urban Level I trauma center located within an academic health system.

Emergency planning efforts must include the potential for an MCI (WHO, 2019). For example, if an agency is using an all-hazards approach to plan for an MCI, measures to address staffing, bed capacity, and supplies must be included. These same needs would exist if the event were a mass shooting or a naturally occurring biological agent. Therefore, planning to improve the overall structure for MCI surge capacity regardless of the reason would be an all-hazards approach. An important document that highlights preparations for MCIs was created for the HHS and is titled *Medical Surge Capacity and Capability: A Management System for Integrating Medical and Health Resources During Large-Scale Emergencies* (Barbera & Macintyre, 2007).

Operational Readiness

Once the potential risks are identified, the agency or organization must develop a plan to prevent, protect, mitigate, respond, and recover from the identified risks, which assures operational readiness (FEMA, 2016b). Local communities are responsible and must take action to assure their emergency preparedness efforts use an all-hazards approach ranging from local to global levels (WHO, 2017a). These arrangements include "political commitment, coordination, risk assessment, infrastructure, preparedness and response plans, financing, human resources, equipment, exercises, and knowledge" (WHO, 2017a, p. 4). One key consideration during the development of an operational plan is making sure that the process involves all stakeholders and does not occur in a silo. In addition, during a disaster response, resources are often limited and the role of the private sector on all levels is vital (WHO, 2017a). The agency must work with stakeholders to identify and build on existing capacities while planning for specialized preparations needed for the entire life cycle of the possible crisis (FEMA, 2016b; WHO, 2017a). Reducing the number and severity of emergencies is essential and requires a tremendous investment, including reinforcement of societal systems to improve access and availability of the community's everyday health infrastructure (WHO, 2017a).

Resources and Logistics

Investing in the local health system community resources and logistics is essential to the success of an emergency response. Health care staff members are a tremendous resource, and a response cannot be completed without adequate staffing. The plan should include an adequately staffed health care workforce that is sufficiently trained with competencies and mixed skills (WHO, 2017a). Resource and logistical capacities of medical inventory and interconnected supply chains also need to be considered when developing an operational plan. COVID-19 was a prime example of the importance of planning for the interconnected nature of the health care system, with health care entities competing directly for essential PPE and other medical supplies (Ranney et al., 2020). Some of the other health system issues required in the operational plan are (CMS, 2019; TJC, 2019; WHO, 2017a):

- Health care workforce (trained and equipped on all levels)
- Volunteers (credentialing and standardized training)
- Structurally and functionally safe hospitals and other health facilities
- Alternate care sites (ACS) (a location or site to which the health care agency can evacuate or relocate)
- Medications, inventory, and PPE supplies
- Crisis standards of care (interoperability, ventilator, oxygen, medical supplies, etc.)
- Infection control and disease surveillance
- Diagnostic and laboratory services
- Health service delivery for people affected by the emergency
- Contingency funds for emergency situations and financing for emergency risk

The importance of financial considerations and continuity of operations planning cannot be overlooked (FEMA, 2016b; TJC, 2019; WHO, 2019). The world is just beginning to realize the financial impact of COVID-19 on the health care system (Cavallo & Forman, 2020). Despite the importance of health care preparedness, there is often a decrease in interest and funding soon after the recovery stage, which can impair future responses (Fig. 2.4) (WHO, 2017a).

Personal and Family Preparedness

Emergency preparedness efforts cannot exist without people, and no health care organization can respond without personnel resources. Both personal and family preparedness are essential to the operational response and overall community (Ready.gov, 2020), but they are crucial for

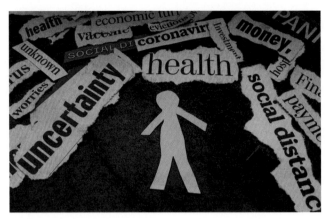

Fig. 2.4   Uncertainty and costs associated with coronavirus. (iStock.com\diegograndi.com)

those required to respond directly to an emergency (California Hospital Association, 2017). For instance, consider the health care worker who is caring for an elderly parent or a child; without a plan to take care of their loved one, this health care worker would not be able to respond. Some steps to take to increase your personal and family preparedness include the following (Ready.gov, 2020):

1. Become familiar with emergency plans in your agency and community.
2. Prepare and practice an emergency plan with your family.
3. Create a family preparedness kit and consider specific needs for your family.
4. Know how you can help or volunteer in your community.
5. Stay informed on all-hazards and seek the most current information on emergency preparedness, basic injury, and disease prevention.

Communication—Incident Management Systems

Communication challenges are often considerable during an emergency response. Each planning agency must consider development of specific measures and programs for training staff on the National Incident Management System (NIMS) and incident command system (ICS) (FEMA, 2019; TJC, 2019). Communication planning is critical to response operations because it outlines the "importance of (1) developing a single set of objectives; (2) using a collective, strategic approach; (3) improving information flow and coordination; (4) creating a common understanding of joint priorities and limitations; (5) ensuring that no agency's legal authorities are compromised or neglected; and (6) optimizing the combined efforts of all participants under a single plan" (FEMA, 2019, p. 11). The agency also must incorporate risk communication into the operational planning. Risk communication is how the agency communicates with people in the community so that they can make informed decisions to address their potential emergency risk (Fig. 2.5) (WHO, 2017b).

Exercises and Lessons Learned

Exercises support emergency preparedness efforts and allow assessment and evidence-based improvement of the EOP (WHO, 2017a). The CMS and TJC require health care agencies to participate in county- and statewide drills and exercises (CMS, 2019; TJC, 2019). Actual responses during which the agency EOP was activated can be used to meet this requirement. Lessons learned during the emergency response provide opportunities to improve the EOP and the overall emergency response (WHO, 2017a).

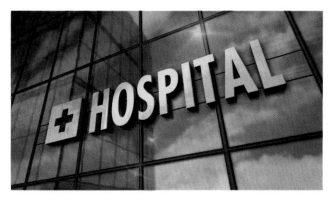

Fig. 2.5 Hospital. (iStock.com\Arkadiusz Warguta)

Case in Point

FORMATION OF A RURAL HOSPITAL HEALTH CARE COALITION

You work in a rural hospital that covers three small counties in your state (total population for the area is 30,000). The closest state health care coalition is located in a large urban county 120 minutes away from your facility. During the COVID-19 pandemic, your facility was the lead for your area's response and does not currently have a local health care coalition. There were many lessons learned from the COVID-19 response and numerous accounts of duplication of services in your area. Nationally and statewide, there has been a 6-month decrease in COVID-19 cases. Your hospital has just appointed you to update your facility EOP and form a new health care coalition that will serve the counties your hospital covers.

Questions for Discussion

1. What is the first thing you should do?
2. Who would you need to involve in your hospital to update the EOP?
3. What stakeholders would you need to seek to serve in your area health care coalition?

Points to Remember

- The importance of emergency planning is often overlooked in nursing and health care. Nurses and other health care providers and agencies need to learn and prepare before the next disaster happens.
- Global and national frameworks guide emergency planners through the process of emergency preparedness planning.
- Local communities are responsible and must take action to assure that their emergency preparedness efforts use an all-hazards approach ranging from local to global levels.
- Nurses must be involved and act because emergency preparedness is a continuous, never-ending process and should remain in the forefront long after a disaster has passed.

Test Your Knowledge

1. The emergency planner understands that global and national frameworks are meant to:
   a. Guide planners through the planning process
   b. Provide specific local community plans

   c. Be followed in the same way in every community

   d. Include all threats and risks the local community may face

2. Which type of approach involves assuring that the emergency response can address any type of situation that can affect society and the health of people?

   a. All-hazards

   b. Mass casualty

   c. Emergency operations plan

   d. Standard operating procedure

3. Which of the following is the potential for an unwanted outcome resulting from an incident or caused by systemic degradation, as determined by its likelihood, associated consequences, and vulnerability to those consequences?

   a. Risk

   b. All-hazards

   c. Mass casualty

   d. Emergency preparedness

4. An emergency planner understands that which of the following reduces loss of life and property by lessening the impact of disasters?

   a. Mitigation

   b. Response

   c. Recovery

   d. Protection

5. An emergency planner understands that planning efforts should be developed to support which of the following levels?

   a. Local

   b. Global

   c. National

   d. Regional

6. A hospital emergency planner is coordinating with a medical supply company when developing the EOP. The planner is doing this for all of the following reasons except:

   a. Abundance of medical supplies

   b. Overlap in the supply chain

   c. Competition securing medical supplies

   d. Secure minimal amounts of PPE

7. Which of the following statements is true?

   a. The CMS and TJC require health care agencies to conduct at least five drills each year.

   b. The CMS and TJC require that exercises that are created by the WHO be used.

   c. An actual emergency response cannot be used to meet the exercise requirements of the CMS and TJC.

   d. An actual emergency response can be used to meet the exercise requirements of the CMS and TJC.

8. What should the emergency planning team do first when developing an EOP?

   a. Conduct a threat and risk assessment

   b. Develop a local health care coalition

   c. Conduct an agencywide drill

   d. Develop a list of operational issues

9. Communication planning is critical to response operations because it outlines the importance of: *(Choose all that apply.)*

   a. Developing a single set of objectives

    b. Improving information flow and coordination

    c. Creating multiple forms to customize for each agency

    d. Optimizing the combined efforts of all participants

10. Which of the following statements is accurate regarding an MCI?

    a. An MCI is the same for any health care agency.

    b. An MCI is declared more often in urban acute care settings than in rural settings.

    c. An MCI is any event that overwhelms the local health care system, as it exceeds the capabilities of that system.

    d. An MCI is declared when the number of victims exceeds 100.

References

Barbera, J. A., & Macintyre, A. G. (2007). *Medical surge capacity and capability: A management system for integrating medical and health resources during large-scale emergencies.* US Department of Health and Human Services, Office of the Assistant Secretary for Preparedness and Response. https://www.phe.gov/Preparedness/planning/mscc/handbook/Documents/mscc080626.pdf.

Barbera, J. A., & Macintyre, A. G. (2009). *Medical surge capacity and capability: The healthcare coalition in emergency response and recovery.* US Department of Health and Human Services. https://www.phe.gov/Preparedness/planning/mscc/Documents/mscctier2jan2010.pdf.

Ben-Ishay, O., Mitaritonno, M., Catena, F., Sartelli, M., Ansaloni, L., & Kluger, Y. (2016). Mass casualty incidents—Time to engage. *World Journal of Emergency Surgery, 11*(8). https://doi.org/10.1186/s13017-016-0064-7.

California Hospital Association. (2017). *Personal preparedness.* https://www.calhospitalprepare.org/personal-preparedness.

Cassell, C. H., Bambery, Z., Roy, K., Meltzer, M. I., Ahmed, Z., Payne, R. L., & Bunnell, R. E. (2017). Relevance of global health security to the US export economy. *Health Security, 15*(6), 563–568. https://doi.org/10.1089/hs.2017.0051.

Cavallo, J. J., & Forman, H. P. (2020). The economic impact of the COVID-19 pandemic on radiology practices. *Radiology, 296*, E141–E144. https://doi.org/10.1148/radiol.2020201495.

Centers for Medicare and Medicaid Services. (2019). Medicare and medicaid programs; regulatory provisions to promote program efficiency, transparency, and burden reduction; fire safety requirements for certain dialysis facilities; hospital and critical access hospital (CAH) changes to promote innovation, flexibility, and improvement in patient care. https://www.federalregister.gov/d/2019-20736.

Federal Emergency Management Agency. (2015). *Effective coordination of recovery resources for state, tribal, territorial, and local incidents.* https://www.fema.gov/media-library-data/1423604728233-1d76a43cabf-1209678054c0828bbe8b8/EffectiveCoordinationofRecoveryResourcesGuide020515vFNL.pdf.

Federal Emergency Management Agency. (2016a). *Emergency Support Function #8—Public health and medical services annex.* https://www.fema.gov/media-library-data/1470149644671-642ccad05d19449d2d-13b1b0952328ed/ESF_8_Public_Health_Medical_20160705_508.pdf.

Federal Emergency Management Agency. (2016b). *National mitigation framework* (2nd ed.). https://www.fema.gov/media-library-data/1466014166147-11a14dee807e1ebc67cd9b74c6c64bb3/National_Mitigation_Framework2nd.pdf.

Federal Emergency Management Agency. (2018). Threat and hazard identification and risk assessment (THIRA) and stakeholder preparedness review (SPR) guide: Comprehensive preparedness guide (CPG) 201 (3rd ed.). https://www.fema.gov/media-library-data/1527613746699-fa31d9ade55988da1293192f1b1 8f4e3/CPG201Final20180525_508c.pdf.

Federal Emergency Management Agency. (2019). *National response framework* (4th ed.). https://www.fema.gov/media-library-data/1582825590194-2f000855d442fc3c9f18547d1468990d/NRF_FINALApproved_508_2011028v1040.pdf.

Office of the Assistant Secretary for Preparedness and Response. (2020). *About ASPR.* https://www.phe.gov/about/aspr/Pages/default.aspx.

Ranney, M. L., Griffeth, V., & Jha, A. K. (2020). Critical supply shortages—The need for ventilators and personal protective equipment during the COVID-19 pandemic. *New England Journal of Medicine, 382*(18), e41. https://doi.org/10.1056/NEJMp2006141.

Ready.gov. (2020). *Make a plan*. https://www.ready.gov/plan.

Ready.gov. (2021). *Community preparedness toolkit*. Ready.gov/community-preparedness-toolkit.

Riley, R. (2010). *Health starts where we learn*. Robert Wood Johnson Foundation. https://www.rwjf.org/content/dam/farm/articles/articles/2010/rwjf69396.

The Joint Commission. (2019). *Hospitals emergency management (EM)*. https://store.jcrinc.com/assets/1/7/cc_hap_em.pdf.

United States (US) Health and Human Services (HHS) Office of the Assistant Secretary for Preparedness and Response (ASPR). (2020). About ASPR. Retrieved from https://www.phe.gov/about/aspr/Pages/default.aspx.

White House Office of Intergovernmental Affairs. (2018). *Recovery through federal-state-local partnership*. https://www.hsdl.org/?view&did=826534.

World Health Organization. (2017a). *A strategic framework for emergency preparedness*. https://www.who.int/ihr/publications/9789241511827/en/.

World Health Organization. (2017b). *Emergency response framework* (2nd ed.). https://www.who.int/hac/about/erf/en/.

World Health Organization. (2019). *Health emergency and disaster risk management framework*. https://www.who.int/hac/techguidance/preparedness/health-emergency-and-disaster-risk-management-framework-eng.pdf?ua=1.

World Health Organization. (2020a, June 17). *About WHO*. https://www.who.int/about.

World Health Organization. (2020b, April 28). *Rolling updates on coronavirus disease (COVID-19)*. https://www.who.int/emergencies/diseases/novel-coronavirus-2019/events-as-they-happen.

CHAPTER 3

Preparedness and Mitigation

Charleen C. McNeill, PhD, MSN, RN ▨ Lavonne M. Adams, PhD, RN, CCRN-K
▨ Rhonda K. Cooke, MD

CHAPTER OUTLINE

Introduction	38	Nurses' Professional Preparedness	49
Systems Preparedness	38	Education for Disaster Response	49
Plan Development and Considerations	39	Culturally Appropriate Preparedness Measures	51
Planning Tools and Resources	39	Nurse Personal Preparedness	51
Types of Plans	40	Preparing Clients with Increased Needs After a Disaster	52
Communication	42		
Disaster Risk Reduction and Mitigation	43	**Case in Point**	55
Resource Management	44	Personal and Professional Emergency Preparedness for Nurses: An Exemplar	55
Blood Products	44	Questions for Discussion	56
Preparedness for Schools of Nursing and Volunteers	45	**Points to Remember**	56
Personal and Professional Preparedness	45	**Test Your Knowledge**	56
Overview of Personal and Professional Emergency Preparedness	45	**References**	58
Personal Preparedness	46		

OBJECTIVES

After reading and studying this chapter, you should be able to:
- Describe the relationship of **preparedness** to disaster risk reduction.
- Identify key elements of surge capacity.
- Differentiate between contingency capacity and crisis capacity.
- Identify your professional emergency preparedness and potential knowledge gaps.
- Identify your personal emergency preparedness plan for potential scenarios.
- Identify client considerations and needs related to emergency preparedness plans.

KEY TERMS

collaboration: Problem solving with others using a network of adaptive capacities and resources such as economic development, social capital, information, and communication to rebuild the community.

disaster risk reduction (DRR): Preventing new and reducing existing disaster risk and managing residual risk, all of which contribute to strengthening resilience and to the achievement of sustainable development.

preparedness: A crucial element in the efforts to mitigate loss, injury, and damage from disaster; requires awareness of disaster risk.

resilience: The ability of a system, community, or society exposed to hazards to resist, absorb, accommodate to, and recover from the effects of a hazard in a timely and efficient manner, including through the preservation and restoration of its essential basic structures and functions.

surge capacity: Level of resources required to meet the needs of the specific event in a given setting.

vulnerable populations: Those at risk or susceptible to physical or emotional harm.

Introduction

As disasters and public health emergencies occur throughout the world with increasing frequency and impact, the global community has responded by exploring and identifying action steps to improve disaster planning and **resilience** at national, regional, and local levels. Disaster planning efforts are now beginning to place an emphasis on **disaster risk reduction** (DRR), which the United Nations International Strategy for Disaster Reduction (UNISDR) describes as being "aimed at preventing new and reducing existing disaster risk and managing residual risk, all of which contribute to strengthening resilience and therefore to the achievement of sustainable development" (UNISDR, 2017, Disaster risk reduction, para 1). Preparedness is a crucial element of these efforts to mitigate loss, injury, and damage from disaster and requires awareness of disaster risk. This chapter provides an overview of methods and resources available to promote systems, professionals, and personal preparedness. The chapter is divided into two parts, addressing the systems perspective first then moving to personal and professional preparedness.

Systems Preparedness

Disaster preparedness includes efforts undertaken to reduce the effects of disasters, with the goals of preventing or diminishing the impact on **vulnerable populations** and promoting effective response to and recovery from such events (International Federation of Red Cross and Red Crescent Societies [IFRC], 2020). Preparedness is not considered an end point but rather a continuous, integrated process of DRR activities, requiring contributions from multiple areas within the community (IFRC, 2020). Disaster preparedness in health care does not have a specific definition but includes interrelated components that contribute to mitigation of negative consequences following an emergency or disaster event. Components frequently cited as crucial to preparedness include having adequate knowledge and skills; plans, procedures, and mutual aid agreements; sufficient human and physical resources; effective coordination and communication; and intentional community engagement, particularly with vulnerable populations (Heagele, 2017; Verheul & Duckers, 2019).

All disasters begin at a local level. In the context of a disaster or public health emergency, the community may be defined as "any group of people associated by a common tie or interest" (Centers for Disease Control and Prevention [CDC], 2018b, p. 2). Communities are complex systems that may include people directly affected by the event and their families, first responders, health care systems and providers, local governmental entities, nongovernmental organizations (NGOs), educational institutions, local business, and media (CDC, 2018b). Building trust within the community and promoting active community engagement in disaster planning is vital to preparedness (World Health Organization [WHO], 2018a).

PLAN DEVELOPMENT AND CONSIDERATIONS

Planning Tools and Resources

Nurses can be crucial assets in DRR and should be prepared to play an active role in all phases of disasters, including planning and decision making (International Council of Nurses [ICN], 2019). To fully embrace this role, nurses must first become familiar with planning documents and frameworks used within their home countries, regions, states, territories, provinces, and local communities. For example, in the United States, public health nurses must use the National Response Framework (US Department of Homeland Security [DHS], 2019) to articulate and evaluate core capabilities designed to engage the whole community in efforts to achieve the National Preparedness Goal of "a secure and resilient nation with the capabilities required across the whole community to prevent, protect against, mitigate, respond to, and recover from the threats and hazards that pose the greatest risk" (DHS, 2019, p. 1). Additional valuable resources are available from the US Department of Health and Human Services (DHHS) Office of the Assistant Secretary for Preparedness and Response (ASPR) through ASPR's Technical Resources, Assistance Center, and Information Exchange (TRACIE), which serves as a gateway for health care emergency preparedness information, providing stakeholders at all levels and in all sectors with access to information, technical resources such as planning tools and templates, and assistance to support improvement in all phases of disaster-related efforts (ASPR, 2020). The CDC (2019) outlines standards for preparedness and response capabilities of public health departments and offers multiple resources to promote effective emergency preparedness and response at the state, local, tribal, and territorial levels.

The WHO (2017) provides a variety of resources, including benchmarking tools and a strategic framework, to aid countries around the world in efforts to strengthen public health capacities. An additional resource is the Sendai Framework for Disaster Risk Reduction (UNISDR, 2015), a voluntary United Nations agreement that is a key aspect of UNISDR's efforts toward DRR, with goals of reducing disaster risk and promoting resilience. The Sendai Framework encourages enhancement of DRR capacities by ensuring a role for multihazard management of disaster risk for scenarios in any location, of all scales, across all sectors, and of any ensuing environmental, technological, and biological risks and health impacts (Aitsi-Selmi & Murray, 2016). Fig. 3.1 provides an example of a framework integrating health into DRR strategies. The next step is for nurses to operationalize relevant response frameworks throughout all phases of disasters, which will entail identifying and planning how to mobilize resources necessary to mitigate the effects of an emergency or disaster event. Because all disasters begin at a local level, nurses who are well connected in the community are crucial assets in maximizing effectiveness of the local planning process. Awareness and use of international frameworks such as the Sendai Framework does not supersede awareness and use of frameworks commonly used within a nurse's home country.

Nursing experts recommend that effective disaster planning include complex issues such as provision of mass care under austere conditions, consideration of behavioral health services and psychosocial support throughout the disaster cycle, identification of and planning for vulnerable populations, and implementation of effective systems to maximize professional and volunteer participation in disaster situations (Association of Public Health Nurses [APHN], 2013; Jakeway et al., 2008). The ICN asserts that nurses' capabilities have not been fully used in disaster planning and advocates for nurses to equip themselves to participate fully in all phases of disasters and in policy making that promotes DRR (ICN, 2019). Nurses' active engagement in disaster planning can aid emergency planners who do not have experience as health care providers to develop cohesive, proactive plans that reflect appropriate and clearly identified health priorities (Veenema et al., 2016).

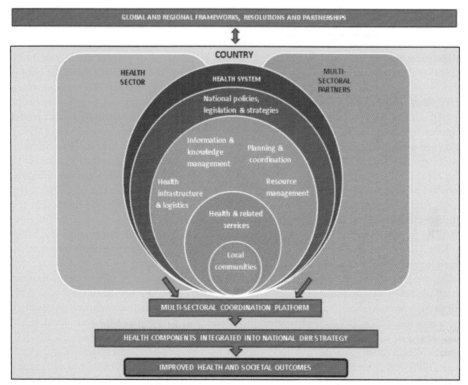

Fig. 3.1 Framework integrating health into disaster risk reduction (DRR) strategies and illustrating the use of partnerships across all levels and systems. (From Aitsi-Selmi, A., et al. [2016]. Reducing risks to health and wellbeing at mass gatherings: The role of the Sendai Framework for Disaster Risk Reduction. *Int J Inf Dis, 47*, 101–104.)

Types of Plans

Disaster risk is defined by the UNISDR as "the potential loss of life, injury, or destroyed or damaged assets which could occur to a system, society or a community in a specific period of time, determined probabilistically as a function of hazard, exposure, vulnerability and capacity" (UNISDR, 2017, Disaster risk reduction, para 1). Comprehensive mitigation and preparedness approaches will entail all-hazards planning, agent-specific planning, and contingency planning. Effective preparedness planning requires identification of and preparedness planning for all hazards likely to occur in a given locale and making an effort to minimize vulnerability and risk of exposure. It is vital to be aware of potential exposure to hazardous materials such as chemical or radioactive compounds, fuel, or agents of bioterrorism (e.g., anthrax), each of which would require a specific response to counteract damage from that agent. In the event that exposure does occur, contingency planning is necessary to address distribution of casualties in light of capacity.

Capacity, and the related concept of **surge capacity**, does not have a single definition or measurement standard; however, key components typically agreed upon are referred to as the 4 S's of staff, "stuff," structure, and systems. *Staff* is the personnel needed to manage an event, *stuff* refers to necessary supplies and equipment, *structure* refers to facilities, and *systems* are policies and procedures (Hick et al., 2009; Watson et al., 2013). Effective preparedness plans must consider the level of capacity required to meet the needs of the specific event in a given setting. Several areas of capacity must be considered: conventional, contingency, and crisis. When the needs of the event

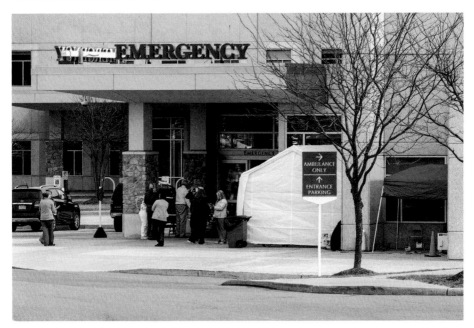

Fig. 3.2 Tents set up for COVID-19 testing in Reading, Pennsylvania. Efforts to prevent COVID-19 positive patients from potentially transmitting the virus to other patients in the emergency department resulted in the need to set up an area outside the facility for testing. (iStock Stock photo ID: 1213482448)

can be met with the amount of staff, supplies, and space consistent with daily institutional operations, conventional capacity is used. An example of this is when a mass casualty incident triggers activation of an institutional emergency operation. When the demand for staff, supplies, and space needed to treat patients exceeds what is available for daily institutional operations but has limited or no impact on the institution's typical patient care practices, contingency capacity is used. Contingency practices can be used on a temporary basis during a major event or in a sustained fashion when incident demands outpace community resources. When space, staff, and supplies have been adapted to provide sufficient care during a catastrophic disaster but are inconsistent with usual standards of care, crisis capacity is being used. This occurs when the event is severe enough that standards of care must be adapted to "provide the best possible care to patients given the circumstances and resources available" (Hick et al., 2009, p. S60).

It is important to note that an event can trigger different effects in different institutions, depending on size, role in the community, and functional ability of community infrastructure; contingency or crisis care may be reached even if an event does not overwhelm assets in all of the areas (Hick et al., 2009). Effective systems preparedness requires that health care facilities consider protection and allocation of resources in the event that contingency or crisis plans must go into effect. In-hospital considerations may include placing limitations on elective procedures to ensure that resources such as personal protective equipment (PPE) are available for critical situations and limiting visitors to decrease risk of exposure to pathogens. Triage may need to be set up outside the hospital to streamline direction to the most appropriate treatment area or to prevent mixing infectious or contaminated patients with those who are noninfectious or noncontaminated (Fig. 3.2). Preparedness for contingencies and crises extends to care facilities and settings outside the hospital, particularly if the number of patients within the hospital overwhelms the system; alternate care sites may need to be sought. For example, outpatient care centers or surgical centers may be helpful to care for patients with lower acuity needs.

Once made, preparedness plans must be tested to ensure that participants are familiar with their roles and to identify gaps and areas for improvement. Chapter 14 provides further details about disaster exercises.

COMMUNICATION

Broad community engagement during the planning cycle is crucial and entails more than message delivery on the part of disaster planners. It requires listening and responding to community needs, connecting with segments of the community that are harder to access, implementing community input into decision making, and ensuring meaningful roles for the community during the response phase (CDC, 2018b). Building a strong base of positive, supportive relationships with stakeholders is vital to the success of the plan. Community stakeholders include but are not limited to local governments and their offices of emergency management (OEMs), public health departments, NGOs or community service organizations (particularly those with a specific mission related to humanitarian disaster response or recovery), and community faith-based organizations (CFBOs). Various communication approaches include strategic emergency risk communication (WHO, 2018a), crisis communication (CDC, 2018a), and crisis emergency risk communication (CERC). Each type of communication requires an understanding of the community, with consideration given to all segments of the community including their unique structures, cultures, and lifestyles (WHO, 2018a). Communication techniques range from delivery of printed messages, media presentations, press conferences, social media use, mass communication such as phone auto-dial or email and text alert notification systems. The best dissemination approach is based on the nature of the event and the community's specific characteristics. Effective communication plans should be designed to anticipate the occurrence of rumors and various communication challenges, with clearly identified methods to dispel misinformation and manage challenges.

The specific approach to plan communication ultimately will rely on several factors, including the availability and quality of information, time frame in which decisions must be made, and potential impact of decisions. Risk communication provides an opportunity for experts and those whose survival, health, or socioeconomic well-being are threatened to mitigate effects of hazards through real-time exchange of information and ideas that promotes informed decision making (WHO, 2018b). The community's response does not necessarily have to be immediate. A step beyond risk communication is crisis communication, a process in which an organization or entity conveys facts to the community about an emergency involving the organization that is beyond its control and requires an immediate response (CDC, 2018a). The most critical level of communication is CERC, which requires urgent communication from experts (who themselves may be affected by the event) and immediate response to an emergency for which limited information is available. Despite the limits of imperfect or incomplete information and narrow time frames, CERC messaging still must be designed to "explain, persuade, and empower decision-making" (CDC, 2018a, p. 4) on the part of affected community members. Examples of decisions that individuals may need to make during situations requiring CERC are:

- "Should I seek medical treatment?"
- "Do I need to treat my drinking water?"
- "Should I evacuate my home?"
- "Should I keep my child home from school?" (CDC, 2018a, p. 4)

Systems preparedness requires consideration of communication within and between organizations or agencies and agreement on who is in charge of the situation, particularly in an event involving multiple agencies. In the event of a disaster, a clear reporting structure (sometimes referred to as "command and control") must exist to ensure a coordinated response through the efficient flow of crucial information for operational and logistic decision making. Responders from outside an organization, such as fire, rescue, and law enforcement, also must be aware of the reporting structure, communication approaches, and overall emergency plans. Examples of approaches to multiagency response coordination are the incident command system (ICS) and National Incident Management System (NIMS) in the United States.

DISASTER RISK REDUCTION AND MITIGATION

A crucial element in the disaster cycle is resilience, which UNISDR (2017) defines as "the ability of a system, community, or society exposed to hazards to resist, absorb, accommodate to and recover from the effects of a hazard in a timely and efficient manner, including through the preservation and restoration of its essential basic structures and functions." Members of resilient communities play significant roles when rebuilding after a disaster through **collaboration** and problem solving with others and through a network of adaptive capacities and resources such as economic development, social capital, information, and communication (Moore et al., 2013; Norris et al., 2008; Uscher-Pines et al., 2013) (Fig. 3.3). Development of such networks requires engagement of a broad range of stakeholders over time because no single entity can preserve and restore community systems after a disaster, and successful relationships are not likely to be built on the day of a disaster. When nurses know the community well, they are ideally positioned to facilitate community-partnered collaboration through previously established connections to community health-related networks and resources vital to developing emergency preparedness plans and policies (APHN, 2013). Effective disaster plans consider risks from multiple likely hazards as well as local context and resources (Chandra et al., 2013; Pfefferbaum et al., 2015). Thus, it is crucial for nurses to develop a thorough understanding of the community's disaster risks as well as ongoing awareness of resources to promote resilience.

As resilience becomes better understood, nurses can serve as champions for "dual-purpose opportunities" that strengthen the community against future hazardous events while also enhancing general community health and well-being (Plough et al., 2013). When such activities take place, they should also address the needs of populations within the community that face particular challenges during disaster recovery, including economically, physically, and age-vulnerable individuals (Heagele, 2017). Nurses can play a key role in increasing public sensitivity to such issues and in promoting interprofessional collaboration among multiple entities, including public health departments, emergency management departments, health care organizations, and CFBOs (Adams, 2016; Heagele, 2017), to protect community members and ensure that their unique perspectives on disaster resilience and preparedness can be addressed (Rooney & White, 2007). Vulnerable populations within the community must be clearly identified through analysis of individual and household determinants, community characteristics, and community infrastructure (Bergstrand et al., 2015). To connect effectively with members of vulnerable populations, it may be useful to collaborate with NGOs that routinely interact with them, such as community centers, home health agencies, senior centers, mobile meal services, and CFBOs (Heagele, 2017).

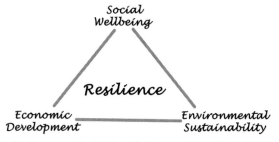

Fig. 3.3 Components of resilience contributing to resilient communities. (iStock Stock photo ID: 825420246)

Such entities often effectively buffer against health disparities, providing information, supplies, direct services, and access to diverse community populations (Acosta et al., 2013; Adams et al., 2018; Heagele, 2017, Plough et al., 2013). They can be highly effective partners in promoting health and disaster risk reduction because of their familiarity with the community's culture and resources; ability to communicate effectively with their constituents; and commitment to engage in community dialogue, disaster planning and decision making; and action (Adams et al., 2018).

RESOURCE MANAGEMENT

Resource management preparation requires consideration of surge capacity; specifically, whether, the affected community or organization is able to "obtain adequate staff, supplies and equipment, structures and systems to provide sufficient care to meet immediate needs of an influx of patients following a large-scale incident or disaster" (Adams, 2009, para 30). The key elements of surge capacity are interwoven with each other and can be complicated by other factors such as finances, transportation, and logistics. A recent illustration of challenges to surge capacity is the COVID-19 pandemic. Among its challenges were:

- A global supply chain disruption that limited availability of PPE (supplies, systems).
- The lack of PPE, leading to staff concerns about safety as well as potential cross-contamination and infection of patients and staff (supplies, staff).
- Illness decreasing availability of staff (staff).
- Variations in approach to testing and use of testing systems, limiting the ability to contain viral spread (systems).
- The increase in patients, limiting available hospital beds for all patients (structure).
- The increase in patients requiring ventilators, leading to a potential shortage of ventilators (supplies).

An ongoing challenge to surge capacity and resource management involves blood products. The next section addresses this highly specialized resource.

Blood Products

During mass casualty events, blood components currently on the shelves are used for bleeding patients, most of whom receive the majority of blood products during the immediate resuscitation period. The time required for blood component collection, processing, infectious disease testing and quarantine, and transport means that products collected after the disaster will not be available until at least the third day post collection. During past events, blood donors have overwhelmed blood collection facilities, drawing blood donor center personnel away from dispensing blood products and ultimately resulting in wastage of components (Schmidt, 2002). This reality highlights the necessity of a stable and robust nationwide blood supply.

In a mass casualty event, all blood products are needed: red blood cells for acute blood loss and to maintain blood volume; plasma for coagulation support, to reverse anticoagulation, and to treat dilutional coagulopathy in patients who have received large amounts of donor components; and platelets to assist clotting, particularly in patients who take antiplatelet medications. When available, cryoprecipitate may be used to supply coagulation factors with less volume compared to plasma. The urgent need for numerous blood components to be transfused quickly in multiple patients presents challenges to the hospital laboratory in general and the blood bank in particular. To dispense emergency-release, uncross-matched products, laboratory computer systems require a patient to be registered, even if only as a John or Jane Doe. To dispense cross-matched and type-specific products, the patient needs a confirmed blood type, preferably drawn prior to receipt of donor blood components, and testing for antibodies to common red blood cell antigens. Patients commonly develop antibodies as a result of pregnancy or from previous transfusions. A positive antibody screen will complicate provision of compatible products in some patients and can result in serious, or even life-threatening, hemolytic reactions if red blood cells positive for the implicated antigen are transfused before antibody identification. Level I trauma centers and some smaller community hospitals have massive transfusion protocols (MTPs) to provide blood components in fixed ratios in a streamlined manner. However, even at facilities with MTPs in place, blood component demand for multiple patients may outstrip the ability of available transfusion service personnel to dispense sufficient products quickly. Depending on the available inventory of specific blood components, demand may exceed supply. Most hospitals keep only a small inventory of group O, Rh-negative red blood cells, and these may be reserved for trauma patients whose ABO type is unknown and women of childbearing age (to prevent maternal alloimmunization). Group O, Rh-negative donors make up only 7% of the donor population (American Red Cross, 2020a), but their red blood cells are the type most needed by emergently bleeding patients who present to a hospital. Increasingly, lean laboratories have limited staff on weekends and overnight shifts, who may cover multiple laboratory areas, particularly at smaller community hospitals.

Disaster preparedness and mass casualty drills are informative and often highlight obstacles to timely blood provision in emergency situations. Delays in registration and proper identification of patients, confusion when multiple unidentified unconscious patients arrive in close proximity, and emergency department staff who are caring for multiple critical patients at one time strain hospital resources, alter established protocols, and often provoke "shortcuts" to processes that protect patient safety. When a patient is bleeding out on the emergency department floor, it may be difficult to understand the blood bank's demand to immediately send a sample for blood typing and antibody screening. However, if specimens are not drawn until after the patient has received multiple donor components, the testing performed will not truly be testing the patient's blood, and it may be impossible to determine the patient's original blood type. This can delay the provision of type-specific blood products and further exhaust the limited hospital supply of valuable group O, Rh-negative red blood cells.

PREPAREDNESS FOR SCHOOLS OF NURSING AND VOLUNTEERS

A disaster or emergency event may strain a community's ability to meet health needs effectively. Community preparedness should thus consider how to expand capacity by developing systems that promote effective collaboration among first responders, health care professionals, and volunteers. Nurses can support community capacity through advocacy of stronger, better coordinated volunteer systems that allow timely deployment of human resources, liability protection, and loss reduction of those who respond (Veenema et al., 2016). Nurses also can play a key role in promoting interprofessional and interagency training and exercises and in engaging those who can assist with such activities, including nurses who are either retired or not employed full-time, students, and volunteers (Jakeway et al., 2008). Although including prelicensure students as part of community surge capacity can be challenging, successful models of community-academic partnerships exist (Adams et al., 2015).

Personal and Professional Preparedness

OVERVIEW OF PERSONAL AND PROFESSIONAL EMERGENCY PREPAREDNESS

Personal emergency preparedness involves being ready for emergencies wherever nurses frequently spend time. This might include one's place of employment, home, car, or anywhere else frequented. The US Ready Campaign (Ready.gov, 2021) prescribes four steps to personal emergency preparedness: Be Informed, Make a Plan, Build a Kit, and Get Involved. These tenets of personal emergency preparedness emphasize the need to know what risks exist locally to facilitate an understanding of what might need to be done before, during, and after an emergency. As stated earlier in this chapter, nurses must know how to obtain information during emergencies. Awareness of how emergency alerts are delivered locally is critical to staying informed, as some governments use multiple delivery systems (text, radio, internet, and television sources) to inform the public. Nurses also must understand the local risks and hazards of the area in which they live so they can plan appropriate response measures. Having an emergency supply kit facilitates the ability to quickly evacuate or shelter in place, depending on the nature of the emergency or disaster. Planning family responses to disruptions in routines is also important. The dynamic within and needs of every family are different and require variations in the plans made and contents of emergency supply kits. Consideration must be given to the needs of each member of the family when crafting response plans and building emergency supply kits to ensure that they are tailored to specific needs. Contents of emergency supply kits are discussed in greater detail in the Personal Preparedness section. The fourth tenet of the US Ready Campaign (Ready.gov, 2021) is to Get Involved before an emergency happens. This tenet involves the entire community's participation, working together to make their community safer and more resilient, and is integral to systems preparedness. Nurses can get involved by volunteering at work, where they can practice essential skills or volunteering in the community to support response efforts (e.g., emergency response shelters).

Professional preparedness involves "the knowledge, skills, abilities, and comprehensive functions required for preparedness and response to natural or man-made emergencies and disasters" (Pourvakhshoori et al., 2017, p. 40). The ICN (2019) provides guidance on the core competencies of disaster nursing (discussed in detail in Chapter 6), which outline the skills and knowledge that enable nurses to respond to a disaster. Nurses must seek continuing education opportunities (online or locally delivered courses) and practice opportunities (e.g., drills and exercises) to fully prepare themselves to respond in a disaster. We provide further details of professional preparedness in the Nurses' Professional Preparedness section.

PERSONAL PREPAREDNESS

Individuals all over the world live and work in varying geographical locations and encounter a multitude of varying risks and hazards. It is important that people assess the areas in which they live and work to facilitate an understanding of the risks and hazards they might encounter and the measures to mitigate them. Recent events provide insight into potential risks faced around the world, including droughts, earthquakes, fires, floods, severe weather events, terrorism, and the pandemic spread of infectious diseases. Such varying risks may require different preparedness measures to increase personal, family, and community resilience. Individuals should speak with emergency preparedness experts and other leaders in their community to learn what risks might exist in their communities and how to best prepare for them. It is also prudent to prepare for risks that might exist at or near their place of work, as the risks at their places of employment might be different than those encountered in the communities in which they live.

Governments frequently provide education on recommended actions to prepare for emergencies. For example, the Swedish government published an emergency preparedness brochure, "If Crisis or War Comes," and created a website (www.dinsakerhet.se/) containing this and other frequently updated information (Swedish Civil Contingencies Agencies, n.d.). Lithuania has taken similar measures, creating their own emergency preparedness website (Lietuvos Respublikos Krašto Apsaugos Ministerija, 2017), as has the United States (American Red Cross, 2020b; Ready.gov, 2019), Australia (Australian Red Cross, 2020), Europe (European Civil Protection and Humanitarian Aid Operations, 2019), and many other countries. All citizens have a shared

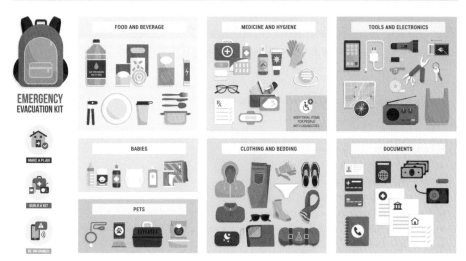

Fig. 3.4 Emergency evacuation kit. (iStock Stock illustration ID:1146891343)

responsibility to determine what guidance exists in their location, review it, and ensure that they prepare themselves, their homes, and their families for emergencies per the recommendations of experts in their countries.

As stated, nurses should be prepared for an emergency in all places they frequent, adhering to the four tenets of preparedness: Be Informed, Make a Plan, Build a Kit, and Get Involved (Ready.gov, 2021). However, the importance of emergency supply kits and the supplies within it should be emphasized, as this is an important component of preparedness and a foundational recommendation for emergency preparedness. Fig. 3.4 provides an illustration of what is frequently recommended in an emergency supply kit for personal use. Although each nation may vary in terms of recommended supplies in emergency supply kits, emergency supply kits typically include enough food and water for each person in the home to sustain them for the recommended period of time. In addition, emergency supply kits should contain money, flashlights or torches, candles, batteries, first aid supplies, hygiene supplies, and other supplies indicated by risk assessment of the area or recommended by governments. See Box 3.1 for further details on items frequently recommended in disaster supply kits.

Families should know how much food, water, and supplies, including medical supplies, are needed for all members of the family to sustain themselves for the recommended period of time. Further, understanding that each member of the family may have increased needs that require consideration when stocking emergency supply kits containing necessary items is also critical. For example, a family with infants will need to consider including formula, baby food, and diapers in the kit. A family caring for an aging parent will need to consider the parent's medications, physicians, equipment, and other possible needs when stocking emergency supply kits. A subsequent section in this chapter, Preparing Clients With Increased Needs After a Disaster, contains more specific recommendations for individuals or their family members who have increased needs or medical vulnerabilities. Finally, pet preparedness is important, as adequate food and medicine for pets also should be a part of an emergency preparedness kit.

Being prepared for an emergency is not simply purchasing a list of recommended items, although items to maintain health while nurses, clients, and their families either evacuate or shelter in place (based on recommendations for the specific hazard or imminent threat) are important. Members of a community, including nurses, also must be aware of resources in their area. Preparedness plans should include a plan for communicating with members of the family after a

---

BOX 3.1 ■ Disaster Supply Kits

Frequently Recommended Items in a Basic Disaster Supply Kit
- One gallon of water per person per day
- Nonperishable food (for all members of the family, to include formula for infants)
- Battery-powered or hand-crank radio to receive weather alerts
- Flashlight
- First aid kit
- Extra batteries
- Whistle (to signal for help)
- Dust mask (to help filter contaminated air)
- Plastic sheeting and duct tape (to shelter in place)
- Personal sanitation items (e.g., garbage bags)
- Personal hygiene items (including feminine hygiene supplies and diapers and baby wipes, if needed)
- Wrench or pliers (to turn off utilities)
- Manual can opener (for food)
- Multipurpose tool (e.g., a tool that serves several functions in a single unit)
- Local maps
- Cell phone with chargers and a backup battery
- Mess kit (e.g., a collection of silverware and cookware used when camping)
- Disposable cups, plates, and utensils (including baby bottles, if needed)
- Prescription and nonprescription medications
- Any other medical equipment needed (e.g., eyeglasses or contact lenses, hearing aids, syringes)
- Extra money
- Pet food and supplies, if needed (including food, water, bowl, leash, collar, and medications as needed)
- Important family documents, such as insurance policies, identification, and bank account records saved electronically or in a waterproof, portable container
- Paper and pencils
- Books, games, puzzles, or other activities for children
  Each country has recommendations appropriate for that area based on risk assessments. The above items are typical contents frequently recommended.

Adapted from Ready.gov. (2020). *Build a kit*. https://www.ready.gov/kit; and American Red Cross. (2020). *What do you need in a survival kit?* https://www.redcross.org/get-help/how-to-prepare-for-emergencies/survival-kit-supplies.html

---

disaster, an evacuation plan that all members of the family are aware of, a plan to shelter in place if need be, and a way to receive emergency alerts and communications. Community members, including nurses, should develop relationships with other members of their community as frequently it is the community members themselves who provide assistance to one another after an emergency until further aid can arrive. Knowledge of where local emergency shelters are typically located in the community is also important. Again, speaking with emergency management professionals and other local community leaders can increase knowledge of recommendations and community resources.

NURSES' PROFESSIONAL PREPAREDNESS

Education for Disaster Response

Nurses are often at the front lines of disaster response, providing care to populations affected by disasters and emergencies, often at great risk to personal health. Events in response to the COVID-19 pandemic highlight the important role nurses all over the world play in disaster response as well as the personal risks they encounter (ICN, 2020). Health care leaders assume that nurses will report to work after a disaster, but evidence suggests that the number of nurses who will show up after a disaster is related to the type of disaster (Adams & Berry, 2012; Milburn & McNeill, 2017) and their knowledge of the disaster type (Chilton et al., 2017; McNeill et al., 2020).

Chapter 6 provides details on the role of the general professional nurse in accordance with the ICN disaster nursing competencies (ICN, 2019). Items comprising each domain provide a critical infrastructure to begin efforts to improve competencies and disaster response. Nurses must endeavor to seek education to become competent in each domain. Many countries have formal education programs where nurses can educate themselves about disaster nursing competencies. Education related to disasters, whether part of a formal degree program, certificate, or continuing education, is essential to nurses becoming professionally prepared for disasters and emergency events. Education is most effective if it addresses how to work as part of a multidisciplinary team with licensed personnel from other professions and unlicensed personnel. Although "just in time" (JIT) training may be necessary to respond to an immediate event to enhance surge capacity, a more systematic approach of continuing education beyond mandatory requirements and ongoing participation in disaster exercises is more likely to enhance a nurse's confidence in being able to respond and perform effectively in a disaster. Table 3.1 provides several examples of current

TABLE 3.1 ■ Disaster Education Resources

Resource Name	Description of Resource	Resource Access URL
The International Federation of Red Cross and Red Crescent Societies (IFRC)	Certified professional development courses include master's level online courses in global health, master's in global health, master's level short course in humanitarian shelter coordination, online course in humanitarian diplomacy, master's level short course in shelter and settlements in emergencies (natural disasters), online course in global trends in international migration, online certificate program in disaster management, online postgraduate certificate in social and voluntary sector leadership.	https://www.ifrc.org/en/ get-involved/learning-education-training/ certified-professional-development-courses/
World Health Organization Regional Office for Europe	Online education in the areas of Prevent, Prepare, Respond, and Recover.	http://www.euro.who. int/en/health-topics/ health-emergencies/ pages/about-health-emergencies-in-the-european-region/ emergency-cycle
National Center for Disaster Medicine and Public Health	Free online disaster health core curriculum course intended for an interdisciplinary health care audience.	https://www.usuhs. edu/ncdmph/core-curriculum

(continued)

TABLE 3.1 ■ Disaster Education Resources —cont'd

Resource Name	Description of Resource	Resource Access URL
Office of the Assistant Secretary for Preparedness and Response–Technical Resources, Assistance Center, and Information Exchange (ASPR-TRACIE), Emergency Preparedness Information Modules for Nurses in Acute Care Settings (EPIMN)	Series of modules designed for nurses in acute care settings.	https://asprtracie.hhs.gov/technical-resources/resource/7209/emncy-preparedness-information-modules-for-nurses-in-acute-care-settings
Centers for Disease Control and Prevention	Free toolkits and educational resources for radiological planning and response, including exposure, decontamination, clinician response, and handling decedents.	https://www.cdc.gov/nceh/radiation/emergencies/toolkits.htm
Institute for Public Health, University of Hawaii at Mānoa's Pacific Emergency Management, Preparedness, and Response Information Network and Training Services (Pacific EMPRINTS) Program	Pacific EMPRINTS includes courses on bioterrorism; chemical terrorism; disaster mental health; disaster preparedness and response; geographic information systems; infectious diseases; medical reserve corps; natural disasters; radiological, nuclear, and explosive threats; and vulnerable populations.	https://iph.sdsu.edu/courses/online.php
Preparedness and Emergency Response Learning Centers (PERLC)	The PERLC Training Catalog features more than 400 online trainings and other learning materials to help public health professionals and their partners prepare for and respond to emergencies.	https://perlc.nwcphp.org/
Public Health Foundation, TRAIN Learning Network	TRAIN Learning Network is a trusted leader in providing training and other learning opportunities to public health, health care, behavioral health, preparedness, and other health professionals and comprises state and federal TRAIN affiliates that operate branded TRAIN web portals and work together to coordinate and share workforce training efforts. Government agencies, academic institutions, and other nationally recognized and respected organizations post content to the TRAIN Learning Network in order to disseminate and track their trainings to the health workforce. There are TRAIN learners in all US states and territories, as well as in 177 other countries. Anyone can register as a learner on TRAIN at no cost and access thousands of openly available course offerings, most of which are free.	https://www.train.org/main/help/about

training that nurses can access, with brief descriptions of those resources. However, nurses should also seek information on locally delivered courses and simulations to further their education in disaster nursing competencies.

Because disasters comprise both natural and human-made occurrences that could happen at any time and location, nurses must be aware of current social, political, and climatological events as they evolve around them, regardless of their practice area. Nurses should maintain current licensure and practice certifications and other knowledge, skills, and abilities required in their practice area at all times in advance of increased needs created by disasters or emergencies. Nurses in all practice areas should be competent in surveilling for communicable diseases and the implications they might have for particular client demographics. For example, pathogens may be more dangerous to one age group than another or more dangerous to people who have underlying conditions. Nurses in the community are well positioned to educate more vulnerable clients about preventive measures, potentially preventing hospital admission. It is important that all nurses understand the nuances of communicable diseases and other types of disasters and be prepared to respond to them using the appropriate level of PPE; and, also to facilitate an understanding of which clients are most at risk.

Culturally Appropriate Preparedness Measures

Because disasters occur all over the world and frequently overwhelm system capacities, requiring external assistance, nurses should be prepared to provide cultural and linguistically competent assistance. There are five elements of cultural competency within disaster preparedness (DHHS, 2015). These efforts are a part of nurse preparedness, as they must be done in advance of a disaster to the extent possible. The first element is to be aware of and accept cultural differences. As external support after a disaster might include responders who are racially, ethnically, or linguistically different than the survivor, it is important that nurses responding be self-aware, assessing their own potential biases and stereotypes. Doing this will improve response efforts without minimizing cultural beliefs and norms of the affected populations.

The second element of cultural competency within disaster preparedness is being aware of one's own cultural values. Honestly assessing personal prejudices and cultural stereotypes by assessing oneself can help nurses become aware of their own personal cultural values and biases (DHHS, 2015). It is critical for nurses to recognize and respect cultural differences and to understand their own biases and beliefs to effectively serve affected communities with diverse populations.

The third element of cultural competency is to understand and manage the "dynamics of difference" (DHHS, 2015). People of different cultures may express themselves and interpret information in various ways. It is important for nurses to learn how various cultures express themselves and interpret information and the potential implications for care. The fourth element of cultural competency within disaster preparedness is the development of cultural knowledge. This can be done by learning the health- and illness-related beliefs, customs, and treatments of various cultural groups in your region, but also in any region you may travel to as a part of disaster response. The fifth element of cultural competency within disaster preparedness is the ability to adapt activities to fit different cultural contexts. This involves adapting and modifying services rendered to fit the cultural context of the survivors, community members, and patients to whom you are providing service. An example of this is the use of interpreters during interviews when the nurse and client do not speak the same language.

NURSE PERSONAL PREPAREDNESS

Current research indicates that nurses report to work after a disaster because of a perceived duty to care, a belief that it is the morally right thing to do, and ethical imperatives (McNeill et al., 2020). However, in responding to a disaster, nurses may find themselves balancing competing demands, including the obligations they have to patients, themselves, and their families, potentially affecting their perceived duty to care (American Nurses Association, 2017). There is evidence that nurses who were more personally prepared for a disaster had a higher perceived duty to care (McNeill et al., 2020), and that personal preparedness also affects the number of nurses indicating that they would report to work after a disaster (McNeill et al., 2020; Patel et al., 2017). This demonstrates the interconnectedness of professional and personal disaster preparedness. These links between personal and professional preparedness for emergencies underscore the importance of ensuring that nurses are personally prepared for emergencies, so they are able to report to work and professionally prepared so they are competent to do so. As such, it is imperative that nurses follow all personal preparedness guidelines as described to ensure adequate capacity to provide care for clients after a disaster.

PREPARING CLIENTS WITH INCREASED NEEDS AFTER A DISASTER

Nurses must endeavor to facilitate personal emergency preparedness in their clients. Nurses should provide education on basic emergency preparedness kits as outlined as part of their normal education practices with their clients. However, nurses must alter preparedness education for clients or their caregivers to include any chronic disease, any access or functional needs, or any vulnerabilities clients might have. Mounting evidence supports that emergency preparedness education provided by health care professionals significantly increases preparedness levels among these vulnerable populations (Killian et al., 2017; McNeill et al., 2018; Olympia et al., 2010). Theoretically, improved preparedness prior to a disaster will facilitate greater resilience after a disaster, though this has not been tested. Several populations require specific consideration in disaster plans. Although the following examples do not constitute an exhaustive list, populations requiring specific consideration might include anyone with a chronic disease, anyone with access or functional needs, children, elderly persons, pregnant women, people with mental health illnesses, those who are cognitively impaired, and those with low health literacy. Caregiver education should always be included.

Preparedness among vulnerable clients requires specific consideration of exactly what contributes to their vulnerability and may include several vulnerabilities or chronic underlying conditions. For example, chronic diseases that require specific medications or treatments must be considered. Clients who frequently seek health care services for their disease or condition should keep a copy of their insurance paperwork in their emergency supply kit and identify alternate health care providers in areas they may evacuate to, particularly for those undergoing specialized care or treatment regimens. Clients who undergo hemodialysis or peritoneal dialysis will need a copy of their physician's orders with the details of their hemodialysis, including volume of dialysate, dextrose concentration of the dialysate, and duration of the exchanges. In addition, hemodialysis clients might want to consider identifying an alternate dialysis facility in another region to which they may evacuate if the need arises. If a client has diabetes, foods in the emergency supply kit should include those that will maintain stable glucose levels and plenty of water. Syringes, glucometers, insulin, coolers, ice packs, needles, alcohol wipes, and any other equipment needed to maintain normal glucose levels should be included in an emergency supply kit for those with diabetes.

Clients who are dependent on electricity should contact their local power or utility companies and notify them of their critical need for electricity to power medical equipment or to maintain thermostasis. If a client has financial resources to purchase a backup generator, this would be prudent. If they are not able to purchase a backup generator, extra batteries may be a feasible alternative for equipment that can be powered by batteries. If available in the area, recommend that the client get on the priority list for restoring power after an outage. Finally, advise electricity-dependent clients or their caregivers to get to a health care facility if they no longer have access to power and their conditions are worsening.

Some clients may be caregivers for patients at home on ventilators, or they may be oxygen-dependent themselves. If a client is oxygen-dependent, associated medical equipment might require electricity. If this is the case, the guidance for electricity-dependent clients should be followed. If a client has portable oxygen, they should maintain extra bottles of oxygen in their emergency supply kit. However, because portable oxygen bottles contain finite volumes, consideration should be given to having a refill system in the home. If clients use an oxygen concentrator, they should request an emergency portable oxygen supply that does not require electricity (e.g., an emergency tank). As with electricity-dependent clients, advise clients whose conditions are worsening to get to a health care facility if they no longer have access to oxygen.

Those with other chronic medical conditions that require specialized treatment, such as pregnancy, complex wound care, plasmapheresis, and cancer treatments, should identify alternative care sites in advance of an emergency. Further, it is important that these clients maintain a copy of their records and their physicians' orders detailing the current treatment regimen should these clients need to use alternative treatment sites. Any client who uses durable medical equipment (DME) should maintain a list of all medical equipment; the settings for each piece of equipment; type, model and make of equipment; and the suppliers' phone numbers and addresses for each item.

Consideration of a client's immune system is also important when supplying emergency preparedness kits. Because the immune system helps the body fight infections and other diseases, those with weakened immune systems, potentially occurring in clients with cancer, HIV/AIDS, diabetes, transplanted organs, multiple sclerosis, lupus, and other diseases are at increased risk for infections and diseases of opportunity. Immunocompromised or potentially immunocompromised clients or their caregivers should take precautions to minimize increased risk to the extent possible. Measures to decrease risk will vary by hazard (e.g., pandemic versus earthquake or flood), so prescribed protections should be crafted in consultation with the client's physician based on individual client conditions and needs.

Many clients take daily medications to maintain health, even if they are not dependent on electricity, medical equipment, or treatments. Review the recommendations by governing authorities for your area regarding how much medication you should stockpile, but typically clients should keep at least a 7-day supply of prescription medications. Clients should maintain a list of all prescription and over-the-counter medications, including dosage amounts and known allergies. Nurses also should instruct clients or their caregivers to review expiration dates for medications and rotate them, so that their emergency supply medications do not expire. For clients with mental impairment, nurses should instruct caregivers to rotate these medications or consider performing this function themselves, if appropriate. In addition, keeping copies of prescriptions also is prudent. Consideration must be given to appropriate storage requirements for each of the medications taken. For example, some medicines require cooler temperatures, whereas others are damaged by sunlight. Nurses should consider components of an emergency supply kit required to properly store medications (e.g., coolers, ice packs) and advise families to include such additional supplies as appropriate.

Elderly clients might have multiple considerations aside from medications, lowered immune systems, and chronic disease, even if they are relatively healthy. For example, DME is important to maintain independence and should be considered in emergency supply kits. Clients should be instructed to make a list of all DME including canes, walkers, nebulizers, hearing aids, eyeglasses, scooters, wheelchairs, prosthetics, orthotics, specialized beds and mattresses, and any other equipment used to maintain health, independence, and function. The list should include the item, any settings, the supplier or manufacturer and their address and phone number, and any physician orders required.

Nurses with pregnant clients should instruct them to speak with their health care provider regarding any prenatal needs they might have associated with individual health conditions. For example, clients with gestational diabetes, hypertension, or hyperemesis gravidarum may require medications to maintain health throughout their pregnancy. Prescriptions for medications, including prenatal vitamins, should be considered in the emergency response kit. Nurses also should teach pregnant clients when they should seek immediate medical care (e.g., bleeding, decreased movement of the baby, severe nausea or vomiting, rupture of membranes, persistent headache, flu symptoms).

Families with children should consider educating their children on disasters (earthquakes, hurricanes, tornadoes, thunderstorms, etc.) in an age-appropriate manner. Teaching children how to safely use emergency phone numbers such as 911 and in which situations it is appropriate is also prudent. Instructing families to role-play disasters in a nonthreatening way can help reduce panic and anxiety should a disaster happen. Books and games are an important component of disaster supply kits for children to reduce boredom and anxiety after a disaster. It is also a good idea to instruct parents on supportive behaviors for children who might act out due to anxiety about impending disasters or in the aftermath of a disaster.

Nurses who have clients either with cognitive impairment or providing care for a family member with any type of cognitive impairment should be instructed that times of upheaval and stress can be particularly difficult. People with Alzheimer disease or dementia can become extremely upset and confused after a disaster. Nurses should instruct caregivers on the signs of anxiety and agitation and to not leave the person with cognitive impairment alone. The level of cognitive impairment or needs related to the impairment also should be considered in the contents of emergency supply kits. For example, incontinence pads, adaptive feeding devices, an identification bracelet, or a recent picture of the person may need to be included.

It is important for nurses to note that although almost everyone will experience some type of psychological distress after an emergency, those who have been diagnosed with severe mental disorders are particularly vulnerable and require access to mental health care after an emergency (WHO, 2019). Clients who have severe mental disorders or are providing care to someone with a severe mental disorder should be instructed to seek care for urgent mental health problems should a disaster happen. Nurses also should consider becoming proficient in delivering psychological first aid in communities affected by disaster.

For nurses with clients who have low health literacy, breaking down larger concepts into smaller, concrete steps can help facilitate understanding of preparedness recommendations. This becomes complicated when the client with low health literacy has increased medical needs, is vulnerable, or has access or functional needs. It is not always apparent that a client has low health literacy, so nurses must be aware of signs indicating low health literacy. For example, things that might indicate a client cannot read could include not filling out required forms, noncompliance with medications, inability to name medications or explain purpose, inability to read pill labels, not following through with instructions given, and not asking questions or asking very few questions (Agency for Healthcare Research and Quality, 2017). Emergency preparedness for these clients is the same as for other clients, but guidelines and plans should be articulated in a simple manner. Use clear, easy-to-follow instructions when educating clients with low health literacy, and instruct their caregivers to do the same.

Many types of access and functional needs (e.g., pediatrics, geriatrics, disabilities, chronic illness, psychological needs, assistive devices or equipment) of clients and their potential implications for emergency preparedness are discussed in this chapter, but there are far more that require purposeful considerations (e.g., aphasia, speech or hearing impairment, bathing, dressing, transferring) in emergency preparedness plans. Nurses must assess each client and the structural or access issues they may face and assist them in determining ways to either overcome those issues in the face of an emergency or mitigate their impact after a disaster. As stated, many clients may have a caregiver. Caregivers should always be consulted and included in emergency preparedness plans. Caregivers are familiar with the needs of the client and typically will aid the client through the disaster. Nurses must educate caregivers on what steps must be taken for the person they provide care to in the interest of emergency preparedness. Caregivers must understand that they should have an emergency supply kit and make emergency preparedness plans not only for themselves but also for those to whom they provide care.

Case in Point

PERSONAL AND PROFESSIONAL EMERGENCY PREPAREDNESS FOR NURSES: AN EXEMPLAR

A registered nurse, who primarily works in the emergency department (ED) at a large, urban hospital, becomes aware of a newly identified illness spreading across countries around the globe. To maintain awareness of current health-related information, the nurse frequently visits experts' websites created by health agencies to monitor health statistics and emerging diseases and provide expert guidance to health care providers. The nurse learns that the virus continues to spread and many countries have high levels of infection and mortality rates. As a result, many governments are mandating quarantines and orders for people to shelter in place, particularly for those with chronic underlying conditions as they are at greatest risk for dying from this new illness. As the nurse notes predictions that the illness will reach her country, she begins thinking of the impact it could have and what she might need to do to prepare.

The nurse is a single mother of two children, but her retired parents lived close by. The nurse's oldest child has autism, is easily upset at changes in his routine, and experiences frequent seizures. The nurse is extremely concerned that if she goes to work in the ED, one of the patients visiting the ED might have the illness and she then would bring it home to her children. Further, she is concerned that if she visits her parents, she might infect them. However, the nurse also believes it is her duty to provide care to the sick and this is something she is committed to doing, even in these circumstances. The nurse decides that should the infection spread to her city, she will have her children stay with her parents to prevent her from potentially transmitting the infection to her family. She discusses this plan with her parents, who agree to provide care if it becomes necessary. In addition, she speaks to her children, who are 8 and 10 years old, about what is happening with the virus and that she wants to make sure they do not get sick. She explains in an age-appropriate manner that she will not get sick because she has the proper equipment at work, but that she doesn't want them to get sick so she will have them stay with their grandparents for a while and talk to them as often as she can. The children are very excited to spend time with their grandparents and are proud that their mother is taking care of sick people.

Over the next couple of weeks, she begins to craft her emergency preparedness plans with her children in mind and sets aside oral medications for her son with autism, as well as her son's doctor's name, address, and telephone number; a copy of the prescriptions her son needs; information on what constitutes an emergency in terms of his seizures; and information on actions her parents should take if her son has a seizure while in their care. The nurse packs clothes, personal hygiene items, books, and toys for both of her children in an emergency supply kit. She also puts together a kit for herself with enough clothes, scrubs, personal hygiene items, and other supplies so that she can sleep at the hospital if necessary. She attends JIT training conducted by her hospital to ensure that she knows what is required to take care of patients who have contracted the illness. Because the nurse has no siblings, she also thinks of her parents; her father is 75 years old with type 2 diabetes and hypertension, and her mother is 72 years old and hearing impaired. She calls her parents to discuss their preparedness plans and to determine if they have enough food, water, and medications for themselves as well as her children to last for 30 days per the most recent expert recommendations. Her parents state that they do not have enough to last for that long and remind her that they are on a fixed income and do not have enough money to buy that much food, though they could refill their medications. The nurse asks her parents to refill their medications and goes to the grocery store to get enough food for her parents and her children to last at least 30 days, and delivers it to them to store for use in case it is needed.

The illness arrives in her city with rapidly increasing rates of infection. The schools close, but the nurse needs to continue working, especially since the number of visits to the ED has been increasing dramatically and some of her coworkers haven't reported to work in the previous days so the ED is short staffed. The nurse takes her children and all their emergency supplies as well as their schoolwork to her parents' home. The nurse double-checks her parents' supplies and makes sure there is enough for at least a month and tells them that she will see them all soon and will drop off additional supplies as needed. Two days later, the government issues an order for everyone in the city to shelter in place. The nurse is considered an essential employee, so she continues to report to work every day but things are getting increasingly hectic. Shifts off become less frequent because nurses are also becoming infected and unable to work. The influx of patients and the decreasing number of nurses able to work means that every available member of the health care team must work as much as they can. So, the nurse takes her own emergency preparedness supplies to work with her so she can sleep there between shifts. The nurse is able to provide care for her patients and get enough rest for herself, all the while speaking with her family every day yet having decreased the chance she will transmit the virus to them.

Questions for Discussion

1. What are three professional preparedness activities this nurse demonstrated prior to going to work for an extended period of time?
2. How did the nurse's activities relate to quarantine mandates for herself, her children, and family members?

Points to Remember

- All disasters begin at the local level.
- All community plans must be congruent with the regional, state, federal or country, or tribal plan that applies where the community is situated.
- A broad range of community stakeholders and networks must be engaged in planning to promote resilience.
- Community members must understand the local risks and hazards of the area in which they live.
- Preparedness among vulnerable clients requires specific consideration of all factors and conditions that contribute to their vulnerability.
- Personal and professional preparedness are interrelated and critical to a nurse's ability to respond to a disaster.

Test Your Knowledge

1. What type of capacity is required when space, staff, and supplies have been adapted to provide sufficient care during a catastrophic disaster but are inconsistent with usual standards of care?
   a. Conventional capacity
   b. Surge capacity
   c. Contingency capacity
   d. Crisis capacity

2. Preparedness plans should include all of the following except:
   a. Where local municipalities will provide food immediately after the emergency
   b. A plan for communicating with family members after a disaster
   c. Knowledge of where local emergency shelters typically are located in the community
   d. An evacuation plan all members of the family are aware of
3. Which of the following are elements of cultural competency within disaster preparedness? *(Choose all that apply.)*
   a. Be aware of and accept cultural differences
   b. Be aware of one's own cultural values
   c. Understand and manage the "dynamics of difference"
   d. Adapt activities to fit different cultural contexts
4. Considerations for the emergency preparedness plans of independent older clients with diabetes would not include:
   a. Glucometers
   b. A caregiver
   c. Coolers
   d. Syringes
5. A tornado and severe thunderstorm sends dozens of injured people to the emergency department of a small hospital. Driving conditions are becoming hazardous due to flooded roads, and multiple hospital personnel report having difficulty getting to work. Administrators are likely to be most concerned about which element of surge capacity?
   a. Supplies
   b. Staff
   c. Systems
   d. Structures
6. A hospital setting up a tent outside the emergency department to serve as an initial triage area is an example of which element of surge capacity?
   a. Staff
   b. Supplies
   c. Structures
   d. Systems
7. Actions that a health system can take to promote disaster preparedness and mitigate loss and harm to vulnerable populations include: *(Choose all that apply.)*
   a. Getting to know and actively engaging with community partners
   b. Assuming that all essential staff will report to work after a disaster
   c. Limiting communication about disaster plans to administrators and managers
   d. Routinely reviewing disaster plans, procedures, and mutual aid agreements
8. A nurse participating in the development of a disaster plan that uses principles of disaster risk reduction should expect the plan to include actions that:
   a. Strengthen community resilience
   b. Focus primarily on a single preexisting disaster risk
   c. Separate community development from disaster planning
   d. Can be used in only one setting
9. Which of the following might be signs that a client has low health literacy? *(Choose all that apply.)*
   a. Asking a lot of questions when receiving instructions
   b. Noting poor handwriting on completed forms
   c. Inability to explain the purpose of their medications
   d. Not following through on instructions

10. Which disaster education resource is designed specifically for nurses in acute care settings?
    a. The International Federation of Red Cross and Red Crescent Societies (IFRC)
    b. World Health Organization Regional Office for Europe
    c. ASPR-TRACIE EPIMN
    d. Preparedness and Emergency Response Learning Centers (PERLC)

References

Acosta, J. D., Chandra, A., & Ringel, J. S. (2013). Nongovernmental resources to support disaster preparedness, response, and recovery. *Disaster Medicine and Public Health Preparedness*, *7*(4), 348–353. https://doi.org/10.1017/dmp.2013.49.

Adams, L., & Berry, D. (2012). Who will show up? Estimating ability and willingness of essential hospital personnel to report to work in response to a disaster. *OJIN: The Online Journal of Issues in Nursing*, *17*(2). https://doi.org/10.3912/OJIN.Vol17No02PPT02.

Adams. L. M. (2009). Exploring the concept of surge capacity. *OJIN: The Online Journal of Issues in Nursing*, *14*(2). https://doi.org/10.3912/OJIN.Vol14No02PPT03.

Adams. L. M. (2016). Promoting disaster resilience through use of interdisciplinary teams: A program evaluation of the integrated care team approach. *World Medical & Health Policy*, *8*, 8–26.

Adams, L. M., Reams, P. K., & Canclini, S. B. (2015). Planning for partnerships: Maximizing surge capacity resources through service learning. *Journal of Emergency Management*, *13*(6), 557–564. https://doi.org/10.5055/jem.2015.0265.

Adams, R. M., Prelip, M. L., Glik, D. C., Donatello, I., & Eisenman, D. P. (2018). Facilitating partnerships with community- and faith-based organizations for disaster preparedness and response: Results of a national survey of public health departments. *Disaster Medicine and Public Health Preparedness,*, *12*(1), 57–66. https://doi.org/10.1017/dmp.2017.36.

Agency for Healthcare Research and Quality. (2017). *Health literacy: Hidden barriers and practical strategies.* https://www.ahrq.gov/health-literacy/quality-resources/tools/literacy-toolkit/tool3a/index.html

Aitsi-Selmi, A., & Murray, V. (2016). Protecting the health and well-being of populations from disasters: Health and health care in the Sendai framework for disaster risk reduction 2015–2030. *Prehospital & Disaster Medicine*, *31*(1), 74–78.

American Nurses Association. (2017). *Who will be there? Ethics, the law, and a nurse's duty to respond in a disaster.* https://www.nursingworld.org/~4af058/globalassets/docs/ana/ethics/who-will-be-there_disaster-preparedness_2017.pdf

American Red Cross. (2020a). *Why is type O blood so important: Here's why blood type matters.* https://www.redcrossblood.org/donate-blood/blood-types/o-blood-type.html

American Red Cross. (2020b). *How to prepare for emergencies.* https://www.redcross.org/get-help/how-to-prepare-for-emergencies.html

Association of Public Health Nurses, Public Health Preparedness Committee. (2013). *The role of the public health nursing in disaster preparedness, response, and recovery: A position paper.* http://www.quadcouncilphn.org/wp-content/uploads/2016/03/2014_APHN-Role-of-PHN-in-Disaster-PRR-Ref-updated-2015.pdf

Australian Red Cross. (2020). *Preparing for emergencies.* https://www.redcross.org.au/prepare

Bergstrand, K., Mayer, B., Brumback, B., & Zhang, Y. (2015). Assessing the relationship between social vulnerability and community resilience to hazards. *Social Indicators Research*, *122*, 391–409. https://doi.org/10.1007/s11205-014-0698-3.

Centers for Disease Control and Prevention. (2018a). Introduction. *Crisis and emergency risk communication (CERC) manual.* https://emergency.cdc.gov/cerc/ppt/CERC_Introduction.pdf

Centers for Disease Control and Prevention. (2018b). Community engagement. *Crisis and emergency risk communication (CERC) manual.* https://emergency.cdc.gov/cerc/ppt/CERC_CommunityEngagement.pdf

Centers for Disease Control and Prevention. (2019). *State and local readiness: Tools and resources.* https://www.cdc.gov/cpr/readiness/toolsandresources.htm

Chandra, A., Williams, M., Plough, A., Stayton, A., Wells, K. B., Horta, M., & Tang, J. (2013). Getting actionable about community resilience: The Los Angeles County community disaster resilience project. *American Journal of Public Health*, *103*(7), 1181–1189.

Chilton, J., McNeill, C., & Alfred, D. (2017). Survey of nursing students' self-reported knowledge of Ebola virus disease, willingness to treat, and perceptions of their duty to treat. *Journal of Professional Nursing, 32*(6), 487–493. https://doi.org/10.1016/j.profnurs.2016.05.004.

European Civil Protection and Humanitarian Aid Operations. (2019). *Disaster preparedness.* https://www.redcross.org.au/prepare.

Heagele. T. (2017). Disaster-related community resilience: A concept analysis and a call to action for nurses. *Public Health Nursing, 34*(3), 295–302.

Hick, J. L., Barbera, J. A., & Kelen, G. D. (2009). Refining surge capacity: Conventional, contingency, and crisis capacity. *Disaster Medicine and Public Health Preparedness, 3, Suppl 1*, S59–S67.

International Council of Nurses. (2019). *Nurses and disaster risk reduction, response and recovery.* https://www.icn.ch/sites/default/files/inline-files/PS_E_Nurses_and_disaster_risk_reduction_response_and_recovery.pdf

International Council of Nurses. (2020). *ICN COVID-19 update: Strong national nursing associations providing vital lead during COVID-19 crisis.* https://www.icn.ch/news/icn-covid-19-update-strong-national-nursing-associations-providing-vital-lead-during-covid-19

International Federation of Red Cross and Red Crescent Societies. (2020). *Disaster preparedness: Working with communities to prepare for disasters and reduce their impact.* https://media.ifrc.org/ifrc/what-we-do/disaster-and-crisis-management/disaster-preparedness/

Jakeway, C. C., LaRosa, G., Cary, A., & Schoenfisch, S. (2008). The role of public health nurses in emergency preparedness and response: A position paper of the Association of State and Territorial Directors of Nursing. *Public Health Nursing, 25*(4), 353–361.

Killian, T., Moon, Z., McNeill, C., Garrison, B., & Moxley, S. (2017). Emergency preparedness of persons over 50 years old: Further results from the health and retirement study. *Disaster Medicine and Public Health Preparedness, 11*(1), 80–89. https://doi.org/10.1017/dmp.2016.162.

Lietuvos Respublikos Krašto Apsaugos Ministerija. (2017). *Ką turime žinoti apie pasirengimą ekstremalioms situacijoms ir karo metui.* https://kam.lt/lt/katurimezinoti.html?__cf_chl_jschl_tk__=17f77cc7088c4 3a40064fbc9a1b506c8e4a68d39-1584899125-0-Af4vmxkEi8Dsm--4_8h0iKqFpYvv2mTlNZeM_-luA_qEpcwwNIQvPJJctwZWxYkKtJDlcIzi9L1IAsJbyILLgK8YR9PJWsxSYZXgLokD2vw pCl_9IeIsXXHfkD1TfP2vTkDf79n3osxB7FgwHvprYUGGiJnFOx5uohJOWAS8cREHn-bIkEN6Qw2g1lPxYCNJ304tSC6zGQWtFUyHChrSw26nwnsHWaIm2Un5nAqgxU_ Tg-y1jBiYA4f7fRX8T77tEnWzkP8-w_KScDDfjKXyjWrRSESc6YlXAQYaL FcEImQquNHtt4nFzdbJ5CVzZhRitHATQu8JrH0D4VR_VZtisKW_W7otnzzi-vzWAMdX1fUwV

McNeill, C., Alfred, D., Nash, T., Chilton, J., & Swanson, M. S. (2020). Characterization of nurses' duty to care and willingness to report. *Nursing Ethics, 27*(2), 348–359. https://doi.org/10.1177/0969733019846645.

McNeill, C., Killian, T., Moon, Z., Way, K., & Garrison, B. (2018). The relationship between perceptions of emergency preparedness, disaster experience, health-care provider education, and emergency preparedness levels. *International Quarterly of Community Health Education, 38*(4), 233–243. https://doi.org/10.1177/0272684X18781792.

Milburn, A. B., & McNeill, C. (2017). Quantifying supply of home health services for public health emergencies. *Home Health Care Management & Practice, 29*(1), 20–34. https://doi.org/10.1177/1084822316658868.

Moore, M., Chandra, A., & Feeney, K. C. (2013). Building community resilience: what can the United States learn from experiences in other countries? *Disaster Medicine and Public Health Preparedness, 7*(3), 292–301. https://doi.org/10.1001/dmp.2012.15.

Norris, F. H., Stevens, S. P., Pfefferbaum, B., Wyche, K. F., & Pfefferbaum, R. L. (2008). Community resilience as a metaphor, theory, set of capacities, and strategy for disaster readiness. *American Journal of Community Psychology, 41*(1–2), 127–150. https://doi.org/10.1007/s10464-007-9156-6.

Office of the Assistant Secretary for Preparedness and Response. (2020). *ASPR technical resources, assistance center, and information exchange (TRACIE).* https://asprtracie.hhs.gov/

Olympia, R. P., Rivera, R., Heverley, S., Anyanwu, U., & Gregorits, M. (2010). Natural disasters and mass-casualty events affecting children and families: A description of emergency preparedness and the role of the primary care physician. *Clinical Pediatrics, 49*(7), 686–698. https://doi.org/10.1177/0009922810364657.

Patel, R., Wattamwar, K., Kanduri, J., Nahass, M., Yoon, J., Oh, J., … Lacy, C. R. (2017). Health care student knowledge and willingness to work in infectious disease outbreaks. *Disaster Medicine and Public Health Preparedness, 11*(6), 694–700. https://doi.org/10.1017/dmp.2017.18.

Pfefferbaum, R. L., Pfefferbaum, B., & VanHorn, R. L. (2015). Community resilience interventions: Participatory, assessment-based, action-oriented process. *American Behavioral Scientist, 59*(2), 238–253. https://doi.org/10.1177/00027642145502958.

Plough, A., Fielding, J. E., Chandra, A., Williams, M., Eisenman, D., Wells, K. B., … Magna, A. (2013). Building community disaster resilience: Perspectives from a large urban county department of health. *American Journal of Public Health, 103*(7), 1190–1197.

Pourvakhshoori, S., Khankeh, H. R., & Mohammadi, F. (2017). Emergency and disaster preparedness in nurses: A concept analysis. *Journal of Holistic Nursing and Midwifery, 27*(1), 35–43.

Ready.gov. (2019). *Emergency response plan.* https://www.ready.gov/business/implementation/emergency

Ready.gov. (2021). About the Ready Campaign. https://www.ready.gov/about-us

Rooney, C., & White, G. W. (2007). Narrative analysis of a disaster preparedness and emergency response survey from persons with mobility impairments. *Journal of Disability Policy Studies, 17*(4), 206–215.

Schmidt. P. J. (2002). Blood and disaster—Supply and demand. *New England Journal of Medicine, 346*(8), 617–619.

Swedish Civil Contingencies Agencies. (n.d.). *Important information for the population of Sweden: If crisis or war comes.* https://www.dinsakerhet.se/siteassets/dinsakerhet.se/broschyren-om-krisen-eller-kriget-kommer/om-krisen-eller-kriget-kommer---engelska-2.pdf

United Nations International Strategy for Disaster Reduction. (2015). *Sendai framework for disaster risk reduction 2015–2030.* http://www.wcdrr.org/uploads/Sendai_Framework_for_Disaster_Risk_Reduction_2015-2030.pdf

United Nations International Strategy for Disaster Reduction. (2017). *UNISDR terminology section: Online glossary.* https://www.undrr.org/terminology/

US Department of Health and Human Services. (2015). *Cultural and linguistic competency in disaster preparedness and response fact sheet.* https://www.phe.gov/Preparedness/planning/abc/Pages/linguistic-facts.aspx

US Department of Homeland Security. (2019). *National response framework.* https://www.fema.gov/media-library-data/1582825590194-2f000855d442fc3c9f18547d1468990d/NRF_FINALApproved_508_2011028v1040.pdf

Uscher-Pines, L., Chandra, A., & Acosta, J. (2013). The promise and pitfalls of community resilience. *Disaster Medicine and Public Health Preparedness, 7*(6), 603–606. 10.107/dmp.2013.100.

Veenema, T. G., Griffin, A., Gable, A. R., MacIntyre, L., Simons, N., Couig, M. P., … Larson, E. (2016). Nurses as leaders in disaster preparedness and response—A call to action. *Journal of Nursing Scholarship, 48*(2), 187–200. https://doi.org/10.1111/jnu.12198.

Verheul, M. L., & Duckers, M. (2019). Defining and operationalizing disaster preparedness in hospitals: A systematic literature review. *Prehospital and Disaster Preparedness, 35*(1), 1–8. https://doi.org/10.1017/S1049023X19005181.

Watson, S. K., Rudge, J. W., & Coker, R. (2013). Health systems'"surge capacity": State of the art and priorities for future research. *The Milbank Quarterly, 91*(1), 78–122.

World Health Organization. (2017). *A strategic framework for emergency preparedness.* https://extranet.who.int/sph/sites/default/files/document-library/document/Preparedness-9789241511827-eng.pdf

World Health Organization. (2018a). Communicating risk in public health emergencies: A WHO guideline for emergency risk communication (ERC) policy and practice. https://www.who.int/risk-communication/guidance/download/en/

World Health Organization. (2018b). *Risk communication FAQ.* https://www.who.int/risk-communication/faq/en/

World Health Organization. (2019). *Mental health in emergencies.* https://www.who.int/news-room/fact-sheets/detail/mental-health-in-emergencies

CHAPTER 4

Disaster Response, Triage, and Decontamination

Joanne C. Langan, PhD, RN, CNE ▓ Rhonda K. Cooke, MD ▓ Helen
Passafiume-Sandkuhl, RN, MSN, CEN, TNS, SANE, FAEN, CHEP

CHAPTER OUTLINE

Introduction	63	Start	74
Reporting and Notification	63	Reverse Triage	74
Authority During a Disaster	63	Provision of Blood Components	74
Hospital Emergency Command System	64	Patient Tracking	77
Interagency Coordination	64	Identification	77
Disaster Response Committee and Plan	65	Confidentiality	77
Management of Events	66	Reunification Centers	77
Surveillance	67	Transfer to Alternative Care Sites	78
Determining Capacity	67	Transfer to Morgue	78
Decontamination Basics	68	**Case in Point**	**78**
Communication During a Disaster	68	Release of a Biological Agent in a	
Casualty Management	**69**	Domed Stadium	78
Preparations for Care	69	Questions for Discussion	78
Staff	72	**Points to Remember**	**78**
Triage	73	**Test Your Knowledge**	**79**
Three-Level Triage	73	**References**	**80**
Five-Level Triage	74		

OBJECTIVES

After reading and studying this chapter, you should be able to:

- Describe and discuss the persons or agencies that must be notified when there is suspicion of a terrorist event.
- Discuss the optimal makeup of a disaster response committee that will plan a coordinated institutional response.
- Discuss the necessary changes in the triage process during a mass casualty event.
- Explore the possible methods of meeting the increased need for medications, equipment, and supplies during a mass casualty event.

- Discuss the multidisciplinary health care team's strategies to safeguard the health of populations.
- Discuss the measures in place to promote, protect, improve, and restore the well-being of the health care team.

KEY TERMS

chain of command: Delineation of authority.

communicable disease: An illness caused by direct or indirect transmission of an infectious agent or toxins from an infected individual, animal, vector, or the inanimate environment to a susceptible animal or human host.

disaster response committee: Group responsible for developing the disaster response plan. In health care, it consists of administrators, management, ancillary support persons, nurses, physicians, and members of the community response agencies.

force protection: All measures taken by administrators to promote, improve, conserve, and restore the mental and physical well-being of members across the range of health care providers, military, or any other sectors related to health care activities or operations.

hospital (emergency) incident command system (H[E]ICS or HICS): A hospital-based incident command system used as a framework for reporting and communicating. The system assigns specific roles to individuals in an effort to create a distinct chain of command that is temporarily enacted in response to a disaster situation.

incident command system (ICS): A framework for reporting and communicating through which specific roles are assigned to individuals in an effort to create a distinct chain of command that is temporarily enacted in response to a disaster situation. It provides standardization through consistent terminology and established organizational structures. A subset of the National Incident Management System.

isolation: Used to separate ill persons who have a communicable disease from those who are healthy.

National Incident Management System (NIMS): An overarching framework that provides a common, nationwide approach to enable the community to work together in managing threats and hazards. NIMS applies to all incidents regardless of cause, size, location, or complexity.

presentation: Clusters or groups of symptoms causing patients to seek medical care. Presenting symptoms aid in forming a clinical picture.

quarantine: Used to separate and restrict movement of well persons who may have been exposed to a communicable disease to see if they become ill.

redundancy: Backup or alternate systems to provide needed services such as communication.

Strategic National Stockpile: The nation's largest supply of potentially life-saving pharmaceuticals and medical supplies for use in a public health emergency.

surge capacity: Estimation of the maximum patient load for which responding hospitals and agencies can provide care after a mass casualty event. It includes beds, staffing, equipment, and Emergency Medical Services (EMS) systems. When determining required beds for decontamination and hospitalization, the estimation accounts for a capacity of 500 acutely ill adult patients per million population.

surveillance: The process of collecting and analyzing data to detect a trend in the health of the population.

universal identification card: Credentialing of health care workers that includes qualifications, education, and skills.

Introduction

Hospitals and nurses face a serious challenge in preparing for the very real possibility of an event, natural or human-made that results in large numbers of victims needing emergency care. During such events, health care systems are challenged to optimize their performance and use their valuable resources efficiently. Nurses must rise to this challenge and assume leadership roles in preparing for the unexpected. This chapter reviews infrastructure and policy that address disaster response, the coordination of efforts on many levels, and what nurses must know and do to become contributing members of disaster response efforts.

How prepared is your health care system for a mass casualty event? The American Hospital Association states that hospitals are preparing in advance for possible natural and human-made events. They are increasing their preparedness efforts for mass casualty events of any scope. Hospital systems are collaborating closely with other essential agencies such as police, fire, search and rescue, and other public safety entities. The goal is to be prepared to respond with personnel and resources.

Reporting and Notification

AUTHORITY DURING A DISASTER

The chain of authority in your community must be defined prior to a mass casualty event. Each major jurisdiction must have a plan that can be implemented within a defined region of authority. The key to success is the coordination of efforts of all who respond to an event.

When large numbers of casualties are anticipated, all responding agencies should be aware of other agencies' roles and coordinate their efforts to avoid duplication of services or unnecessary use of resources. The incident command system (ICS) was developed as an interdisciplinary agency coordination tool. The priorities of the ICS are life safety, incident stability, and property conservation. Communication among agencies and the community involves adoption of the ICS that is already in place in the community to ensure effective communication and use of the same terminology. Using the terminology in the ICS ensures that those who offer aid in the response effort understand the roles and duties of each service area regardless of geographical location or nation. The ICS defines the chain of authority during the event, thus supporting a safe and coordinated response. It is the model for command, control, and coordination of the response. The chain of authority is different from the normal day-to-day structure; it requires interagency cooperation and promotes a cohesive response of team members from multiple agencies.

The incident commander is the first responder on the scene, although once a higher-ranking responder or one with specialized training arrives that person will likely assume command of the situation. For example, when a situation involves hazardous materials, the use of qualified personnel is essential to contain the noxious materials.

Responsibilities of the incident commander may include:

- Assume command
- Assess the situation or event
- Implement the emergency management plan
- Determine response strategies
- Activate resources
- Order an evacuation
- Oversee activities
- Determine the conclusion of the incident

Health care professionals should be familiar with the specialized terminology and processes associated with the ICS in their area. Each responder should know their role once the ICS is activated. The importance of incident command in health care settings is more fully explained in the next section.

HOSPITAL EMERGENCY COMMAND SYSTEM

In 2013 The Joint Commission (TJC) identified the need to remove the Emergency Management section from the "Environment of Care" chapter and create a new chapter concentrating on the importance of preparedness and emergency management in health care settings. This change was necessary to address both the six functional areas of emergency management and annual review of the Emergency Operations Plan and Hazard Vulnerability Analysis.

The six critical areas of emergency response according to TJC are:

- Communication (EM.02.02.01)
- Resources and assets (EM.02.02.03)
- Safety and security (EM.02.02.05)
- Staff responsibilities (EM.02.02.07)
- Utilities management (EM.02.02.09)
- Patient clinical and support activities (EM.02.02.11) (California Hospital Association, 2017).

In addition, on September 8, 2016, the Centers for Medicare and Medicaid Services (CMS) published the "Emergency Preparedness Requirements for Medicare and Medicaid Participating Providers and Suppliers: Final Rule" in the *Federal Register*. The purpose was to establish national emergency preparedness requirements to ensure adequate planning for both natural and human-made disasters and coordination with federal, state, tribal, regional, and local emergency preparedness systems. The significance of government entities supporting disaster preparedness and public health emergencies cannot be overemphasized. This regulation became effective on November 16, 2016 (Centers for Medicare and Medicaid Services, 2019).

Interagency Coordination

Within each city or jurisdiction, health care agencies or institutions should plan how their roles will complement each other. Health care facilities must develop their plan to work seamlessly with the higher authorities in the state or region for the most efficient use of resources. Local response is required at the time of the event and those officials will be on-site prior to the arrival of more distant assistance. The local responders will serve as valuable resources for health care facilities during and after a disaster. Plans must be developed that cover specific instances in which supplies and personnel will be available to assist at collaborating institutions. Large-scale events may need the assistance of larger entities such as the Federal Emergency Management Agency (FEMA) (Fig. 4.1).

Personnel who respond to disaster sites must be able to provide response coordinators with verification of their credentials or license to practice. It is common for well-meaning citizens to respond to disaster areas eager to help, but these citizens can become a liability if they are not legally sanctioned to perform the necessary duties. Most licensed responders who are associated with a sanctioned entity will be welcomed to help in the relief effort but must be formally registered at the relief site. Volunteer health care providers can be a very valuable component in a disaster relief effort (Fig. 4.2).

Nurses may choose to seek education and training in advanced techniques in forensics and victim identification methods, for example. Agencies that are able to accept large numbers of victims have a mission and purpose when a surge of casualties is expected. Nurses who seek this advanced education and knowledge strengthen the assets of their respective agencies.

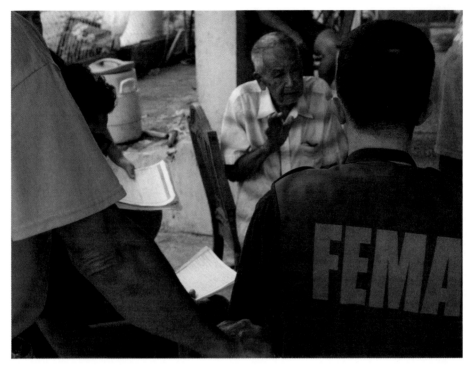

Fig. 4.1   FEMA in Naguabo, Puerto Rico. (https://www.fema.gov)

DISASTER RESPONSE COMMITTEE AND PLAN

A team effort is vital for a smooth implementation of the response plan. Acknowledging the superior and selfless efforts of all involved encourages others to contribute to the plan. Each person has a role during a disaster response and must handle the responsibilities that that role entails. Furthermore, each person must be aware of everyone else's roles and be able to rely on their contributions for a successful disaster response. Coalitions of responders should foster relationships before they are needed, when temperaments are cool and stress is reduced. Coalitions of first responders and health care professionals assist affiliated organizations to access clinical capabilities needed to respond effectively to disasters and public health emergencies (US Department of Health and Human Services [DHSS], 2021a).

The disaster response committee is also responsible for developing a response plan. Response plans maximize the use of available resources across large areas of states and countries (DHHS, 2021b). On a local level, individual agency plans must be coordinated with the regional plan. For example, if a large hospital reaches capacity and load balancing is necessary, it must be clear where the overflow victims will be sent.

During a disaster response, diverse planning committee membership is very important. Diverse members contribute a fresh perspective on the system, as well as significant information about what is expected of first responders. Those who work exclusively within a hospital or within the community may be unaware of others' efforts, the constraints that guide clinical practice, and the resources all can access. Working collaboratively enables understanding, provides a realistic perspective, and reduces the indecisiveness of where to send patients. Mutual support results in a smooth transition from ground zero to the acute care setting, and continuous dialogue reduces

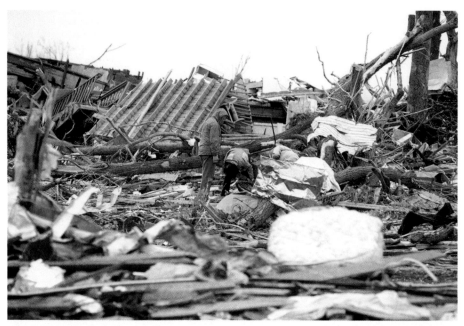

Fig. 4.2 People search for personal items only a few days after a deadly F5 tornado in Joplin, Missouri. (iStock.com\eyecrave)

the risk of miscommunication during a disaster. When large numbers of victims rely on the health care system, it is important that all responders are familiar with the roles of other responders to avoid conflicts or duplication of effort. Agreeing on what is possible in the field and how those efforts will be continued in an acute care or alternate care setting facilitates the effective and efficient use of resources.

Key disaster response plan questions include:
1. Who is in charge?
2. What are the responsibilities of those in charge?
3. What kinds of injuries or illnesses can the receiving agency expect?
4. When can the agency expect the arrival of the first victims or patients?
5. Who must come to the hospital for the most effective response?
6. How many nurses and physicians will be available?
7. What working relationships with other agencies are needed to facilitate the response?
8. What types of communication networks must be activated?

MANAGEMENT OF EVENTS

Before an incident, it is important to evaluate an institution's or agency's plan for the physical flow of patients. After an event, one's response is based on the answers to several questions: Where does triage occur? Where does decontamination occur? What security is necessary? All responders must be familiar with the host agency's flow pattern during a mass casualty event. If victims are being transported haphazardly to various departments, a traffic jam or bottleneck can result. All victims should go in one direction when leaving the emergency department (no victims return) and be moved as they progress through the treatment series to the next area. Potential bottleneck areas are x-ray, computed tomography (CT), ultrasound, and laboratory areas. In addition, areas in which intensive interventions such as airway management, table thoracotomy, and blood transfusions are performed may slow the flow of patients. Assign someone who does not have direct patient care responsibilities to manage the response and provide them with two-way radios or walkie talkies.

When considering the flow of patients and decontamination corridors, an important response need when bioterrorism is suspected is the ability to quarantine or isolate suspected victims. In other disasters, such as bombings or earthquakes, a small percentage of victims are admitted to the hospital. Most victims are treated and sent to their homes or to designated shelters. However, after the release of a biological agent, victims are sick and often require hospitalization. Without rapid identification of suspicious cases and isolation of these victims, the institution, health care providers, and other patients are at risk. If the onset of a bioterrorism event is insidious and community health care providers do not recognize the illness pattern or diagnostic clues, large numbers of casualties will result along with widespread panic. To prevent the spread of the disease-causing agent, standard precautions include handwashing; personal protective equipment (PPE) such as gloves and masks, eye protection, face shields, and gowns; and isolation or cohort placement (DHHS, 2020). Additional considerations in the management of the event include proper treatment and disinfection of equipment and the environment, postmortem care, notifying the pathology department, and possible further decontamination of patients and the environment.

SURVEILLANCE

Surveillance is a concept usually associated with the public health department.

Within the hospital, it is imperative to collect data related to the number of patients seen in the emergency department (ED) and how many are admitted with specific symptoms. This surveillance is typically supervised by the infection prevention or infection prevention and control department. There is a process in place to regulate the type of information that is reported by the clinical laboratories as results are confirmed. A syndromic surveillance process permits easy identification of trends or symptoms; presentations that are not typically seen in such numbers; or a larger than normal number of persons arriving at EDs, clinics, or health care providers' offices with similar symptoms or complaints. The first case identified is the sentinel event, the case or symptoms that first trigger an alarm.

Many disasters will not be announced with events as dramatic as those that occurred on September 11, 2001, and that involved victims from around the world. Careful observations and assessments by nurses and health care professionals will be key components in identifying the occurrence of terrorism and the specific type of event. Identification of suspicious illnesses or side effects of toxic agents within an institution cannot stop there. A thorough examination of the extent of the problem, number of occurrences, and disposition of the victims must be reported to the appropriate authorities so that the public can be protected and appropriate interventions can be provided to the victims and to the community as a whole.

DETERMINING CAPACITY

Those in authority must be able to quickly determine overall hospital capacity, status of critical care beds, how many casualties they can handle, how many operating rooms are available, and how many ventilators are available. Surge capacity is an estimation of the maximum patient load for which responding hospitals and agencies can provide care following a mass casualty event. It includes beds, staffing, equipment, and Emergency Medical Services (EMS) systems. When considering needed beds, surge capacity may be estimated to include a bed capacity of 500 acutely ill patients per million population for hospitalization and decontamination. Hospitals should be prepared to answer the following questions: Which patients can be discharged from the ED and inpatient floors quickly? Is it possible to relocate patients internally to provide additional space for victims or patients? Are nearby schools and hotels appropriate to provide efficient and necessary space for victims? How long will it take to prepare an appropriate triage area, and how much time is needed to set up a decontamination area? How many staff members can be recalled quickly? Nurses must take an active role in preparations to meet the increased needs following a disaster and increase the surge capacity of health care agencies and institutions.

DECONTAMINATION BASICS

Protection of staff and agency may involve decontamination. If contamination is suspected, victims should not be brought into the hospital until they have been decontaminated. Decontamination is the physical process of removing harmful substances from personnel, equipment, and supplies whenever there is a risk of secondary exposure from a hazardous substance. First, immediate evacuation efforts should be undertaken to remove victims from the source of contamination. Those victims who are ambulatory must be directed toward the decontamination process. The personnel performing decontamination must be wearing the appropriate level of PPE for the suspected contaminants (Fig. 4.3).

Personnel should remain alert, move upwind from the source, evacuate the area or go inside, close windows and doors, cover their mouths and noses, rinse copiously if splashed with an agent, and report all suspicious situations and objects. The decontamination process varies depending on the contaminant. Although water showers are frequently used (Fig. 4.4), dry (powder form) decontamination supplies must also be available. The decontamination area must have running water for showers and necessary ventilation. In addition, it is ideal that the area be at least 100 meters from the ED entrance and downwind from the hospital (Box 4.1).

Decontamination is used primarily for chemical warfare. It is not needed for covert bioterrorism events. A possible exception is an overt anthrax attack in which the toxins may mimic chemical exposures and warrant decontamination until the agent is known (Fig. 4.5).

COMMUNICATION DURING A DISASTER

Effective communication is vital during a disaster. Those involved in the disaster response must be able to communicate with each other and coordinate their efforts. If utilities are disabled or destroyed, many forms of traditional communication are lost. Today, more than ever, society is dependent on technology for communication and will be at a loss if common communication systems are disabled.

The communication system that will be used during a mass casualty event must be tested when lives are not depending on it. During this collaborative exercise, potential problems can be identified in advance. One method used is local planning committee drills to answer three key questions: How will we communicate? With whom should one communicate? What do authorities expect from each person? During or after a disaster, the communication system used may be different from the one used on a day-to-day basis. When this happens, a multitiered plan is activated and the needed equipment is moved to the triage area.

Despite planning prior to a disaster, the situation can become even more complicated and direct communication difficult if the health care providers must use PPE. Once a formerly easily recognizable colleague disappears into a cumbersome protective suit, accented with boots, heavy gloves, and a gas mask, verbal communication may be difficult or impossible. Methods of easily identifying each professional must be used to avoid needless movement and searching for a specific type of worker. For example, fluorescent signs or vests can be color coded according to role, such as doctors, nurses, and administrators, to quickly differentiate people.

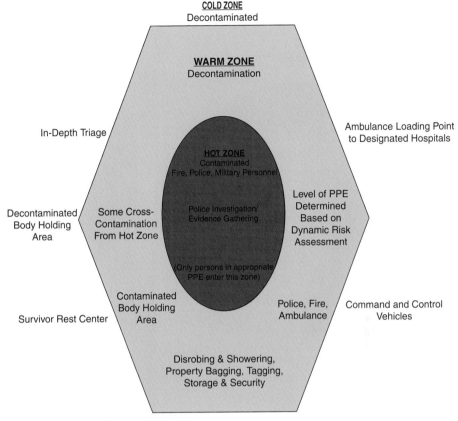

Fig. 4.3 Contamination/Decontamination Zones.

Each health care provider who may be an initial contact point for victims of bioterrorism should be familiar with their responsibility to report and with the person identified as the next contact. It may be easier to provide key personnel with a communication algorithm that can be carried at all times. Include appropriate telephone numbers. The entire communication plan should be easily available, but knowing the next step is critical and may result in a smooth response when suspicious incidents occur. Keep in mind that situations may change rapidly. For example, during the COVID-19 pandemic, changes occurred and information was updated daily or, in some cases, hourly. Numerous communications can overwhelm the ability of health care providers to review and respond appropriately. If health care agencies, health science centers, and schools of nursing and medicine, for example, appoint a "point person" who has the expertise to sift through information and provide employees and students with the most salient and evidence-based information, positive progress can be toward effective casualty and illness management.

Casualty Management

PREPARATIONS FOR CARE

Certain types of injuries can be anticipated depending on the type of event. For example, conventional weapons generally result in blast and penetration injuries. It is more difficult to anticipate

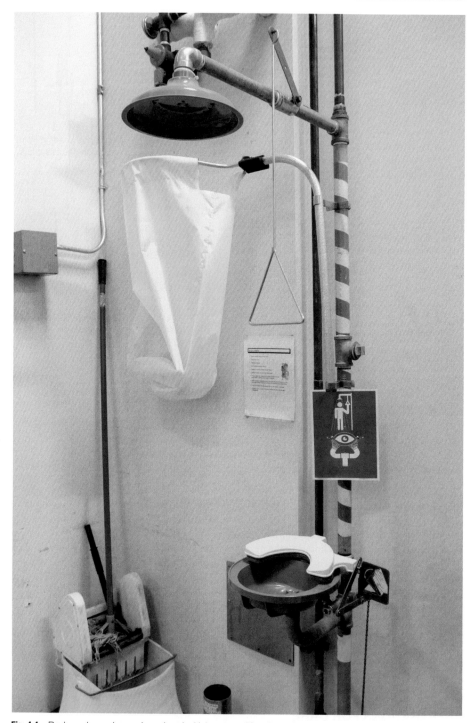

Fig. 4.4 Body and eye shower in a chemical laboratory. (iStock.com\marcduf)

> ## BOX 4.1 ■ Decontamination Considerations and Process
>
> Terrorist organizations throughout the world have used a variety of chemical, biological, and radiological weapons (collectively known as HAZMAT/weapons of mass destruction [WMD]) to further their agendas. The possibility of such incidents requires first responders to prepare for such incidents, which can affect individuals or inflict mass casualties.
>
> Incidents involving HAZMAT/WMD are complicated because victims may become contaminated with the hazardous material. The purpose of decontamination is to make an individual and/or their equipment safe by physically removing toxic substances quickly and easily.
>
> 1. Set up the decontamination and support areas
> 2. Conduct decontamination triage (for mass casualty incidents)
> 3. Decontaminate the victims
> 4. Segregate victims for observation or treatment
> 5. Release the victims afterwards
>
> ### Cold Weather Considerations
>
> Even in cold weather conditions to temperatures as low as 36° F, it is still most efficient to conduct decontamination outdoors using the water deluge method. Below 36° F, the removal of clothing and a dry decontamination method (such as blotting with paper towel) for the removal of liquids is recommended, followed by a water shower deluge at a heated facility.
>
> When using wet decontamination methods outdoors in cold weather, watch the victims for signs of hypothermia, including:
>
> ■ Severe shivering
> ■ Pallor in adults and flushed skin in children
> ■ Decreased hand coordination
> ■ Confusion
> ■ Slurred speech
> Note that children and elderly are at increased risk for hypothermia.
>
> Victims exhibiting signs of hypothermia may need to be treated both for exposure to the HAZMAT/WMD and exposure to the cold.
>
> ---
>
> Modified from US Department of Health and Human Services, Chemical Hazards Emergency Medical Management. (2021). Decontamination procedures. Retrieved from https://chemm.nlm.nih.gov/decontamination.htm#:~:text=%20Decontamination%20Procedures%20%201%20Step%201%3A%20Set,the%20water

injuries with an unknown or unrecognized chemical or biological agent. For this reason, a high index of suspicion may alert health care providers to the risk of contamination from chemical or biological agents sooner and decrease the overall number of injured or exposed. If the disaster is an industrial accident, the chemical may be known. In a terrorist attack, there may be a period when the agent is unknown but the institutions must be prepared to provide care. A mass transportation accident, a building collapse, a natural disaster such as an earthquake or a tornado all pose unique challenges to preparation and care. Maintaining contact with first responders on the scene of the event will enable the hospital or agency to prepare for the specific victim injuries seen with that type of disaster. Infectious diseases such as COVID-19 also present some unique challenges. Screening and testing of suspected cases present difficulties in providing adequate collection materials such as swabs, viral transport media, test kits, and laboratory reagents.

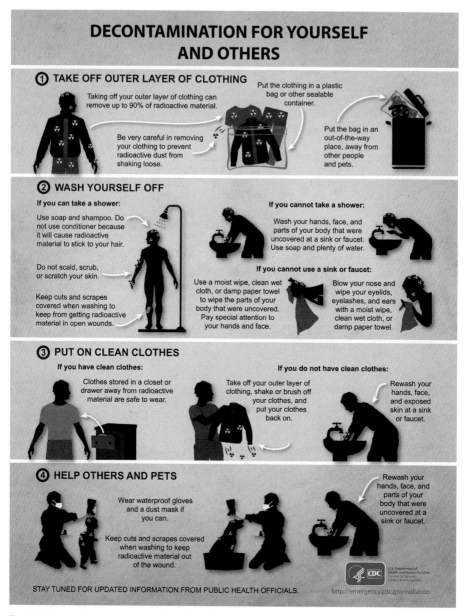

Fig. 4.5   Infographic on decontamination. (https://www.cdc.gov/)

STAFF

A specific community's needs and resources will determine the use of paid professional nurses or volunteers following a disaster or public health emergency (Fig. 4.6). The person in charge should plan for at least two shifts a day. In addition, plan for the protection of staff during decontamination and when caring for victims of biological agents. The California Emergency Medical Services Authority (EMSA, 2018) offers recommendations and education modules for hospitals

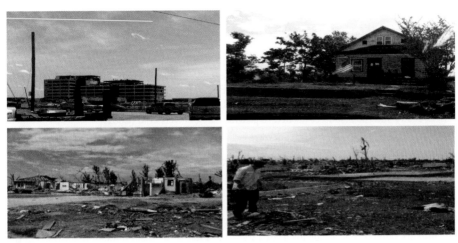

Fig. 4.6 Joplin tornado response. Volunteers assist in clean-up effort. (Used with permission Rachel Bené.)

that provide practical information for staff protection, decontamination, and evidence collection as well as an algorithm for setting up a decontamination area.

Maintaining the chain of evidence is an important responsibility after a terrorist event. Although patient care is the primary function of health care providers, management of evidence may be required as well. If victims can undress without assistance, direct them to place their valuables in a clear plastic bag with photo identification that is visible from the outside. Any assistive devices, including glasses, canes, or hearing aids, should remain with the victim during decontamination. Clothing should be placed in a prelabeled paper bag. If there is risk of secondary contamination due to the agent, place this paper bag in a clear plastic bag. Specific information should be included on the bag, such as name, date of birth, medical record number, date, time, any decontamination that was necessary, and the geographical site where the incident or contamination occurred. The same procedure is followed if the staff removes the victim's clothing. If possible, it is helpful to take a photo of the victim before undressing and then place this photo in the bag. Ideally, bags are stored without touching each other. Security or police officers should supervise this process, if possible (EMSA, 2018).

TRIAGE

Triage comes from the French word meaning "to sort." It is the continuous process in which priorities are reassigned as needed treatments, time, and conditions of the victims change. Victims are quickly assessed and assigned a priority or classification for receiving treatment according to the severity of the illness or injury. Triage involves balancing human lives with the realities of the situation, such as available supplies and personnel. Professional nurses perform triage every day in every ED through careful assessment and prioritizing of care. Personnel assigned to triage are expected to function independently yet as an integral part of a coordinated effort. Several types of triage exist.

Three-Level Triage

In the past, the Emergency Nurses Association manual described systems having three-, four-, and five-category models for triaging casualties. The three-level system groups victims as follows:
Category 1: Life threatening
Category 2: Emergent
Category 3: Stable, nonurgent

Research has suggested that this three-level model has lower reliability and efficacy (Travers, Waller, Bowling, Flowers, & Tintinalli, 2002).

Five-Level Triage

The five-level model is generally thought to be safer and more stable than the three- or four-level models. It categorizes patients according to the Emergency Severity Index (ESI) and includes specific questions asked about the victim, with the answers fitting into an algorithm based on patient acuity and the resources needed to provide care (Travers et al., 2002).

Start

Another form of triage is the Simple Triage and Rapid Treatment (START) technique, which is a specific triage method used to evaluate patient respiratory, circulatory, and neurological function and categorize each into one of four care categories (DHHS, 2021c) (Fig. 4.7).

Reverse Triage

The primary difference of triage associated with a disaster is the magnitude of the event and the focus on saving the greatest number of lives. Following a mass casualty event, nurses should expect a reverse or upside-down triage. In a normal situation, severely injured or ill patients are treated first, with less serious injuries or illnesses treated afterwards. In a mass casualty event, this is reversed. Victims who are most severely injured—those who require large amounts of supplies and health care provider time with little chance of surviving—are treated last. After a mass casualty event, victims are grouped into four classifications (Table 4.1).

Nurses at each health care facility must be knowledgeable about their institution's triage procedures, enabling them to respond quickly and effectively when a mass casualty event occurs and to provide guidance to other personnel. The specific procedures for prioritizing patient needs must be familiar to them and readily available to all responders as wall charts and as portable or individual prompt or cue cards.

PROVISION OF BLOOD COMPONENTS

During mass casualty events, blood components on the shelves are used for bleeding patients, most of whom receive the majority of blood products during the immediate resuscitation period. The time required for blood component collection, processing, infectious disease testing and quarantine, and transport means that products collected after the disaster will not be available until at least the third day post collection. During past events, blood donors have overwhelmed blood collection facilities, diverting blood donor center personnel away from dispensing blood products and ultimately resulting in waste of blood components (Schmidt, 2002). This reality highlights the need for a stable and robust nationwide blood supply.

In a mass casualty event, all blood products are needed: red blood cells for acute blood loss and to maintain blood volume; plasma for coagulation support, to reverse anticoagulation, and to treat dilutional coagulopathy in patients who have received large amounts of donor components; and platelets to assist clotting, particularly in patients who take antiplatelet medications. When available, cryoprecipitate may be used to supply coagulation factors with less volume compared to plasma. The urgent need for numerous blood components to be transfused quickly in multiple patients presents challenges to the hospital laboratory in general and the blood bank in particular. To dispense emergency-release uncross-matched products, laboratory computer systems require the patient to be registered, even if only as a John or Jane Doe. Transfusing emergency products is a risk for patients who may have antibodies, but in cases of severe bleeding, transfusion of blood products may be necessary. To dispense cross-matched and type-specific products, the patient

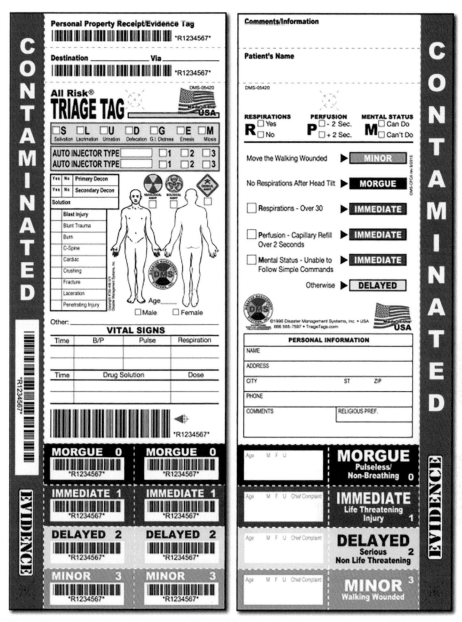

Fig. 4.7 Examples of triage tags. (Courtesy Disaster Management Systems, Inc., Pomona, CA.)

needs a confirmed blood type preferably drawn prior to receipt of donor blood components, and testing for antibodies to common red blood cell antigens. Patients commonly develop antibodies as a result of pregnancy or from previous transfusions. A positive antibody screen will complicate provision of compatible products in some patients and can result in serious or even life-threatening hemolytic reactions if red blood cells positive for the implicated antigen are transfused before

TABLE 4.1 ■ Triage Classifications: Mass Casualty Event

Survivor Classification	Treatment Needs and Location
Class I	Minor professional treatment needed
	Handled in outpatient or ambulatory setting
Class II	Injuries require immediate life-sustaining treatments
	Moderately injured victims
	Initial treatment requires minimum of time, personnel, and supplies
Class III	Victims' definitive treatment can be delayed without jeopardy to life or loss of limb
Class IV	Victims with wounds or injuries requiring extensive treatment beyond the immediate medical capabilities
	Treatment of these victims jeopardizes other victims
	Victims need large amounts of supplies and personnel

Adapted from Clarkson, L., & Williams, M. (2019). *EMS mass casualty triage*. National Center for Biotechnology Research. Retrieved from https://www.ncbi.nlm.nih.gov/books/NBK459369/

antibody identification. Level I Trauma Centers and some smaller community hospitals have massive transfusion protocols (MTPs) to provide blood components in fixed ratios in a streamlined manner. However, even at facilities with MTPs in place, blood component demand for multiple patients may outstrip the ability of available transfusion service personnel to dispense sufficient products quickly. Depending on the available inventory of specific blood components, demand may exceed supply. Most hospitals keep only a small inventory of group O, Rh-negative red blood cells, and these may be reserved for trauma patients whose ABO type is unknown and for women of childbearing age. These women are at heightened risk if exposure to blood causes an antibody to form, so-called alloimmunization. Any red blood cell antibody that forms can put future pregnancies at risk for hemolytic disease of the fetus and newborn (HDFN), in which maternal red blood cell antibodies (specific for red cell antigens that are paternally inherited) cause the potentially life-threatening destruction of fetal and newborn red cells (Fung et al., 2017). Group O, Rh-negative donors make up only 7% of the donor population. However, their red blood cells are the type most needed by emergently bleeding patients who present to the hospital during the interval in which their specific blood type has yet to be determined. Increasingly, some laboratories have limited staff on weekends and overnight shifts; these staff members may cover multiple laboratory areas, particularly at smaller community hospitals. This type of "lean" staffing further complicates a sudden influx of large numbers of bleeding patients.

Disaster preparedness and mass casualty drills are informative and often highlight obstacles to timely blood provision in emergency situations. Delays in registration and proper identification of patients, confusion when multiple unidentified unconscious patients arrive in close proximity, and ED staff who are caring for many critical patients at one time strain hospital resources, alter established protocols, and often provoke "shortcuts" in processes developed to protect patient safety. When a patient is bleeding out in the ED, it may be difficult to understand the blood bank's demand to immediately send a sample for blood typing and antibody screening. However, if specimens are not drawn until after the patient has received multiple donor blood components, the testing will not truly be performed on the patient's blood, and it may be impossible to determine the patient's original blood type or antibody status. This can delay the provision of type-specific blood products and further exhaust the limited hospital supply of valuable group O, Rh-negative red blood cells (Fig. 4.8).

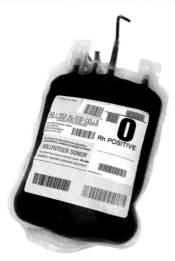

Fig. 4.8 A Life-Saving Unit of Blood. (From Stein, L., & Hollen, C. J. (2021). *Concept-based clinical nursing skills*. Elsevier.)

PATIENT TRACKING

Identification

One of the issues facing all health care facilities is the identification and tracking of patients. If the influx of patients overwhelms the electronic health record (EHR) system, an EHR is not used, or there is no power in the building, pre-assembled medical records should be located throughout the ED or triage area. Staff must be able to identify people as soon as possible after they arrive for care, as patients must be moved rapidly and efficiently through the triage and decontamination areas and into the facility for indicated treatments and procedures. The prepared medical records are opened using an identification system. The system does not need to be elaborate. A simple system such as each record containing adhesive number sheets is adequate, so that all treatment information, testing, and follow-up are documented using these numbers. As soon as possible, the facility can return to using more traditional identification procedures, such as EHRs, if power is available or its typical patient identification and tracking system.

Confidentiality

The security and privacy of health data should be protected for all patients. This security of medical information is challenge during an episode of mass casualties. Password protection of patient information needs to be incorporated within the identification and tracking systems. This may be increasingly difficult with larger numbers of casualties and victim information being entered at multiple locations during care by multiple people with access to the patient tracking system.

Reunification Centers

The DHHS (2021d) has an excellent website that offers a great deal of information on family reunification and resources (https://asprtracie.hhs.gov/technical-resources/64/family-reunification-and-support/0).

Most disasters are very frightening experiences; the trauma to individuals escalates when family members are not easily found. Reunification centers provide valuable services in locating lost loved ones and collecting information to aid in this effort.

Transfer to Alternative Care Sites

At times, it will be impossible to treat disaster survivors at the typical or familiar community locations due to the health care agencies having suffered severe damage. Alternative care sites are often quickly erected by those who have come to the aid of victims. If the broad-based community plans include these alternative care sites, it is possible that these sites will be well stocked and prepared for a surge of patients. However, even the best plans do not satisfy every disaster situation, which often results in the need for creative problem solving among those with the authority to provide care in available often quickly constructed shelters. If the community's care sites are able to care for patients, they often come to realize that some patients no longer have homes in the wake of the disaster. These families will have to seek temporary shelter where it is available and safe. Keeping track of these survivors, who are now essentially homeless, poses another challenge to officials who would like to reunite family members and support communication with distant family members.

Transfer to Morgue

An unfortunate reality of many disasters and public health emergencies is the need to create morgue space for human remains. The goal is to return these remains to family members when possible for humanitarian and legal reasons. This is yet another type of reunification, albeit a very tragic result of disaster response efforts.

Case in Point

RELEASE OF A BIOLOGICAL AGENT IN A DOMED STADIUM

It is 3:00 p.m on a Sunday afternoon. The city's professional football team is playing, and the domed stadium is filled to capacity (55,000). The EMS personnel on-site have called to report that they have seen 12 persons exhibiting symptoms of watery eyes, coughing, shortness of breath, hypertension, fever, and prostration. Family members of the victims have begun to talk with other spectators, and people have begun to respond to the news of a possible biological agent and are hurrying from the area. EMS suspects that many of these people will be coming to the hospital. You are the charge nurse in the ED.

Questions for Discussion

1. What is the first thing you should do?
2. Describe the process of activating the disaster response plan.
3. What departments and services should be notified?

Points to Remember

- As a professional nurse, you are expected to recognize and report clusters of patients who report to the health care facility with suspicious signs and symptoms of a disease outbreak.
- An effective disaster preparedness, response, and recovery team consists of multidisciplinary members, including safety and security, fire, police, infection control officers, and representative health care providers (nurses, physicians and laboratory, pharmacy, nutrition, and plant management).
- Basic triage means the sorting of patients based on illness or injury. Reverse triage occurs during mass casualty events when the least injured are treated first to do the greatest good for the greatest number.

- Stockpiling of necessary medicines, equipment, supplies, and shelter provisions is a proactive means of preparing for potential disasters and public health emergencies.

Test Your Knowledge

1. Important members or groups to include when selecting for the disaster response committee include: *(Choose all that apply.)*
   a. Nursing
   b. Medicine
   c. Infection control
   d. Safety and security
2. If a bioterrorism event is suspected, the first notification entity is:
   a. Emergency department and infection control
   b. Law enforcement and fire department
   c. Local health department
   d. American Red Cross
3. The system used for analyzing data to track a perpetrator to limit further damage to persons or property is the responsibility of:
   a. The Director of Nursing
   b. The FBI
   c. The Medical Director
   d. The Security Detail at the scene
4. Which of the following reflect basic decontamination principles? *(Choose all that apply.)*
   a. The person who will care for the hospitalized patient will decontaminate the patient.
   b. The person who decontaminates patients will stay in that area for the entire shift.
   c. The person who decontaminates patients also will be decontaminated.
   d. The person who cares for the patient in the hospital will remain in the clean area.
5. After a mass casualty event or a drill, which of the following should take place? *(Choose all that apply.)*
   a. A careful review of actions or inactions should occur.
   b. The deficient team members should be transferred to less stressful areas.
   c. A no-blame climate should permeate the debriefing session.
   d. An action plan should be developed to strengthen identified areas of weakness.
6. A method of sorting disaster victims and prioritizing their care after a mass casualty event when there are limited resources of personnel and equipment is called:
   a. Triage
   b. Mitigation
   c. Reverse triage
   d. Response and recovery
7. Which of the following blood products may be used during emergency transfusion support? *(Choose all that apply.)*
   a. Red blood cells
   b. Plasma
   c. Platelets
   d. Cryoprecipitate
8. What type of red blood cell is needed when an emergency patient is a woman of childbearing age and her blood type is unknown?
   a. Group O, Rh-positive
   b. Group O, Rh-negative
   c. Group A, Rh-positive
   d. Group AB, Rh-negative

   9. In hemolytic disease of the fetus and newborn (HDFN), what is the source of the potentially life-threatening antibodies?
   a. Maternal
   b. Paternal
   c. HLA
   d. Neonatal
   10. Why is it critical that severely bleeding patients have their blood drawn prior to receiving donor blood products?
   a. Risk of hemolytic disease of the fetus and newborn (HDFN) during future pregnancies
   b. Patient misidentification
   c. Difficulty in blood typing due to donor red blood cell interference
   d. Need for critical medications

References

California Emergency Medical Services Authority. (2018). *Tactical casualty care and tactical medicine*. Retrieved from https://emsa.ca.gov/tactical_casualty_care_and_tactical_medicine_for_special_operations/

California Hospital Association. (2017). *What are the six critical areas of emergency response according to The Joint Commission (TJC)?* Retrieved from https://www.calhospitalprepare.org/post/what-are-six-critical-areas-emergency-response-according-joint-commission-tjc

Centers for Medicare and Medicaid Services. (2019). *Emergency preparedness rule*. Retrieved from https://www.cms.gov/Medicare/Provider-Enrollment-and-Certification/SurveyCertEmergPrep/Emergency-Prep-Rule

Fung MK, Eder AF, Spitalnik SL, Westhoff CM. *AABB technical manual*. 19th ed. : AABB; 2017.

Schmidt PJ. Blood and disaster—Supply and demand. *New England Journal of Medicine*. 2002;346(8):617–619.

Travers DA, Waller AE, Bowling JM, Flowers D, Tintinalli J. Five-level triage system more effective than three-level in tertiary emergency department. *Journal of Emergency Nursing*. 2002;28(5):395–400.

US Department of Health and Human Services. (2020). *What is the difference between isolation and quarantine?* Retrieved from https://www.hhs.gov/answers/public-health-and-safety/what-is-the-difference-between-isolation-and-quarantine/index.html

US Department of Health and Human Services. (2021a). *Regional disaster health response system: An overview*. Retrieved from https://www.phe.gov/Preparedness/planning/RDHRS/Pages/rdhrs-overview.aspx

US Department of Health and Human Services. (2021b). *Strategic national stockpile*. Retrieved from https://www.phe.gov/about/sns/Pages/default.aspx

US Department of Health and Human Services. (2021c). *Chemical hazards emergency medical management: START adult triage*. Retrieved from https://chemm.nlm.nih.gov/startadult.htm

US Department of Health and Human Services. (2021d). *Topic collection: Family reunification and support*. Retrieved from https://asprtracie.hhs.gov/technical-resources/64/family-reunification-and-support/0

CHAPTER 5

Recovery: Promoting Behavioral Health

Dorcas McLaughlin, PhD, APRN, PMHCNS-BC ◼ Jody Spiess, PhD, RN, GCPH ◼ Janice L. Palmer, PhD, RN, CNE

CHAPTER OUTLINE

Introduction 82

Neurobiology of Stress 83

Population Exposure Model 85

Phases of Disaster Responses 86

Resiliency 89

Early Intervention and Triage 89

Protecting from Further
  Threat and Distress 90

Helping to Locate Family Members 90

Sharing Experiences and
  Validating Emotions 91

Facilitating a Sense of Being in
  Control 91

Linking Survivors with Support and
  Resources 92

Stabilizing the Family Unit 92

Promoting Community Support 92

Crisis Intervention 92

Crisis Counseling Assistance and
  Training Program 93

Six-Step Crisis Intervention Model 94

Crisis Assessment and Intervention 94

**Adverse Behavioral Health Outcomes
and Therapies** 97

Emotions 97

  Stress 97

  Grief 98

  Anger 99

  Shame 99

  Survivor's Guilt 100

Behavioral Health Disorders 100

  Acute Stress Disorder 100

  Post-Traumatic Stress Disorder 101

  Major Depressive Disorder 101

  Substance Use Disorders 101

Select Post-Traumatic Distress Disorder
  Therapies 101

  Cognitive Behavioral Therapy 101

  Expressive Art Therapy 102

Vulnerable Populations 102

Children 102

Older Adults and Those with Cognitive
  Impairment or Disabilities 103

People of Diverse Cultural Backgrounds 104

People with Low Socioeconomic Status 104

Vicarious Traumatization 104

Self-Care 105

Case in Point 106

Boston Marathon Bombing: Survivor
  Experiencing Symptoms of Acute
  Stress Disorder 106

  Questions for Discussion 107

Points to Remember 107

Test Your Knowledge 107

References 108

After reading and studying this chapter, you should be able to:
- Describe the neurobiology of stress and trauma
- Compare and contrast the psychological responses of survivors in each phase of a disaster and various intervention methods
- Examine ways to promote recovery before and after disaster, including prevention, psychological first aid, triage, crisis assessment and intervention, and follow-up
- Discuss ways to help survivors cope with loss
- Describe adverse behavioral health outcomes postdisaster among individuals and families
- Explore psychological interventions to facilitate recovery in survivors after disasters
- Identify vulnerable or at-risk groups for adverse behavioral health outcomes
- Describe vicarious traumatization and methods to prevent and alleviate symptoms

crisis: A life event that occurs when stressors are overwhelming and usual problem-solving and coping skills are inadequate.

crisis intervention: Short-term, action-oriented intervention with the goals of reducing distress, restoring a person to the predisaster level of functioning, and preventing adverse behavioral health outcomes.

psychological first aid: An early intervention to help people in the immediate aftermath of a disaster to reduce distress and facilitate adaptation and coping.

recovery: Actions taken to restore the physical, psychological, social, environmental, and economic well-being of individuals and the community to facilitate return to the predisaster level of functioning.

resilience: The ability to "bounce back" or prepare for, adapt to, and rapidly recover from a disastrous event and resume a productive life.

stress: The response of the body to any external or internal demands for change and adaptation.

vicarious traumatization: Negative psychological responses from repeatedly hearing firsthand accounts of disasters and trauma, which causes effects similar to direct exposure to the events. Also referred to as compassion fatigue.

vulnerability: Greater risk of negative experiences, effects, and reactions before, during, and after a disaster.

Introduction

Every year people all over the world are affected by human-made and natural disasters. Disasters result in extensive damage and suffering, seriously disrupt the lives of those affected, and exceed the usual coping resources of some. Behavioral health issues are regarded as a major concern following disasters. Study findings indicate that psychological traumas, as compared to physical injuries, comprise the greatest health risks for disaster survivors with ratios ranging from 4:1 to as much as 50:1 (Substance Abuse and Mental Health Services Administration [SAMHSA], 2016). In the immediate aftermath of a disaster, most people manifest stress reactions; however, even when these stress reactions are extreme, they are not considered pathological. Although some survivors have more long-term behavioral health needs, the vast majority of disaster survivors show considerable strength and resilience.

As the largest group of health care professionals, nurses often play an integral role in the disaster recovery process. In addition to treating physical injuries, nurses address the emotional, social, and cultural dimensions associated with disasters. Therefore, nurses need to develop the interpersonal skills to assist survivors to cope and also to be aware of their own risk for vicarious traumatization as they care for others.

This chapter explores frameworks for understanding recovery, including the neurobiological stress responses to disasters, phases of disaster response, guidelines for assessment, and behavioral health interventions to promote recovery. Assessment, planning, and pertinent interventions are integrated throughout since these steps of the nursing process proceed quickly and together in times of disasters. The final section focuses on the assessment of adverse behavioral health outcomes, interventions to promote recovery, and self-care.

Since the beginning of time, disasters have caused chaos and turmoil affecting the health and well-being of individuals and communities. Originally, natural disasters such as famines, earthquakes, and wildfires were the focus of attention. However, more recently human-made disasters such as mass violence; wars; oil spills; and diseases such as SARS, Ebola, and COVID-19 have become more prevalent, mandating greater attention to the recovery process. The recovery process focuses on the safety and stabilization of individuals and communities and returning to a new normal.

Disasters are stressful experiences that threaten life, safety, health, and well-being. Stress is the response of the body to any external *(outer)* or internal *(inner)* demands for change and adaptation. In disasters, people adapt with an array of physical and psychological reactions that vary in severity and type. Table 5.1 summarizes the common physical, emotional, behavioral, and cognitive reactions to disasters and traumatic events. Some individuals express these reactions immediately, whereas others may express them weeks, months, or years later. See Box 5.1 for examples of the reactions of tornado survivors in Joplin, Missouri. Unrelenting high levels of stress resulting in persistent epinephrine surges may lead to or exacerbate a wide range of physical and behavioral health problems such as cardiovascular and respiratory complications, difficulty sleeping, feelings of anxiety, and post-traumatic stress disorder.

Neurobiology of Stress

Understanding the neurobiological underpinnings of stress and trauma provides nurses with a conceptual framework for understanding the physiological reactions and behavioral health

TABLE 5.1 ■ **Common Stress Reactions to Disasters and Traumatic Events**

Physical	Emotional	Behavioral	Cognitive
Heart palpitations	Fear and terror	Crying easily	Confusion
Rapid breathing	Anxiety	Irritability	Memory impairment
Tension	Numbness	Aggression	Intrusive thoughts
Agitation	Grief and sadness	Hypervigilance	Nightmares
Lightheadedness	Anger	Suspiciousness	Flashbacks
Fatigue	Helplessness	Avoidance	Distorted time
Sleep disturbances	Hopelessness	Isolation	Dissociation
Body aches and pain	Shame	Withdrawal	Worry
Appetite changes	Guilt	Relationship conflicts	Self-blame
Startle response	Mood swings	Impaired functioning	Self-doubt

BOX 5.1 ■ Examples of the Range of Experiences of Disaster Survivors

Individuals who experience direct exposure to the disaster

"I remember walking back to my house and I know I saw people gravely injured but I couldn't tell you, I couldn't tell you what they looked like. I couldn't tell you who they were. I know they were my neighbors ... my brain shut it off" (Langan et al., 2017, p. 62).

"I ... think you go through an inventory, you know what's here, what's not here, what's important, and what's not important ... you answer the most important questions first. You know: Where am I gonna sleep tonight? What am I going to eat tomorrow? Is my house livable? Is my car drivable ... After the tornado, you start to take an inventory" (Langan et al., 2017, p. 62).

First responders and health care personnel who participate in rescue and recovery activities

"I knew that I was safe, my daughters were safe, everyone in my family was safe. Then I knew I had to deal with what I saw later. I am sure that is part of nursing mode to know you just have to deal with, face things head on and process what you saw later" (Langan et al., 2017, p. 62).

Community, including those who converge, who altruistically offer help, and who share the grief and loss or are in some way involved

"Coping with stress is not an issue for me at this time. It comes later for me ... Right after the tornado ... I headed straight towards the hospital. I had to hike in through the neighborhoods that had been hit ... Well the memories are there. It's a blur, the stress was there but you didn't stop to evaluate your stress" (Langan et al., 2017, p. 62).

Individuals who are upset or psychologically distressed

"... the only thing that was left in my house was the deck. It was intact, everything else was completely destroyed and we were sitting there, we were just crying and crying and crying ... So I just kind of disengaged myself from relationships, people who you know I used to talk to on a daily basis ... I would kind of blow them off" (Langan et al., 2017, p. 62).

Quotes are from research of tornado survivors in Joplin, Missouri, as reported in Langan, J., Palmer, J. L., Christopher, K., & Shagavah, A. (2017). Joplin tornado survivors, hospital employees and community members: Reflections of resilience and acknowledgment of pain. Health Emergency and Disaster Nursing, *4*, 57–65. https://doi.org/10.24298/hedn.2016-0004

---

responses commonly observed in survivors. In extremely stressful or life-threatening disasters, pandemics, or traumas, the body continually adapts and changes in response to signals from the external environment and internal bodily sensations. In response to this sensory input, the body automatically initiates a multitude of physiological adaptations to expedite the likelihood of survival (van der Kolk, 2014).

Sensory information enters the body through the eyes, ears, nose, tongue, and skin and is sent to the thalamus, an area of the brain that acts as a relay station. Then the thalamus directs the information to the amygdala, an area of the brain that interprets the sensory input and evaluates the situation as dangerous or safe. With the help of the hippocampus, an area of the brain adjacent to the amygdala, new experiences are compared with previous experiences to assist with the appraisal. If the amygdala appraises the situation as dangerous or threatening, within milliseconds distress signals are sent to the autonomic nervous system (ANS) and the hypothalamus to stimulate a defensive survival response and ready the body for mobilization or action. In addition, the thalamus relays the sensory information to the prefrontal cortex to facilitate conscious processing of the experience. Because the amygdala processes the sensory information so much faster than the prefrontal cortex, the body automatically initiates the defensive survival response before conscious awareness (van der Kolk, 2014).

The ANS plays a crucial role in survival. It controls all automatic functions of the body, such as heartbeat, body temperature, rate of breathing, and digestion. It consists of an extensive network of interconnected neurons throughout the brain and body that operates automatically by sending signals to glands, smooth muscles, and the heart to regulate states of arousal and calming. The ANS has two main divisions—the sympathetic and parasympathetic nervous systems—that regulate energy levels and homeostasis in the body. The sympathetic nervous system (SNS) functions as an accelerator or stimulator by arousing and mobilizing the body for action. In contrast, the parasympathetic nervous system (PNS) acts as a decelerator or inhibitor by calming, conserving, and restoring the body. These two ANS divisions work together to ensure that the body responds appropriately to situations that arise.

In moments of extreme stress, the sympathetic and parasympathetic nervous systems precipitate an automatic, involuntary, physiological survival response known as fight, flight, freeze, or faint. This response involves a complex set of interactions among multiple parts of the brain, the ANS and the body. The first line of survival is an SNS arousal or mobilization response resulting in fight or flight. When threatened with danger, the SNS signals the adrenal medullary system and the hypothalamic-pituitary-adrenal (HPA) axis to release a cascade of biochemical changes to arouse the body for mobilization. The adrenal medullary system secretes epinephrine and norepinephrine for an immediate response to the threat or danger. If energy triggered by the release of epinephrine and norepinephrine is not sufficient to resolve the distress, the HPA axis signals the release of cortisol, which further mobilizes the body for action. Cortisol increases the amount of energy needed by raising glucose levels to fuel the body and to sharpen mental activity in the brain. At the same time, cortisol shuts down body systems not immediately necessary for responding to the threat, such as the digestive system and immune response. These biochemical changes activate SNS arousal, including pupil dilatation, airway expansion, increased muscle tone, rapid heart rate, and release of glucose from fat storage sites. However, when fight or flight is not possible, the PNS activates a last-resort defensive survival response, freezing or fainting, resulting in immobility or collapse. With a surge of acetylcholine, the PNS inhibits the SNS, causing a decrease in heart rate and blood pressure. If blood flow is restricted to the brain, consciousness may be lost and fainting may occur due to the disruption of signals to maintain muscle tone. The freeze-or-faint survival response may range from a partial freeze, such as the inability to move body parts or think clearly, to a full body freeze and collapse (van der Kolk, 2014).

For most survivors, stress reactions are transient and normal functioning returns quickly, especially with support from family friends, and the community. However, for other survivors recovery is slower and functioning may be impaired in their personal, family and work lives. Risk factors that may contribute to more symptomatic stress reactions in survivors after disasters and trauma include severity of exposure, meaning attributed to the disaster or trauma, level of personal maturity, predisaster level of functioning, cultural influences, and limited availability of support systems and resources. Box 5.2 lists symptomatic stress reactions to disasters and traumatic events that require behavioral health evaluation.

Population Exposure Model

The *population exposure model* provides guidance in predicting and understanding the variability of responses of individuals and communities (Federal Emergency Management Agency [FEMA], 2016). According to this model, individuals with the greatest direct experiences associated with a disaster are likely to be the most affected physically and psychologically. As a tornado survivor in Joplin, Missouri, explained: "I see it like ripples in the pond when you drop that stone. Everyone [in the tornado area] is affected and no one doubts that or questions that in any way. But there is a difference in experience depending on what ripple you were in" (Langan, Palmer, Christopher, & Shagavah, 2017, p. 62). The population exposure model consists of a series of concentric circles representing survivors most affected at the center and moving outward to survivors with lower impact (Fig. 5.1). However, since disaster exposure intersects with individual and community vulnerability risk factors, it is important not to assume that all survivors on the outer circles of the

---

BOX 5.2 ■ Symptomatic Stress Reactions to Disasters and Traumatic Events

- Significant disorientation to time, place, person, place
- Suicidal or homicidal thoughts, plans, attempts
- Flashbacks, terrifying nightmares, intrusive thoughts.
- Hearing voices, seeing visions, bizarre thoughts
- Feeling out of body, feeling unreal, numbness, dissociations

- Extreme restlessness, agitation, aggression, violence
- Debilitating anxiety, panic, fear of another disaster
- Problematic substance or alcohol abuse
- Inability to care for self or provide basic needs
- Pervasive feelings of hopelessness, helplessness, despair

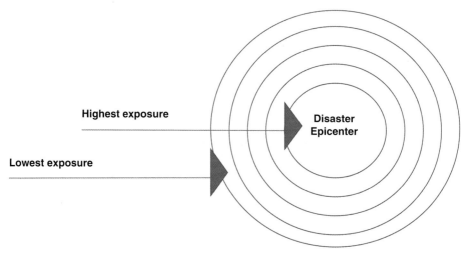

Fig. 5.1 Population exposure model FEMA, 2016.

model will be affected only minimally and that two individuals with a shared level of exposure will be affected similarly.

Phases of Disaster Responses

A disaster may be described as a sequence of phases in which various psychological responses are manifested in individuals and the community as a whole. The first phase, the *predisaster phase*, focuses on preparedness. The next four phases, *impact, heroic, honeymoon,* and *disillusionment phases*, address response efforts. The final phase, the *reconstruction phase*, emphasizes recovery with the hope of returning to the predisaster state of function or adapting to a new sense of normality (FEMA, 2016). See Fig. 5.2 for a graphic illustration of the phases of disasters and the corresponding psychological reactions. The normality or predictability of the response and recovery of individuals, groups, and the community are discussed next.

The *predisaster phase* consists of recognizing that a disaster could occur, a *warning*, or that a disaster is approaching, a *threat*. Responses among those at risk for disaster range from active planning and protective measures to denial of the reality of a threat. There has been a dramatic surge of interest in the psychological impact of disasters on people, especially in the wake of the

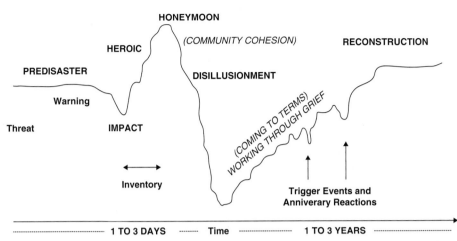

Fig. 5.2 Phases of disaster FEMA, 2016.

COVID-19 pandemic, recent terrorist attacks, and mass violence. The destruction of the World Trade Center, the bombing at the Boston Marathon, the shooting at the Pulse nightclub in Orlando, and terrorist actions in other communities make us acutely aware of our own vulnerability. These atrocities shatter our belief that the world is a predictable, safe place. The unpredictability, lack of control, and malevolence associated with terrorist attacks and mass violence are more disturbing to behavioral health than natural disasters related to weather changes or geophysical forces (Riaz et al., 2015). Anticipating disasters can be stressful, and those who do not heed warnings may experience feelings of guilt or shame (FEMA, 2016). The increased media attention to these tragedies has increased our awareness of their far-reaching behavioral health effects and the need for psychological preparedness.

The *impact phase (first hours or days after a disaster)* is a period of chaos and disorganization (Fig. 5.3). This phase is variable, depending on the degree of life threat, the number of deaths and injuries, and the extent of destruction to the community. The larger the area of destruction and devastation, the more adverse the physical and psychological effects will be (FEMA, 2016). Reactions in this phase vary from panic and hysteria to clarity. Family members may be displaced or separated, resulting in increased anxiety and distress. The decision to leave pets behind or hand them off to strangers can affect a survivor's decision to evacuate or leave a potentially dangerous situation and cause distress. Even during the impact phase, most survivors show a great deal of strength and resilience. Positive responses include efforts to cope physically and emotionally and altruistic efforts to help others.

During the *heroic phase (hours to weeks after a disaster)*, survivors may act heroically by helping their neighbors and loved ones even at the risk of injury to themselves. Likewise, natural leaders and rescue workers from the affected community begin to appear and attend to the physical and psychological needs of others (Math, Nirmala, Maoirangthem, & Kumer, 2015). Rescuers do everything possible to prevent loss of life and property; efforts focus on stabilizing the situation. During the heroic phase, a number of crises may arise, affecting physical or emotional health, employment, or financial stability. Although survivors and disaster rescue workers are likely to experience normal to severe stress responses, most do not develop long-term physical health problems or adverse behavioral health disorders (Goldmann & Galea, 2014; Math et al., 2015). The helping response at this time should be supportive counseling and, if necessary, referral and treatment.

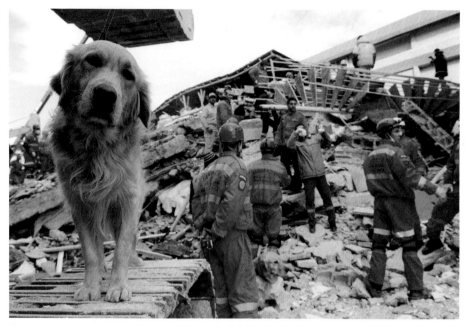

Fig. 5.3   Chaos, disorganization, and heroic rescue after an earthquake. (iStock.com\deepspace)

In the immediate aftermath of a disaster, survivors often go through a *honeymoon phase (first few days to weeks after impact)*. The outpouring of community support lifts spirits, and optimism is high concerning the promise of government aid. Survivors are grateful to be alive. The main concern in this phase is meeting basic needs, but some survivors may not understand the full extent of the emotional turmoil resulting from the situation. The community is thankful for the attention and presence of disaster response personnel, and people naturally gather to demonstrate mutual support, share experiences, and make meaning out of what has happened (FEMA, 2016; Math et al., 2015).

However, in the weeks that follow, survivors may experience the *disillusionment phase* when making a more realistic appraisal of the full extent of loss, the financial resources needed to rebuild, and the likelihood that things will never completely return to the way they were prior to the disaster. Survivors take inventory and begin to comprehend the losses sustained. The suddenness, multiple losses, and violent deaths often lead to complicated mourning. Both women and men may weep as they focus on the immediate past and how they managed to survive and become aware of the full impact of the event. Masses of people converge on the disaster site and may inadvertently create additional problems. Some wish to help, others search for loved ones, and many are curious. The media also bring in crews to report on the event. Survivors attempt to re-establish contact with family and community.

The *reconstruction phase* or *recovery (months or in some cases 2 to 3 years after the disaster)* is the prolonged period of returning to the predisaster level of functioning. Individuals and communities on their way to healing attempt to bring their lives and activities back to normal. Clean up of debris, rebuilding of physical structures, and implementation of long-term recovery programs occur. Survivors begin to solve their own problems and work to rebuild the community. This rebuilding and recovery process may continue for years after a disaster (FEMA, 2016). The emotional, cognitive, behavioral, and spiritual effects of devastation and implications for the future must be dealt with through interventions with individuals, families, and community groups. The emergence of disaster trauma may become evident and require high levels of intervention. Survivors in the recovery process begin to put the disaster behind them and look toward the future. The reconstruction or recovery phase may last for several years.

Resiliency

Many survivors show resilience and adaptation following disasters. According to Richardson, Neiger, Jensen, and Kumpfer (1990), individuals may recover from a disaster with one of four levels of resiliency. Some will have higher levels of resiliency, referred to as *resilient reintegration*, as they find and appreciate new strengths. An older adult tornado survivor in Joplin, Missouri, expressed this with the following quote: "During the past year it seems like I'm in better health than some of my children ... I have coped and helped support them ... Anyone that needs assistance, just give me a call" (Langan et al., 2017, p. 62). Some individuals experience a return to their baseline level of resiliency, referred to as *homeostasis*. Other individuals struggle to cope and adapt and experience a lower level of resiliency *(reintegration with loss)*, and some experience *dysfunctional reintegration*. Individuals with higher levels of resiliency experience the distress associated with disasters for a shorter time and return to predisaster functioning more quickly. Protective factors including social support, coping style, community response, higher income and education, and successful mastery of past disasters and traumatic events may moderate behavioral health problems. Positive coping strategies, such as humor or assertiveness, along with availability of recovery services and expressions of care, concern, and understanding from recovery services personnel are also protective factors.

The aim of many disaster preparedness and recovery plans is to decrease the severity of the impact of disasters through building resilience in individuals and communities. Resilience is generally defined as the ability to "bounce back" or prepare for, adapt to, and rapidly recover from a disastrous event and resume a productive life. It is important to consider that only a small proportion of people exposed to a disaster develop significant behavioral health complications (FEMA, 2016). For example, Langan et al. (2017) found that only approximately 10% of the Joplin tornado study participants continued to have low or concerning levels of resilience 3 years postevent. In other words, nurses can expect recovery of the behavioral health of most survivors and should convey a sense of hope.

As noted, survivors vary enormously in the ways they respond to disasters. Often confused by their reactions, survivors are uncertain about the best way of adapting to their distress. It is essential to communicate that stress reactions in the immediate aftermath of a disaster, such as anxiety, sadness, irritability, intrusive thoughts, memory problems, relationship difficulties, sleep disturbances, and appetite changes, are highly prevalent. These are normal reactions to abnormal events. Usually these stress reactions are time-limited and resolve completely (Goldmann & Galea, 2014; Math et al., 2015; Webber & Mascari, 2018).

Early Intervention and Triage

Experts agree that early intervention following disasters can reduce psychological distress and prevent chronic adverse behavioral health problems (Webber & Mascari, 2018). Interventions include acknowledgement of perceptions and the reality of the experiences, assurance about perceived strengths, validation of the ability to survive and manage, education about normal stress reactions, methods to increase self-care and coping skills, and linkage with or referral to services. Frequently, survivors do not see themselves as needing behavioral health services. Often they turn to family members or significant others for assistance in coping with psychological distress following disasters (FEMA, 2016; Langan & Krieger, 2018).

Psychological first aid (PFA) is an early intervention to help survivors in the immediate aftermath of disasters to reduce distress and facilitate adaptation and coping. PFA includes offering compassionate presence, providing psychological support, assisting survivors to cope with normal stress reactions, making referrals when more intensive interventions are needed, and helping survivors return to their predisaster baseline level of functioning. Foundations for providing psychological first aid interventions are based on crisis intervention (Shultz & Forbes, 2013).

Early PFA interventions include establishing trust and rapport and being firm and positive to ensure that persons do not injure themselves. Demonstrate empathy: "You're hurting a lot." Offer presence. Acknowledge and validate the survivor's experience: "I'm sorry this happened to you." "You are alive." "I'm here to help you." The triage process can link those affected with either supportive counseling or, if necessary, emergency behavioral health care. Identify and refer those who are particularly stressed or at risk for adverse behavioral health outcomes to a mental health professional. Medications may be appropriate and necessary. Triage can also ensure that those likely to be at higher risk are linked to follow-up care. Although most survivors experience normal stress reactions, some may need immediate psychological intervention to manage feelings of panic or intense grief. Signs of panic include palpitations, trembling, rapid speech, difficulty breathing, agitation, erratic behavior, and concerns about survival. Signs of intense grief include sobbing, numbness, immobilization, and rage.

Currently the American Red Cross uses Psychological Simple Triage and Rapid Treatment (PsySTART) as the standard of care to rapidly assess and triage disaster survivors. PsySTART, an evidence-based psychological triage and management system, matches survivors who may be at risk for developing behavioral health problems as a consequence of disasters with appropriate levels of care (SAMHSA, 2016). The goal of PsySTART is to provide a way for emergency responders, who may not have a behavioral health background, to rapidly and effectively assess survivors who need referral for more focused behavioral health evaluation or treatment. This rapid triage system helps responders become aware of previous behavioral health care or traumatic exposures that may affect a survivor's response to the current disaster. It is also a way to assess the need for psychological intervention (SAMHSA, 2016).

PROTECTING FROM FURTHER THREAT AND DISTRESS

To ensure physical safety, survivors should be moved away from the site of the disaster. To promote feelings of safety, create a calm and stable environment and provide reassurance by verbally telling survivors that they are in a safe place. To the extent possible, provide personal space and privacy and help survivors secure personal belongings they have brought with them. Protect survivors from disturbing stimuli as much as possible. Greater sensory exposure, such as seeing, smelling, or hearing distressing things, increases the likelihood of adverse behavioral health outcomes. To avoid secondary traumatization, protect survivors, especially children, from onlookers and interviews by media.

HELPING TO LOCATE FAMILY MEMBERS

Connecting survivors with family members, natural support systems, and community resources is essential to promoting healing and recovery. Survivors of a disaster may have lost connection with everything familiar to them. Families will be concerned with the safety of their members, and a desperate search for missing family members is likely (Fig. 5.4). Set up an information center to assist with the registration of those affected by the disaster and to facilitate locating and verifying the personal safety of family members and friends. Children should be reunited with their parents as soon as possible to avoid adverse behavioral health outcomes.

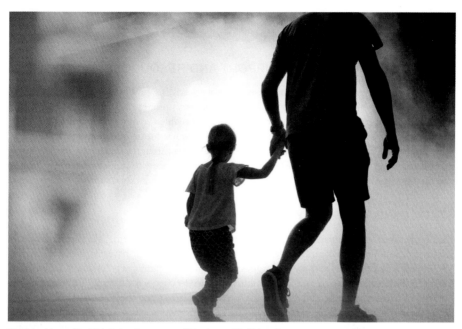

Fig. 5.4 Man with child during fire rescue. (iStock.com\Saklakova)

SHARING EXPERIENCES AND VALIDATING EMOTIONS

Use active listening. Allow time for ventilation of feelings. If the survivor begins to cry, remain with the person and offer a tissue. Avoid attempting to get the person to stop crying or regain immediate composure. Touching or giving a hug has often been a part of consoling and comforting. Sometime touch is appropriate; at other times it may violate a person's personal or cultural boundaries. Before you touch someone, ask: "Would it be all right if I gave you a hug or touched your shoulder?"

People may need to share their experiences with others. As natural groups form, support sharing that occurs spontaneously. This natural sharing of experiences with others in a caring and supportive setting promotes psychological recovery, begins the process of making meaning of the disaster, gives testimony to those affected by the disaster, validates feelings, and generates support from others. However, others may choose not to talk about the disaster because they do not feel ready to face the emotions brought on by discussing their experiences. Avoid probing or forcing survivors to talk about the disaster. Some survivors may not be able to attend to emotional needs because they are busy coping with other consequences of the disaster; therefore, it is important to link survivors to support systems and services that may be accessed later.

FACILITATING A SENSE OF BEING IN CONTROL

Help each person feel a sense of importance and uniqueness. Counteract feelings of powerlessness by helping survivors gain some sense of control over their situation. As soon as possible, encourage survivors to resume daily activities, re-establish social support systems, and participate in resolving problems caused by the disaster. Providing structure can assist the person to shape the stressful trajectory and facilitate a sense of meaning. It is important to help survivors progress from a sense of being a helpless victim to a sense of being a survivor. Promoting a sense of self-esteem, mastery, and ability to reintegrate into the social community enhances the subjective quality of life and increases global sense of well-being and overall psychosocial functioning.

LINKING SURVIVORS WITH SUPPORT AND RESOURCES

As much as possible, identify and connect survivors with existing support systems such as family, friends, neighbors, and clergy. If needed, link survivors with proper referral services that match their needs. Also provide instructions about resources available to vulnerable populations, while continuing to monitor high-risk populations that may require future interventions. In addition, inform survivors about resources and support services offered through social media, such as information and education about the disaster, ways to find and connect with support systems, collection and distribution of material resources, and availability of online emotional support communities.

STABILIZING THE FAMILY UNIT

Family members need reassurance and support, information about normal stress responses, and referral to community services. The devastating effects of disasters may have considerable implications for family dynamics and stability. Disasters often cause family separations, disabilities, or deaths. Relationships may be strained. Children's ability to cope with disaster is affected by the capacity of parents and other adults to handle their own distress and support the child. The stress of the disaster may increase the sense of closeness as family members turn to one another for emotional support. For others, as distress increases, marital conflict and parent-child conflicts become more intense and disruptive. Relocation can also greatly affect the recovery of the family unit.

PROMOTING COMMUNITY SUPPORT

Displacement, relocation, property loss, and unemployment after a disaster are a few factors that disrupt the functioning of the community. Each community responds to disruptions differently and is influenced by its cultural perspectives. Only by understanding the culture of the community can the nurse intervene effectively. Community structure is also altered by the convergence of rescue workers and the media following the disaster and the apparent lack of continued interest and abandonment as those rescue workers and media move on in a few days or weeks. Strong leadership is critical.

Community groups may develop to facilitate support and should be encouraged. Cultural groups within the community may vary in their response; stoicism and resilience may be strong values. Rituals are also an important step in the healing process. Spiritual services, restoration projects, and memorials are ways of providing closure, paying tribute to the courage and suffering of community members, and making meaning out of the disaster (Fig. 5.5). Supportive networks help people in the ongoing recovery process, both through the exchange of resources and practical assistance and through emotional support.

When survivors and rescue workers have opportunities to share their stories, normalization, validation, and empathy are experienced, which facilitates healing and recovery. Mutual support and opportunities to identify further needs also can be provided in supportive or informal groups.

Crisis Intervention

Disasters, by their very nature, precipitate crises. A crisis occurs when stressors are overwhelming and the usual problem-solving and coping skills are inadequate. Initial interventions after a disaster build on crisis intervention as a preventive method to decrease the likelihood of physical and behavioral health problems. Crisis intervention is short term, action oriented, and strength based, with the

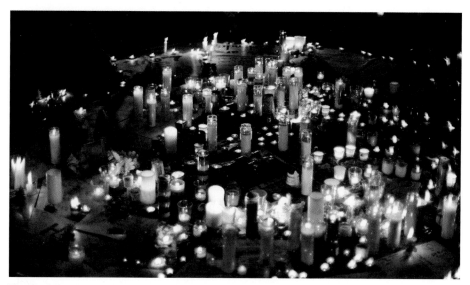

Fig. 5.5 Pulse nightclub vigil in Philadelphia. (iStock.com\BasSlabbers)

goals of achieving stabilization, reducing distress, increasing a sense of empowerment, and returning survivors to their predisaster level of functioning. It attempts to prevent adverse behavioral health outcomes by helping survivors understand that they are experiencing severe stress responses related to extraordinarily uncommon events. Crisis intervention assumes that most disaster survivors are resilient and will return to their predisaster health status. However, crisis intervention workers also recognize that some disaster survivors experience severe stress responses or symptoms and refer these individuals to appropriate treatment services and resources (FEMA, 2016).

CRISIS COUNSELING ASSISTANCE AND TRAINING PROGRAM

The Crisis Counseling Assistance and Training Program (CCP) is a federally funded program that provides survivors of disasters with crisis counseling, psychoeducation programs, and linkage to services and resources. Crisis counseling, which focuses on providing immediate support and behavioral health services, may be delivered in a home, workplace, school, church, or even a coffee shop. The CCP uses a population exposure model to help identify and prioritize disaster survivors who could benefit from crisis intervention. Core principles of the CCP include interventions that are strength based, outreach oriented, diagnosis free, culturally aware, conducted in nontraditional settings, and designed to strengthen existing community support systems. Through a crisis counseling approach, the CCP assists survivors of disasters and trauma to return to some semblance of normalcy. In addition, crisis counseling is valuable because it addresses the needs of the community as a whole (FEMA, 2016).

During disasters and traumatic events, an array of individuals, including behavioral health professionals, police officers, firefighters, rescue workers, physicians, nurses, community volunteers, family, neighbors, friends, and funeral directors, enter the scene and find themselves providing crisis intervention services to survivors. Realizing that comprehensive training is essential to the success of the program, the CCP has developed a series of training modules and courses to prepare individuals and communities with critical information and skills needed to provide quality crisis intervention (SAMHSA, 2016).

SIX-STEP CRISIS INTERVENTION MODEL

Crisis intervention seeks to prevent the onset of diagnosable disorders through early support and intervention. The six-step model of crisis intervention developed by James and Gilliland is very useful for working with survivors who have experienced disasters and trauma. The first three steps focus on *listening;* the last three steps focus on *plans* and *action* (Cavaiola & Colford, 2018). These steps of crisis intervention correspond closely to the nursing process.

1. **Defining the problem:** Define the problem from the individual's perspective.
2. **Ensuring safety:** Assess dangerousness to self or others, including a lethality (suicide) assessment.
3. **Providing support:** Approach the individual and establish rapport. Demonstrate support and caring.
4. **Examining alternatives:** Explore choices and options available to the individual. Identify coping skills and support systems that can be used immediately.
5. **Making plans:** Collaborate with the individual in making a short-term realistic plan. Identify specific action steps to solve the problem.
6. **Obtaining commitment:** Assist the individual in committing to specific action steps that realistically can be accomplished.

CRISIS ASSESSMENT AND INTERVENTION

The art of being present, reflected in the nurse's ability to be approachable, warm, open, receptive, and compassionate provides the emotional holding environment needed by survivors to share their thoughts, feelings, and behaviors associated with the disaster or traumatic event. *"Being with"* the survivor through empathic presence and listening is essential to assist the survivor with the healing process and recovery (Fig. 5.6). Such attentiveness involves *"bearing witness"* to the pain

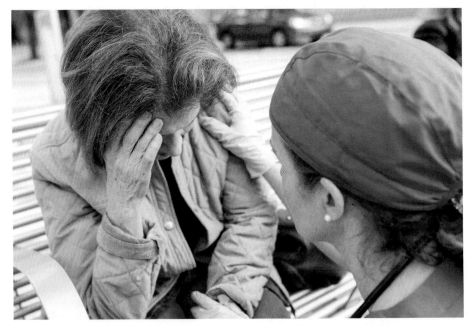

Fig. 5.6   Being with and bearing witness to disaster, loss, and grief. (iStock.com\Juanmonino)

and grief frequently associated with disasters. Since assessment and intervention occur together, both processes are explained simultaneously.

Focus on the immediate problem and the survivor's feelings. Ask: "What happened?" Expect to hear about the survivor's feelings as well as about the event. Remain calm. Take time to listen and convey that even amid the hurry and task demands of the impact, the person is important. Be genuine; show unconditional positive regard and empathy. Assess the level of anxiety and affect. Understand the problem from the survivor's perspective: "What does this event mean to you?" Is the trauma perceived accurately or is it distorted? The perception is the reality for the survivor. Do not argue or try to persuade the survivor differently if the perception is greatly distorted, but assure safety.

Determine situational supports. Ask: "Who are the people you are particularly close to?" or "Who can be called to help you?" The survivor may not have identifying information and may be unable to think of whom to notify. Let the survivor rest. Often, with a little time, the person can recall who could be contacted.

Observe the person to give you a sense of the survivor's ability to handle problems and cope. Ask: "How have you coped with tough times in the past?" "Has anything like this ever happened to you before?" How do you deal with stress?" "What works?" Disorganized thought or speech may not be an indication of the usual pattern of functioning. As anxiety lowers, the person usually can answer questions more accurately.

Another aspect of the assessment process is to assess the client's safety. Ask if the client is suicidal or homicidal. Be specific. Ask: "Do you have any thoughts of hurting yourself or others?" "Have you thought about ending your life?" "Do you have a specific plan?" Convey what you observe: "You sound really angry about .--. What have you thought about doing?" Asking these questions will not precipitate suicide but rather provide an opportunity to talk about feelings and convey the importance of continuing to strive for life.

Assessment of mental state should include potential physiological factors, such as head injury or toxic effects. Refer the survivor to appropriate medical care resources and link the person to ongoing systems of social support. Be sensitive to the impact of the assessment on the acutely traumatized person. When someone has suffered a severe trauma, panic attacks dissociative reactions, or flashbacks may occur. In a panic attack, the person may feel as if they are having a heart attack and a fear of death is expressed. Palpitations, difficulty breathing, and a desire to escape are common. Panic attacks require a direct and structured intervention. Remain with the person and assure safety. Maintain a calm, serene manner. Encourage the person to use deep abdominal breathing and to focus on the breathing, counting to 10, or on an image of a safe place.

Survivors may experience episodes of dissociation and flashbacks when they recall details of the traumatic event. *Dissociation* is a survival response in which a person's thoughts and feelings associated with the disaster or trauma are pushed aside or repressed. The person feels completely unreal or outside of themself and may have periods of amnesia. If the person dissociates during the assessment process, one observable behavior is a blank stare. Eyelashes may flutter and even close. A quick shift in consciousness may happen, in which the person appears to have changed mood or to be asleep. Gently address the person by name, until the eyes open and the person reconnects with the interviewer. The person may comment, "I must have dozed off." Shift the conversation to a less anxiety-laden topic. As trust and rapport develop, the survivor may be able to share more details of the traumatic event. A *flashback* is reliving of the traumatic event during the early post-impact phase or even later. This can happen visually in images, or the event can be re-experienced with sounds, smells, feelings, or other such sensory memories when someone is reminded of the disaster. Not everyone realizes they are suffering from a flashback. Tell the survivor: "It feels real, but it actually isn't happening again." If someone is in the middle of a flashback, help them to "become grounded." Remain calm and speak in a gentle, confident manner. Encourage the person to keep their eyes open, focus on your voice, take slow gentle breathes, put their feet firmly on the ground, and slowly look around the room to establish location and safety. Attempt to differentiate the present environment from the past one by noting details or objects that could not have been nearby when the traumatic event occurred. For example, remind the survivor that you were not present when the trauma occurred. Offer your hand to show support; however, allow the survivor to decide whether to reciprocate.

Interventions aim to help survivors come to terms with loss and other distressing events they have suffered in the disaster. The emphasis of interventions in the early phases of disaster recovery are on enhancing positive coping and facilitating active mastery and involvement in the recovery process. In-depth counseling is not appropriate for most individuals in the earliest stages but should be available for those considered at higher risk of adverse behavioral health outcomes.

Provide support, reinforce adaptive behaviors, and help the person identify strengths. Immediate emotional and social support may counteract long-term adverse effects. Communicate caring and empathy. Some survivors may believe there are no options. Assist survivors to recognize that alternatives are available. Alternatives may include situational supports, such as people known to the survivor who care and would want to help. Assist the survivor to develop some plan of action for possible solutions to the problem. If the solutions are not effective, the nurse and survivor work toward finding other solutions. Restore a sense of control and power by using collaboration in planning. Survivors of disasters and trauma often feel totally out of control. Active roles are important for those affected by disasters because activity counteracts feelings of powerlessness and helplessness that may have occurred during the impact.

Experience indicates that relatively few survivors make use of available behavioral health services post disaster. This may be due to a lack of awareness of the availability of such services, a low perceived need for them, a lack of confidence in their utility, or negative attitudes toward behavioral health care. Thus crisis intervention on location at the time of disaster is important (FEMA, 2016).

Following a disaster, people are generally amenable to a variety of interventions. However, any intervention must always be tailored to the specific person(s) and situation. For example, considerations should include the words used; timing; nonverbal behavior; and the emotional, social, and cultural factors previously described. Crisis intervention guidelines include the following:

1. **Begin with comfort measures, conveying care and consolation** while attending to physical status as necessary. Recognize that the person may be associating this event with other violent situations, which can account for unusual reactions. Listen and observe for such reactions.

2. **Acknowledge and validate or encourage and facilitate expression of feelings** while assisting with physical care or self-help measures and gathering information. Give the person time to express feelings in a way that is comfortable. Ask: "What are you thinking?" or "What are you feeling?"

3. **Acknowledge strengths and coping abilities**. State: "Your reactions are normal." "This is very overwhelming." "You're doing as well as you can." If the person does not express emotions, let the conversation move in the direction comfortable for the person.

4. **Clarify perception of the event, the losses involved, and the realities of the situation** to help gain a more realistic view of possible implications or consequences. If the person is reluctant to talk, you might say, "As a child, you may have been told never to talk, but here it is safe to share as much as you want."

5. **Accept statements that reflect denial or distortion. Do not argue**. State: "This was random bad luck that led to trauma. It didn't happen because of you."

6. **Avoid false reassurance**. Don't say, "This won't happen again" or "It's all going to be all right."

7. **Through repetitive, gentle explanations, relay information, convey hope and the importance of working together, and promote problem-solving abilities**. Say: "It takes courage to share what you just said. I see ways in which we can work to get through this."

8. **Encourage ability to manage; explore prior coping strategies and examine alternative ways of coping.** Review realistic plans to help the person gain a sense of control over future events. Role-playing how to handle situations can be useful.

9. **Involve in activity with specific tasks**, especially related to personal needs but also related to helping others. Set limits and give instructions as needed. Activity can decrease anxiety, and self-help and altruism contribute toward problem solving, increased self-esteem, and a sense of hope and manageability.

10. **Accept suggestions that are useful and relevant** for getting the task at hand done. Collaboration is necessary for completing work but also enhances a sense of normality and positive self-concept and self-confidence, which can strengthen the sense of resilience and coherence.

11. **Foster social relationships and effective use of social support systems or referral agencies.** Encourage seeking and accepting help, as necessary, for current or future needs that are likely to arise. Encourage spiritual expression and participation in group activities, if appropriate.

12. **Clarify continuing decisions and actions while being supportive.** Recognize that outcomes for initial crisis interaction may not be known but that initial crisis intervention is likely to prevent adverse behavioral health outcomes.

13. **Do not retaliate to angry, derogatory, accusatory, or bitter statements; this is a way to cope with feelings.** Do not take the statement personally, but consider if there is any accuracy to the statement. If so, correct actions, procedures, or policies, if possible, or do what is possible to convey caring and genuine concern.

14. **Accept lack of responsiveness to directions given, information shared, comforting expressions, and a caring attitude.** These interventions may be remembered and used later.

Adverse Behavioral Health Outcomes and Therapies

While most persons affected by a disaster spontaneously recover, some survivors will need behavioral health interventions beyond psychological first aid. The impact on survivors varies depending on multiple risk factors, such as exposure to the disaster, previous experiences of disasters or trauma, history of behavioral health problems, gender, and age. Survivors are reluctant to seek behavioral health services in the aftermath of a disaster, typically not contacting formal service agencies except as a last resort. Instead, survivors prefer to turn to family and friends (FEMA, 2016; Goldmann & Galea, 2014; Langan & Krieger, 2018). Certain factors both before and after a disaster contribute to a greater risk for difficulty with recovery postdisaster. Box 5.3 summarizes the risk factors for difficulty with postdisaster recovery. Assess for these risks.

EMOTIONS

During and following disasters, survivors experience strong emotions; this is a natural response to a devastating situation. Listen carefully to survivors' expressions of stress, grief, anger, shame, and guilt that may arise.

Stress

An individual's emotional reaction following a disaster may range from little distress to extreme stress reactions. Many survivors feel nervous, anxious, or irritable. Other symptoms of stress may include physical symptoms such as headaches, fatigue, and pain. In stressful situations, some survivors may abuse alcohol or substances. The following techniques, with rationales, can be used with individuals or a small group to reduce or manage stress:

1. **Deep breathing training:** Teach abdominal breathing to bring about the relaxation response or avoid hyperventilation.

BOX 5.3 ■ Risk Factors for Difficulty With Postdisaster Recovery

- Lack of preparation for disasters
- Severity and duration of exposure and perceived life threat, loss, or injury
- Exposure to massive death, bodily injury, or intentional violence
- Death of loved ones
- Loss of home, valued possessions, or community structures
- Displacement from support systems, stigma, or discrimination experiences
- Extreme fatigue, sleep deprivation, or exposure to other traumas
- Poverty, homelessness, unemployment, marital stress, or family instability
- Guilt feelings or feelings of helplessness or powerlessness
- Elderly or children, especially if separated from loved ones or parents
- Existing or pre-existing psychopathology or developmental disabilities
- History of childhood trauma or abuse
- Occupation of rescue worker or body handler

---

2. **Relaxation training:** Teach systematic relaxation of the major muscle groups to counteract tension associated with anxiety. Avoid beverages, candy, and foods that contain caffeine or other stimulants that interfere with rest and sleep.
3. **Positive self-talk:** Replace negative automatic thoughts with positive thoughts to cope with feelings; enhance self-esteem and coping.
4. **Journals, logs, art, and music:** Express feelings; substitute positive expressions that promote self-esteem.
5. **Thought stopping:** Distraction techniques such as inwardly saying "Stop" to overcome distressing thoughts.
6. **Meditation, visualization, or imagery exercises:** Focus thoughts on a neutral or pleasant object or situation to reduce anxiety, clarify decisions, and enhance self-esteem and hope.
7. **Assertiveness training:** Teach the person how to express wishes, opinions, and emotions without infringing on the rights of others.
8. **Anticipatory guidance:** Discuss potentially anxiety-provoking situations and how they can be handled. The person may also benefit from a short-term anxiolytic medication.

Grief

In situations of disaster and catastrophic loss, the survivor may experience intense feelings of grief. Symptoms of grief include a longing for the loved one, a sense of emptiness, pain or heaviness in the chest, and hopelessness about the future. Individuals may cry easily, lose their appetite, feel restless, and complain of stomach upset or headache (Worden, 2018).

Initially there may be a period of shock, numbness and disbelief, and, to a degree, denial. This initial period usually gives way to intense separation distress or anxiety. The bereaved person is highly aroused, seeking the lost person, particularly if it is not certain that the person is dead or if the body has not been identified. Anger may be expressed toward the deceased for being among those who died. Anger is also directed toward those who may be perceived as having caused or been associated with the death, or who are alive when the deceased is not.

Risk factors for complications of mourning include suddenness or unexpectedness of death, violent or traumatic deaths, multiple losses, other concurrent crises or stressors, and perceived lack of social support (Worden, 2018).

Survivors must come to terms with the loss of their loved one, as well as the manner in which that loss occurred. Traumatic deaths are particularly likely to result in intense and prolonged grief if the death was violent or if it was brought about by a malevolent act or homicide. It is common for survivors to agonize about what their loved ones experienced during their final moments of life. Survivors may experience feelings of rage toward the perpetrator. Death of a child is particularly difficult because people expect to die before their children (Worden, 2018).

Trauma may interfere with the ability to go through the process of mourning. Concerns about seeing the body of the deceased due to injuries sustained in the disaster may prevent the bereaved from viewing the body. Inability to see the body of the dead person may further contribute to risk of adverse outcomes because it interferes with opportunities to say goodbye. Obstacles to a normal response to the death of a loved one may contribute to a feeling of lack of closure or permit fantasies that the deceased person has not died. Legal processes may delay funeral proceedings. Both bereaved and traumatized individuals are likely to experience similar symptoms in terms of intrusive thoughts, avoidance responses, and high levels of arousal.

Psychological interventions to facilitate the normal grieving process include dealing with the circumstances of the death; reviewing the lost relationship; expressing feelings; mourning the deceased; accepting the new realities that result from the loss, including any role or status changes; and dealing with simultaneous life stressors (Worden, 2018).

Several strategies that can be useful in grief counseling are as follows:

1. Use of photographs, possessions, and other symbols of the deceased to promote both acknowledgement of the loss and the development of an internal relationship.
2. Encouragement of creative expression by writing or drawing, which can capture feelings that may be difficult to verbalize.
3. Creation of rituals, dioramas, or a memorial box, which can be a means of remembering or commemorating the dead person or lost object.
4. Promotion of cognitive restructuring, which involves confronting and testing distorted beliefs that may maintain a pathological response.
5. Review of positive and negative aspects of the relationship to assist with grieving.

Anger

Anger is a common and normal feeling following a disaster. The person may cry, blame others, be irritable, curse, pound fists, and proclaim, "The world is unfair" or "You are no help." Sometimes anger is internalized and may be expressed somatically with headaches, sleep disturbances, eating problems, and weight loss. Also indicative of anger are signs of depression, including hopeless statements such as "Why try? It won't make any difference," or despair such as decreased interest in daily activities or other events. Panic attacks may continue but normally lessen over time. Interpersonal relations may be strained or erratic. The person may blame others who are not responsible for what has happened. Severe anger may result in violence toward self (suicide) or others (homicide).

Shame

Survivors may feel shame about their behavior during the disaster or traumatic event, especially when others blame them. Tragedies amplify our awareness that the world is ambiguous and unpredictable. People naturally search for meaning. It is difficult to find meaning in disasters and traumatic events, especially those involving human malevolence. Because of this desperate need to understand traumatic events, which may not have any real meaning, people tend to come up with a reason based on irrational thinking. For example, when something bad happens to someone, people often conclude that the survivor must have deserved what happened. Likewise, survivors, in an attempt to find a meaning for a meaningless tragedy, may blame themselves. Although victim blaming or self-blaming explanations may be inaccurate and personally devastating, it meets the need for understanding the event and maintains the belief that the world is safe and predictable.

Survivor's Guilt

Individuals, both children and adults, may feel guilty for surviving or being uninjured when others were killed or injured, especially when they were unable to rescue someone or when they had to leave someone to die in the disaster. During a disaster, individuals often have to act quickly in order to survive. This can lead to an inaccurate assessment of responsibility for the results of actions taken or not taken during a disaster. Often survivors are particularly troubled by the fact that they were unable to exert control over what was happening. They may ruminate over their own activities or be preoccupied by thoughts about what they feel they should have done. Survivors are often unable to function or to address other issues until they process their guilt feelings. It is therapeutic to repeatedly say, "Whatever decisions you made at the time of the disaster were the right ones because you are alive." Individuals who experience the risks previously listed or repeatedly express anger, shame, or survivor's guilt are at risk for developing acute stress disorder or post-traumatic stress disorder. Linking survivors to support networks and identifying those at risk who may need follow-up services is important. Anger, shame, and guilt can diminish over time and with the assistance of supportive counseling, which involves comforting, reassuring, providing information, and allowing people to discuss their experience, if they feel the need.

Early identification of those at risk for negative outcomes following a disaster can facilitate prevention, referral, and treatment. Screening can be accomplished by brief semistructured interviews and standardized assessment questionnaires. Screening should address the crisis assessment points and risk factors previously discussed. Especially important are acute levels of traumatic stress symptoms, which may predict chronic problems.

Even when those who might benefit from behavioral health services have been adequately identified, factors such as embarrassment, fear of stigmatization, and cultural norms may limit motivation to seek help or pursue a referral. Those making referrals can address these attitudes and attempt to prevent avoidance of needed services.

BEHAVIORAL HEALTH DISORDERS

Disaster survivors may display a wide range of stress reactions and symptoms. Most survivors who experience these stress reactions and symptoms recover without professional intervention, although some survivors develop persistent symptoms that lead to behavioral health disorders (Briere & Scott, 2014; Goldmann & Galea, 2014; Langan & Krieger, 2018; Webber & Mascari, 2018). Severe stress reactions may include acute stress disorders, post-traumatic stress disorders, major depressive disorders, suicidal behavior, anxiety disorders, substance use, grief and bereavement complications, and somatic symptoms (Goldmann & Galea, 2014; Langan & Krieger, 2018; Webber & Mascari, 2018). It is essential to assess for symptomatic stress reactions and make appropriate referrals for survivors presenting with these problems. The most common behavioral health disorders resulting from disaster exposure are discussed next.

Acute Stress Disorder

Acute stress disorder (ASD) describes the acute stress responses that occur in the first 4 weeks following trauma. Typically symptoms begin immediately. Since severe stress responses following a disaster or trauma are often transient in nature, a diagnosis of ASD is not made until at least 3 days of persistent symptoms after exposure to a traumatic event. In addition to trauma exposure, ASD diagnostic criteria include at least nine symptoms from the five categories of intrusion, negative mood, dissociation, avoidance, and arousal. Symptom duration must be a minimum of 3 days up to a maximum of 4 weeks. Furthermore, survivors must manifest significant impairment in functioning. ASD and post-traumatic stress disorder (PTSD) share many of the same symptoms (American Psychiatric Association [APA], 2013). Use of interventions described in a later section can help the person overcome ASD and prevent PTSD.

Post-Traumatic Stress Disorder

Post-traumatic stress disorder (PTSD) is the most commonly studied diagnosis that follows a disaster (Langan & Krieger, 2018). PTSD is characterized by the development of a persistent stress response after a traumatic event and differs from ASD with a later onset. Similar to ASD, the individual experiences or witnesses a traumatic event, such as actual or threatened death, serious injury, or sexual violation. Symptoms are grouped into four categories: (1) presence of intrusive symptoms, (2) persistent avoidance of stimuli, (3) negative alterations in cognition and mood, and (4) marked alterations in arousal and reactivity. Symptom duration must be at least 1 month following the trauma, and symptoms must be severe enough to impair functioning. Symptoms may be acute and occur after the trauma or be delayed (APA, 2013).

Major Depressive Disorder

Major depressive disorder (MDD) is characterized by sadness and loss of pleasure or interest in things once enjoyed, as well as symptoms such as changes in sleep and weight, difficulty concentrating, and irritability (APA, 2013). MDD is the second most commonly studied diagnosis that follows a disaster (Goldmann & Galea, 2014). Survivors, especially if they have experienced significant personal losses or injuries, may be at risk for MDD. Symptoms such as sadness, irritability, loss of energy or appetite, and sleep disturbances are common following disasters and typically resolve within a relatively short period. However, if symptoms persist, the survivor should be referred to a behavioral health professional for assessment of MDD and treatment.

Substance Use Disorders

Substance use disorders are characterized by problematic alcohol or drug use that results in difficulty fulfilling home, work, or school responsibilities; legal issues; relationship problems; risk-taking behaviors; symptoms of withdrawal; and unsuccessful attempts to quit (APA, 2013). Although substance use disorders have been identified in disaster survivors, some evidence suggests that pre--existing substance use disorders may be exacerbated by the disaster or traumatic event, rather than the disaster leading to a new behavioral disorder diagnosis (Goldmann & Galea, 2014). In addition, increased use of alcohol and substances following a disaster may be a coping strategy used by survivors (Goldmann & Galea, 2014). If the use of alcohol or substances becomes problematic, survivors should be referred for further assessment and intervention by a behavioral health professional.

SELECT POST-TRAUMATIC DISTRESS DISORDER THERAPIES

As previously described, PTSD is a behavioral health disorder that may develop after exposure to a disaster or trauma. PTSD includes physical, emotional, behavioral, and cognitive symptoms. Trauma-focused therapies such as *cognitive behavioral therapy* and *expressive art therapy* assist survivors with reprocessing trauma memories to reduce PTSD symptoms (Malchiodi, 2020; Webber & Mascari, 2018). Cognitive behavioral therapy is a traditional talk therapy that challenges and reframes unhelpful or distorted beliefs about traumas (Webber & Mascari, 2018). Expressive art therapy, an embodied experiential therapy, uses creative mediums such as art, drama, music, and dance to explore, express, externalize, and reprocess traumatic experiences (Malchiodi, 2020). These trauma-focused therapies are briefly discussed next.

Cognitive Behavioral Therapy

Cognitive behavioral therapy (CBT) has gained empirical support for treating and preventing PTSD (Goldmann & Galea, 2014; Math et al., 2015; Webber & Mascari, 2018). The goals of

CBT are to teach survivors to identify dysfunctional or automatic thoughts, to weigh evidence for or against these thoughts, and to adopt realistic thoughts that will generate more balanced emotions. CBT techniques include reframing a situation, identifying triggering situations, developing coping methods, and various homework assignments to learn new thought and behavior patterns.

Expressive Art Therapy

Expressive art therapy uses drama, music, painting, sculpture, dance, poetry, freewriting, and storytelling to help survivors express and reprocess their traumatic experiences (Malchiodi, 2020; Webber & Mascari, 2018). Modalities used in expressive art therapy stimulate the senses and assist survivors to reconnect with nonverbal feelings and memories stored in their bodies. By creating some emotional distance and containment with the use of art modalities, expressive art therapy allows survivors to share their unspoken and unspeakable feelings in a safe way. Through sharing of feelings and trauma experiences, survivors feel supported rather than isolated and begin the process of reconnecting with others and the world. In addition, expressive art therapy provides a vehicle for meaning making, which involves survivors reprocessing their experiences and allocating new meaning to the impact of the disaster on their lives.

Vulnerable Populations

Disasters cause disruptions to homes, schools, and workplaces, including death and injuries. Populations at special risk for behavioral health issues include children and adolescents; the elderly, especially the frail elderly; refugee and migrant groups; and the developmentally or mentally disabled. These individuals may perceive the stress associated with a disaster quite differently from others and may be in particular need of help and support. People from diverse cultural background may also respond differently.

Children

The main emotional responses in adults with PTSD are fear, helplessness, and horror. However, PTSD in children manifests with the following variances according to age group (American Academy of Child and Adolescent Psychiatry [AACAP], 2020):
1. Preschool children may experience more temper tantrums, hyperactivity, reversion on toilet training, fearfulness, nightmares, sleep and appetite changes, and clinginess.
2. Younger school-age children may show their feelings through play, be hyperactive or irritable, experience sleep and appetite changes, have lower grades and an inability to focus, and experience physical symptoms of stomachaches and headaches.
3. Older children may experience increased anxiety, panic, depression, and behavior issues such as violence or conflicts with others.
4. Adolescents may experience anxiety, depression, fear of death, a decrease in pleasurable activities, sudden independence, social withdrawal, suicidal thoughts, and substance use or abuse.

The AACAP (2020) recommends that children should be assured of their safety; kept with family; listened to; allowed to express feelings; allowed to cling and grieve over losses, including of material things; included in activities; exposed minimally to news about the event, especially media with violent images; and returned to normal routines and expectations, including regular meal times, as soon as possible.

OLDER ADULTS AND THOSE WITH COGNITIVE IMPAIRMENT OR DISABILITIES

Older adults and those with cognitive impairment or disabilities have also been found to be a high-risk population for disaster reactions and need for interventions. The impact of disaster-related losses has shown that a higher incidence of personal loss, injury, and death are experienced by older adults and medically frail persons (Heagele & Pacquiao, 2019). Individuals may feel that they cannot start over again when loved ones, homes, and prized possessions are lost. They may feel devastated and robbed of what they worked for. If the anger and grief are not resolved, chronic PTSD may occur. Adverse reactions are more intense if survivors view the disaster as preventable. The frailer the person, the more likely the person is to have difficulty coping emotionally with disaster impact or its consequences (Fig. 5.7). Research has shown that older adults are less likely to evacuate and less likely to heed warnings for several reasons, including a false sense of comfort from surviving previous disasters without negative outcomes (Heagele & Pacquiao, 2019). Certain determinants in the elderly may interfere with coping with a crisis or disaster and may contribute to physical injury and to adverse mental health outcomes. A focused review of the literature conducted by Heagele and Pacquiao (2019) found the following determinants of vulnerability:
1. Sociodemographic variables, including advanced age, female gender, low socioeconomic status, low education, language barriers, and experience with disasters.
2. Chronic illnesses, including diabetes, stroke, heart attack, chronic lung conditions, hereditary blood disorders, end-stage renal disease, high blood pressure, arthritis, and dementia.
3. Mobility, cognitive, and sensory deficits. Mobility deficits include inability to evacuate quickly or take cover due to the use of a wheelchair, walker, or cane. Cognitive deficits

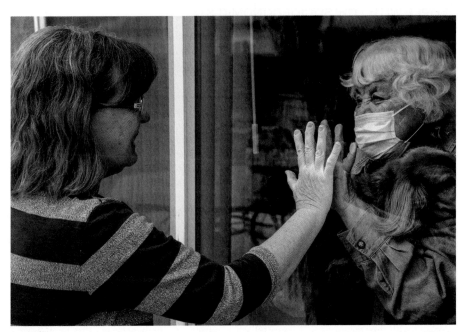

Fig. 5.7   Comfort interventions and communication to the vulnerable during the COVID-19 pandemic. (iStock. com\grandriver)

include memory disorders, dementia, delayed reaction times, and psychological distress. Sensory deficits include the inability to see, hear, taste, or smell.

4. Dependence on others or devices; reliance on others to perform activities of daily living, including help with meals or medical care; and electricity needs, including for supplemental oxygen or refrigeration of medications.

5. Lack of social support. Housebound and socially isolated people are less likely to receive disaster information or resources.

6. Environmental conditions. High-risk geographical conditions include those who are isolated, in urban or flood-prone areas, in areas with a high risk of hurricanes, or near the shoreline. Other environmental conditions include poorly constructed infrastructure, a high level of poverty, limited resources, poor shelter conditions, and poor home conditions.

However, these individuals also have resilience and perseverance that can be tapped into and strengthened to promote resolution and adaptation. Reminiscence and soliciting their insights can strengthen self-esteem and help them resolve to overcome the vicissitudes of the situation.

PEOPLE OF DIVERSE CULTURAL BACKGROUNDS

Cultural factors may be powerful in determining the reaction of the affected person and the response of others. There may be cultural rituals and social traditions that help people deal with grief, the aftermath of disaster, and healing. These need to be understood and supported. Mourning rituals are culture specific. It is essential that cultural issues be taken into account in understanding responses to disaster in different communities and that appropriate, culturally sensitive postdisaster mental health services are provided. Cultural beliefs may also dictate the likelihood of seeking health and support services (Substance Abuse and Mental Health Services Administration, 2018).

PEOPLE WITH LOW SOCIOECONOMIC STATUS

Consequences of a disaster are especially difficult for people who live in poverty, including (1) those who are in acute poverty with limited economic means because of current circumstances; (2) those who are in chronic poverty, with a long history of inadequate economic means for a variety of reasons; (3) those who are homeless and, therefore, often have no ready support system or economic means and now must share shelter space with those who lost their housing in a disaster; (4) migrant workers and their families who may lack housing and transportation to move to another area and are displaced from their marginal employment by a disaster; and (5) refugees seeking a home in a strange land, who fled their home because of persecution and who are again displaced by a disaster without the economic resources or social support systems to provide safety and security. These populations may be adversely affected by disasters because their communities are suffering due to marginal status; inadequate information about the disaster response or ineligibility for disaster relief programs; poor physical health and housing; problems of cultural loss; and ongoing trauma or PTSD, depression, anxiety, and grief. Furthermore, agencies that work with refugees may not have a way to track individuals. Often the adult generations of migrant, refugee, and immigrant populations rely on their children for information and interpretation of announcements or for explanations related to personal or family status or needs. The sense of powerlessness adds to the trauma effects and may be difficult to resolve.

Vicarious Traumatization

Working with disaster survivors is stressful; often nurses are simultaneously suffering a disaster while caring for survivors and working amid disaster impact. Nurses who work with survivors of disasters are at risk for vicarious traumatization or compassion fatigue, which occurs in response to witnessing trauma and listening to survivors' stories of traumatic events. Hearing stories of loss, grief, and devastation can take a toll. These accounts elicit strong feelings. Emotional reactions that overwhelm the nurse may interfere with the ability to function. Nurses who experience vicarious traumatization may experience psychological responses that can be disruptive and painful and can persist after working with trauma victims (Webber & Mascari, 2018).

The nurse, as a member of the rescue and caretaking team, must recognize that health care workers are vulnerable to and may experience any of the reactions to crisis and disaster described earlier (Fig. 5.8). Nurses should (1) observe for signs and symptoms of stress in themselves and each other and seek help as needed; (2) periodically leave the immediate disaster scene and follow the rules established for workers, such as taking time to eat and sleep; and (3) avoid taking on the "martyr role" or engaging in "rescue fantasy."

Nurses should consider limiting their time with disaster victims to defuse the impact. This is especially true for workers assigned to recover human remains, as they can tolerate only a few hours at a time of confronting the horror. They need time away from the work and an opportunity to process what they have witnessed.

Furthermore, disaster recovery work should not be done in isolation. No person can be the only or primary one to assume responsibility or engage in all facets of disaster intervention. A team approach is mandatory; each worker contributes toward the whole recovery effort, both physically and emotionally.

Self-Care

Nurses cannot be totally immune to the effects of helping survivors work through their trauma. However, they can take some steps to provide some degree of protection and relief from becoming overwhelmed and ineffective in their care. It is essential to take time to eat, sleep, and do exercises unrelated to disaster work. Protection against vicarious traumatization involves recognizing the

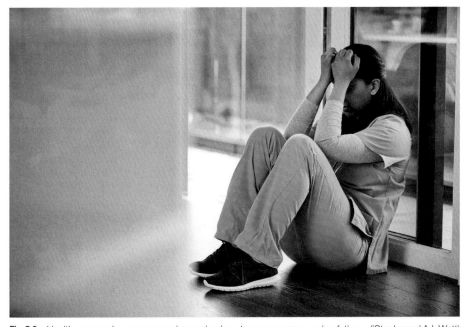

Fig. 5.8 Health care workers may experience vicarious trauma or compassion fatigue. (iStock.com\AJ_Watt)

impact of the trauma on others, including the stories and emotional reactions to personal beliefs and identity; developing a support network; and ventilating feelings in a supportive environment with coworkers and other professionals. Strategies of acting assertively; encouraging goodwill; discharging pent-up emotions; taking mental health breaks by creating a distance or withdrawing self, even if temporarily; and using humor and meditation are helpful. Frequently, nurses and other rescue workers benefit from attending memorial sites. Dioramas to honor the deceased often spontaneously appear as members of the community bring flowers, pictures, and messages of condolence. It is important to allow time for reflecting, giving and receiving support, and releasing pent-up emotions.

Workers should seek and use social support and participate in formal help if stress reactions persist. These strategies can be taught to individuals, families, and groups, as well as applied to oneself and rescue workers. The methods used to cope with crises and the interventions discussed in this chapter can be applied by nurses to themselves as well as taught to survivors.

Case in Point

BOSTON MARATHON BOMBING: SURVIVOR EXPERIENCING SYMPTOMS OF ACUTE STRESS DISORDER

This case is a composite of several survivors of the Boston Marathon bombing (Fig. 5.9).

A 19-year old runner at the 2013 Boston Marathon was injured by flying shrapnel when a homemade pressure cooker bomb detonated near the finish line of the marathon. The bombing embedded two pieces of shrapnel in his body, one in his left leg and the other in his left arm. The survivor was taken to the hospital for treatment of his wounds. After surgery, the survivor remained in the hospital for a couple of days and then was discharged to home. Although the

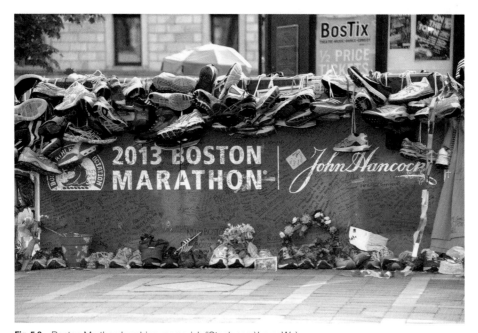

Fig. 5.9 Boston Marthon bombing memorial. (iStock.com\LornaWu)

treatment was painful, the survivor felt very lucky to be alive and to have endured the bombing with minimal injury.

Upon discharge to home, a home health nurse was assigned to visit the survivor for wound assessment and dressing changes. During the home health visit, the parents expressed concern about their son's insomnia and frequent nightmares related to the bombing. The survivor revealed that whenever he ventures outside the house, he experiences heart palpitations, dizziness, sweating, and shortness of breath. He is hesitant to leave the house or engage in any activities. When his parents leave the house, even briefly, to run an errand or visit the neighbors, he calls them, asking them to return.

Questions for Discussion

1. The stress reactions of survivors following disasters are frequently complex. How is this concept expressed in this case?
2. What stress reactions is the survivor exhibiting?
3. What nursing interventions should be implemented?

Points to Remember

- Most people are resilient and return to the level of function that existed prior to the disaster or crisis.
- Disasters, whether of natural or human origin, evoke predictable emotional and cognitive responses in survivors.
- These responses are described in terms of levels of victims, phases of disasters, stress reactions, and phases of and responses to crises, which are inherent in disaster.
- Stress reactions are physical, emotional, behavioral, and cognitive in nature.
- Several factors influence perception and outcome of the disaster.
- Initial interventions aim to promote safety and security by providing survivors with basic needs such as food, medical supplies, and shelter.
- Immediately following the impact phase of a disaster, psychological first aid (PFA) is the preferred intervention. The goals of PFA are to reduce stress reactions, strengthen coping skills, and connect survivors with supportive services and resources.
- Communicating information about the disaster in a calm manner to decrease fear and panic may reduce distress among survivors.
- The therapeutic approaches used by nurses during disasters address the needs of the individual, family, and group.
- Nurses must also recognize the needs of caregivers, including themselves, and use measures to promote self-care and avoid vicarious trauma.

Test Your Knowledge

1. The honeymoon phase in a disaster includes which of the following behaviors?
   a. People do everything possible to prevent loss of life and property.
   b. People complain about the lack of government response but are hopeful for aid.
   c. People are busy solving their own problems.
   d. People experience a sense of optimism and persist in doing what is necessary to meet basic needs.
2. Which of the following is a parasympathetic nervous system response?
   a. Pupil dilation
   b. Increased muscle tone
   c. Decreased heart rate
   d. Release of epinephrine

3. Psychological first aid interventions include: *(Choose all that apply.)*
   a. Providing for psychological needs
   b. Implementing cognitive behavioral therapy
   c. Connecting survivors with family members
   d. Discouraging spontaneous sharing of feelings and experiences

4. One of the most important attributes of the nurse when interviewing a survivor is:
   a. Always be in a position of authority
   b. Keep emotional distance from the survivor
   c. Be a good listener
   d. Maintain control by making all decisions

5. When assessing for suicide, the nurse should: *(Choose all that apply.)*
   a. Directly ask whether the survivor has thoughts of harming self
   b. Be supportive
   c. Ask about suicide only if the survivor brings it up
   d. Ask specific questions about a suicide plan

6. Which of the following are high-risk factors for difficulty with postdisaster recovery? *(Choose all that apply.)*
   a. Exposure to gruesome or massive death
   b. History of mental illness
   c. Use of dissociation during the traumatic event
   d. Mastery of previous traumatic events

7. Which of the following behaviors are associated with unresolved grief after a disaster? *(Choose all that apply.)*
   a. Continued social isolation
   b. Maintenance of the illusion that a person is not dead
   c. Reorganization of behavior directed toward new persons or objects
   d. Development of symptoms similar to those of the deceased

8. Crisis interventions include which of the following? *(Choose all that apply.)*
   a. Assessing accurately the crisis event
   b. Cognitive behavioral therapy to treat post-traumatic stress disorder
   c. Exploring coping mechanisms and realistic problem solving by the survivor
   d. Collaborating with the survivor to form a short-term, realistic plan

9. Which of the following symptoms are reflective of the diagnosis post-traumatic stress disorder (PTSD)? *(Choose all that apply.)*
   a. Re-experiencing distressing thoughts, dreams, or flashbacks
   b. Feeling numb
   c. Being jumpy or easily startled
   d. Fantasizing orientation toward the future

10. Which of these interventions would assist with reducing anxiety? *(Choose all that apply.)*
    a. Abdominal breathing
    b. Replacing negative thoughts with positive thoughts
    c. Relaxation training
    d. Ruminating about the details associated with the disaster or trauma

References

American Academy of Child and Adolescent Psychiatry. (2020). *Disaster and trauma resource center*. Retrieved from https://www.aacap.org/aacap/families_and_youth/resource_centers/Disaster_Resource_Center/Home.aspx

American Psychiatric Association. (2013). *Diagnostic and statistical manual of mental disorders* (5th ed.). https://doi.org/10.1176/appi.books.9780890425596

Briere J, Scott C. *DSM-5 update: Principles of trauma therapy: A guide to symptoms, evaluations, and treatment.* 2nd ed. : Sage; 2014.

Cavaiola, A.A., & Colford, J.E. (2018). *Crisis intervention: A practical guide.* Sage.

Federal Emergency Management Agency. (2016). *Crisis counseling assistance and training program guidance: CCP application toolkit, version 5.0.* Retrieved from https://www.samhsa.gov/sites/default/files/dtac/ccp-toolkit/fema-ccp-guidance.pdf

Goldmann E, Galea S. Mental health consequences of disasters. *Annual Review of Public Health.* 2014;35:169–183. https://doi.org/10.1146/annurev-publhealth-032013-182435.

Heagele T, Pacquiao D. Disaster vulnerability of elderly and medically frail populations. *Health Emergency and Disaster Nursing.* 2019;6:50–61. https://doi.org/10.24298/hedn.2016-0009.

Langan J, Palmer JL, Christopher K, Shagavah A. Joplin tornado survivors, hospital employees and community members: Reflections of resilience and acknowledgment of pain. *Health Emergency and Disaster Nursing.* 2017;4:57–65. https://doi.org/10.24298/hedn.2016-0004.

Langan JC, Krieger MM. Survivor notification of post-disaster mental health services: An integrative review. *Issues in Mental Health Nursing.* 2018;39(7):568–574. https://doi.org/10.1080/01612840.2018.1426065.

Malchiodi CA. *Trauma and expressive arts therapy: Brain, body, and imagination in the healing process.* : Guilford Press; 2020.

Math SB, Nirmala MC, Maoirangthem S, Kumer NC. Disaster management: Mental health perspective. *Indian Journal of Psychological Medicine.* 2015;37(3):261–271. https://doi.org/10.4103/0253-7176.162915.

Riaz MN, Malik S, Nawaz S, Riaz MA, Batool N, Shujaat JM. Well-being and post-traumatic stress disorder due to natural and man-made disasters on adults. *Pakistan Journal of Medical Research.* 2015;54(1):25–28.

Richardson GE, Neiger B, Jensen S, Kumpfer K. The resiliency model. *Health Education.* 1990;21:33–39. https://doi.org/10.1080/00970050.1990.10614589.

Shultz JM, Forbes D. Psychological first aid: Rapid proliferation and the search for evidence. *Disaster Health.* 2013;2(1):3–12. https://doi.org/10.4161/dish.26006.

Substance Abuse and Mental Health Services Administration. (2016). *Stronger together: An in-depth look at selected community-level approaches to disaster behavioral health.* Retrieved from https://www.samhsa.gov/sites/default/files/programs_campaigns/dtac/srb-community-approaches.pdf

Substance Abuse and Mental Health Services Administration Cultural and population sensitivity in disaster behavioral health programs. *The Dialogue.* 2018;14(3-4):1–29. Retrieved from. https://www.samhsa.gov/sites/default/files/dtac/dialoguevol14i3and4compliant-508c.pdf.

van der Kolk B. *The body keeps the score: Brain, mind and body in the healing of trauma.* : Penguin Books; 2014. https://doi.org/10.1080/0092623X.2017.1348102.

Webber J, Mascari JB, eds. *Disaster mental health counseling: A guide to preparing and responding.* 4th ed. : American Counseling Association Foundation; 2018.

Worden W. *Grief counseling and grief therapy: A handbook for mental health practioners.* 5th ed. : Springer Publishing Company; 2018.

Nursing Roles in Disasters and Public Health Emergencies

CHAPTER 6

Role of the General Professional Nurse

Charleen C. McNeill, PhD, MSN, RN ▨ Lavonne M. Adams, PhD, RN, CCRN-K
▨ Lisa S. Conlon, RN, BSc, MN, DN ▨ Donna M. Dorsey, RN, MS, FAAN

CHAPTER OUTLINE

Introduction 112

Global Threats and the Role of the General Professional Nurse 112

Global Threats 112

The Role of the General Professional Nurse 114

Competencies for the General Professional Nurse 116

Domain 1: Preparation and Planning 116

Domain 2: Communication 117

Domain 3: Incident Management Systems 118

Domain 4: Safety and Security 118

Domain 5: Assessment 120

Domain 6: Intervention 120

Domain 7: Recovery 120

Domain 8: Law and Ethics 122

Specialty Areas of Practice for General Professional Nurses and Implications For Disaster Nursing 122

Hospital or Acute Care Nurses 122

Public Health Nurses 123

Institutions of Higher Learning 123

Student Nurses 124

Clinic or Outpatient Care and Health Center Nurses 125

Long-Term Care 125

Volunteers 125

Working in International Emergency Medical Teams 125

Lessons Learned 126

Case in Point 127

Disaster Shelter Milieu 127

Questions for Discussion 128

Points to Remember 129

Test Your Knowledge 129

References 130

OBJECTIVES

After reading and studying this chapter, you should be able to:

- Describe the roles of the Level I general professional nurse during an emergency or disaster event.
- Describe the domains of the International Council of Nurses (ICN) *Core Competencies in Disaster Nursing, Version 2.0.*

- Explain how to demonstrate knowledge within the domains of the ICN *Core Competencies in Disaster Nursing, Version 2.0*.
- Explain how the domains of the ICN *Core Competencies in Disaster Nursing, Version 2.0*, can be implemented into nursing roles during an emergency or disaster event.

KEY TERMS

competencies: The knowledge, skills, abilities, and attributes required to perform one's professional role.

disaster: An occurrence, either natural or human-made, that causes human suffering and creates human needs that victims cannot alleviate, or reduce the risk, without assistance.

emergency medical team: Groups of health professionals who treat patients affected by an emergency or disaster.

first responder: A person who is specially trained to be among the first to arrive after a disaster to provide assistance.

Level I nurse: Any nurse who has completed a program of basic, generalized nursing education and is authorized to practice by the regulatory agency of their country.

Level II nurse: Any nurse who has achieved the Level I competencies and is or aspires to be a designated disaster responder within an institution, organization, or system.

Level III nurse: Any nurse who has achieved Level I and II competencies and is prepared to respond to a wide range of disasters and emergencies and to serve on a deployable team.

Introduction

Nurses are often the first responders during an emergency or disaster event. Therefore, understanding the roles that nurses may be required to undertake during these events is vital. The aim of this chapter is to provide details regarding the roles that nurses may be required to undertake in an emergency or disaster situation. These details and information relate to the International Council of Nurses (ICN) *Core Competencies in Disaster Nursing, Version 2.0* (ICN, 2019a), with information on how the competencies should be achieved and then implemented in practice. This chapter also provides information specifically focused on the roles and responsibilities of the Level I nurse, or general professional nurse (GPN), during a disaster event.

Global Threats and the Role of the General Professional Nurse

GLOBAL THREATS

Currently, nations and states all over the world face a multitude of threats. These threats result in the need for nurses to be aware of risks to themselves, family members, and the community and to acquire knowledge and skills to respond to such events. This knowledge will result in the recognition of potential threats and identify ways to minimize their impact on human life and suffering to the extent possible. Current threats range from the effects of climate change, to infectious diseases and global pandemics, to chemical, biological, radiological, and nuclear attacks, and terrorism. For example, as a result of human interaction in the environment, global warming will likely increase by 1.5°C between 2030 and 2052 (Intergovernmental Panel on Climate Change, 2018; Matthews, Wilby, & Murphy, 2017).

Due to the long-term effects of global warming, trends in weather extremes have already resulted in changes in the frequency and intensity of precipitous events in some regions and droughts in others (Fig. 6.1). Without appropriate intervention, such changes are predicted to continue, as seen in the devastating floods in Myanmar, Haiti, Venice, the Philippines, Puerto Rico, and the

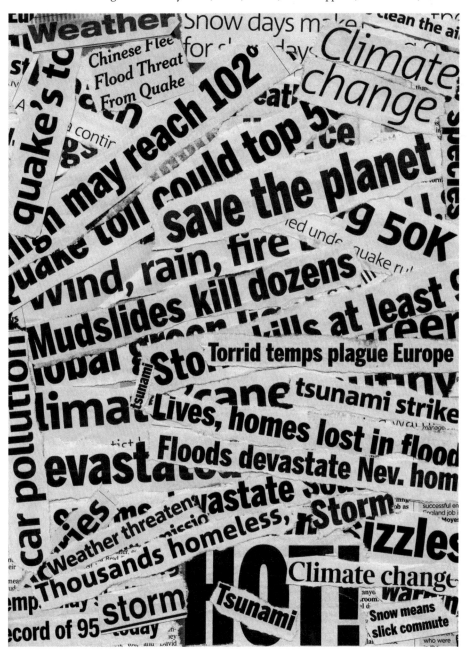

Fig. 6.1 A collage of newspaper headlines focusing on the far-reaching effects of global warming all over the world. (iStock.com\belterz)

Unites States. Conversely, droughts resulting in wildfires have been seen in the United States, New Zealand, United Kingdom, and Australia. Unfortunately, terrorism also looms as a pervasive threat around the world. As a result of the global increase in the number and lethality of terrorist attacks, nations, states, and private citizens must become more involved in a strategic vision to recognize and prepare for such attacks (RAND Corporation, 2019). According to the Nuclear Threat Initiative (NTI, 2018), factors that increase nuclear security against the theft of nuclear materials have deteriorated in 54 countries since 2016. Simultaneously, global terrorist organizations are actively seeking the materials needed to build weapons of mass destruction as well as the knowledge to conduct cyberattacks on nuclear facilities (NTI, 2018). When combined, this highlights that there is an increased threat level for nuclear disasters.

Infectious diseases also pose a significant threat to life and health. In December 2019, the World Health Organization (WHO, 2020a, January 20), China Country Office, became aware of cases of pneumonia of unknown etiology in Wuhan, Hubei Province of China. This was later identified as novel coronavirus 2019-nCoV, or COVID-19. Currently, the pandemic continues, with the number of people infected or dying exponentially increasing daily in many areas (WHO, 2020b). These events demonstrate the need for nurses to gain knowledge of the threats and risks around them and be prepared to respond accordingly.

Nurses frequently have been involved in the response to disasters resulting from multiple threats in an attempt to minimize the impact on human life (ICN, 2006). However, most nurses are not typically involved in decision making at the policy-making level to prevent or decrease the impact of such events. Though underused at present, nurses should be an important resource in the development and implementation of disaster risk reduction, response, and recovery policies internationally (ICN, 2019b). The ICN further supports and encourages the education and training of nurses in disaster risk reduction, response, and recovery and provides guidance to this end (ICN, 2019a). The ICN *Core Competencies in Disaster Nursing, Version 2.0* provides details that can assist nurses with their roles during emergency or disaster events (ICN, 2019a).

According to the ICN, there are three levels of nurses who should achieve competency in disaster nursing at increasing levels of complexity of care, with the focus of this chapter being the Level I nurse or GPN (ICN, 2019b). The levels identified by the ICN are:

- **Level I (GPN):** Any nurse who has completed a program of basic, generalized nursing education and is authorized to practice by the regulatory agency of their country. For example: staff nurses in a hospital, clinic, or public health center; all nurse educators.
- **Level II (advanced or specialized nurse):** Any nurse who has achieved the Level I competencies and is or aspires to be a designated disaster responder within an institution, organization, or system. For example: a supervisor or head nurse; a nurse designated for leadership within an organization's emergency plan; a nurse representing the profession on a hospital or agency emergency planning committee; preparedness and response nurse educators.
- **Level III:** Any nurse who has achieved Level I and II competencies and is prepared to respond to a wide range of disasters and emergencies and to serve on a deployable team. For example: frequent responders to either national or international disasters; military nurses; nurses conducting comprehensive disaster nursing research. Note that specific competencies for the Level III nurse are currently not included in ICN *Core Competencies in Disaster Nursing, Version 2.0* at this time, with many of the competencies expected at this level common across many disaster-associated disciplines (ICN, 2019a).

THE ROLE OF THE GENERAL PROFESSIONAL NURSE

The recently updated and revised ICN *Core Competencies in Disaster Nursing, Version 2.0* delineates eight domains of competency (ICN, 2019a): Domain 1: Preparation and Planning; Domain 2:

Communication; Domain 3: Incident Management Systems; Domain 4: Safety and Security; Domain 5: Assessment; Domain 6: Intervention; Domain 7: Recovery; and Domain 8: Law and Ethics. Table 6.1 provides details of each domain.

As previously mentioned, this chapter focuses solely on achieving the competencies required by a Level I nurse or GPN. Note that the GPN is not expected to be an expert in any particular type of disaster response and should work as a member of a team. Should a GPN encounter a disaster or event in their community, they should use their professional skills (and within their individual scope of practice) and first aid (to the level of the training and expertise) until additional responders arrive and a more formal team response can be derived (ICN, 2019a). It is important to note that nurses whose areas of practice differ (e.g., acute care or emergency department versus outpatient care or clinic setting) from that of others may develop greater proficiency in one competency over another in their everyday clinical practice setting. For example, a nurse working in public health may be more astute regarding disease surveillance and epidemiology, whereas a nurse who works in an emergency department or intensive care unit may be more proficient at responding to trauma and have the skills to deliver more advanced life-saving measures.

As previously stated, a GPN or Level I nurse is "any nurse who has completed a programme of basic, generalized nursing education and is authorised to practice by the regulatory agency of his/her country" (ICN, 2019a). It is imperative that GPNs familiarize themselves with disaster risks in their area and their state's or nation's policies and plans currently in place to respond to them. As the profession of nursing is now very portable, with many nurses working in new countries and environments, nurses new to an area must ascertain what risks are most likely in that area (e.g., flooding, earthquakes, ice storms, tsunamis, droughts, wildfires). It is important to remember that within each state or nation, emergencies and disaster situations are managed differently, and it is incumbent on the nurse to be aware of local risks and hazards. Identifying and using relevant resources such as disaster management plans, health facility disaster management plans, and other reliable resources will facilitate increased knowledge. Many of these resources can be found and accessed on the internet. In addition, speaking with local leaders and experts within the emergency planning sector or speaking with members of the community at large will greatly assist in preparation for future events. Further, it is imperative that all nurses become familiar with their

TABLE 6.1 ■ The Eight Domains Encompassing the Core Competencies in Disaster Nursing

ICN Domain	ICN Domain Description
Domain 1	Preparation and Planning (actions taken apart from any specific emergency to increase readiness and confidence in actions to be taken during an event)
Domain 2	Communication (approaches to conveying essential information within one's place of work or emergency assignment and documenting decisions made)
Domain 3	Incident Management Systems (structure of disaster or emergency responses required by countries, organizations, or institutions and actions to make them effective)
Domain 4	Safety and Security (assuring that nurses, their colleagues, and patients do not add to the burden of response through unsafe practices)
Domain 5	Assessment (gathering data about assigned patients, families, or communities on which to base subsequent nursing actions)
Domain 6	Intervention (clinical or other actions taken in response to assessment of patients, families, or communities within the incident management of the disaster event)
Domain 7	Recovery (any steps taken to facilitate resumption of pre-event individual, family, community, or organization functioning or moving it to a higher level)
Domain 8	Law and Ethics (the legal and ethical framework for disaster or emergency nursing)

Adapted from International Council of Nurses (ICN). (2019a). Core Competencies in Disaster Nursing, Version 2.0. Copyright 2019 by the International Council of Nurses.

organizational response plans and their role within these plans. Participation in emergency drills or tabletop exercises will improve knowledge of and response to disaster events. Tabletop exercises and drills are discussed in more detail in Chapter 14.

COMPETENCIES FOR THE GENERAL PROFESSIONAL NURSE

As stated previously, within the ICN *Core Competencies in Disaster Nursing, Version 2.0*, there are eight domains (see Table 6.1) (ICN, 2019a). Within each domain are the tasks to be navigated to successfully achieve competency within that domain. In the following sections, we describe each of the ICN core competency domains and discuss what GPNs should do to achieve each competency domain.

Domain 1: Preparation and Planning

The Preparation and Planning domain includes actions to be taken prior to an event to increase readiness and confidence in knowing what to do during an event (ICN, 2019a). Preparedness may be the most critical phase of the disaster cycle, as it is through proper planning for appropriate preparation, response, and recovery, that mitigation can more readily occur. Preparation is vital to reduce loss of life and property and facilitates a systematic, controlled manner in response to a disaster or event. It should be noted that there is no single method of preparedness. Therefore, GPNs must become aware of the preparedness measures to meet their personal and professional needs as well as the risks faced in the geographical area in which they live and work.

GPNs possess a wide range of professional knowledge, skills, and abilities that uniquely position them to provide assistance in many areas of preparedness and response plans. GPNs should speak with emergency planning professionals in the organizations where they work to learn about policies and procedures and their role in these organizations. It is also important that GPNs familiarize themselves with local response resources available in their community. Professional preparedness involves achieving competence to practice in a disaster situation as well as knowing and becoming proficient in any organizational response roles assigned to the individual. It is also important that nurses participate in tabletop and other emergency exercises (see Chapter 14) in order to prepare for future events. Without necessary professional preparedness actions, nurses are less likely to respond to disasters appropriately and in a timely manner (Ben Natan, Nigel, Yevdayev, Qadan, & Dudkiewicz, 2014; Errett et al., 2013; Melnikov, Itzhaki, & Kagan, 2014), or they may lack confidence in responding effectively (Labrague et al., 2017).

Actions taken to increase readiness and confidence in knowing what to do during an event do not necessarily include actions taken for a specific emergency. Rather, these actions generally include steps to increase knowledge that would apply to many disaster events, both natural and human-made. For example, GPNs should learn how to conduct surveillance for infectious diseases and the processes associated with such surveillance. A critical component of infectious disease surveillance is maintaining current, real-time awareness of what diseases and associated clinical presentations are being noted in the local area or region. Detailed, real-time information regarding infectious disease outbreaks can be found on the internet. For example, the WHO provides current, detailed information on disease outbreaks at https://www.who.int/emergencies/disease-outbreak-news. This is one example of the steps to increase general knowledge and confidence in knowing what to do during a disaster. Chapter 3 provides detailed insight on how to become personally and professionally prepared to respond in a future disaster.

It is also vital that GPNs maintain and develop a general personal, family, and professional preparedness plan. This is described in detail in Chapter 3, but the importance of being prepared and the need to undertake planning measures cannot be overstated. GPNs must differentiate between personal and professional preparedness and understand that, as a first responder, it is important to achieve preparedness in both areas. Personal preparedness involves having a personal emergency response plan that includes all family members for whom a GPN is responsible. Without adequate personal preparedness measures, nurses may be less able to respond in their professional role, or their response time may be prolonged (Nash, 2015). GPNs must consider any special requirements that they or their family members have that warrant extra consideration during a disaster or emergency situation. For example, if a GPN provides care for the young, disabled, or elderly, it may be necessary to consider additional equipment or items needed as a part of the personal preparedness plan. This may include medical equipment (e.g., nebulizers, medications, diapers), or it could be as simple as making copies of medical orders or finding alternative sites for needed procedures (e.g., dialysis, wound care) in the event of an evacuation.

Domain 2: Communication

The Communication domain for a GPN includes approaches to convey essential information within one's place of work or emergency duty assignment and the necessary documentation of decisions made during the event (ICN, 2019a). Tasks necessary to successfully achieve competency in this domain include learning to use disaster terminology correctly in communication with all responders and receivers and communicating disaster-related priority information promptly to designated individuals. In addition, the GPN must demonstrate basic crisis communication skills during emergency or disaster events, using available multilingual resources to provide clear communication with disaster-effected populations, and adapt documentation of essential assessment and intervention information to the resources and scale of the emergency (ICN, 2019a).

Six (6) principles of crisis and emergency risk communication are (1) be first, (2) be right, (3) be credible, (4) express empathy, (5) promote action, and (6) show respect (USDHHS, 2018). For the GPN, *being first* on the scene would involve communicating information quickly and accurately in a time-sensitive manner, knowing what information is essential, and knowing to whom this information should be reported. This would include communicating with other members of the team and communicating identified health or environmental risks to the appropriate authorities (e.g., the health department). *Being right* includes providing information that demonstrates accuracy and establishes credibility, and *being credible* requires individuals to demonstrate honesty and truthfulness. *Expressing empathy* in a fast-paced environment one may encounter in a disaster situation, means addressing what people are feeling and highlighting the need for the building of trust and rapport. *Promoting action* highlights the need to give people meaningful things to do in order to assist them to become calm, reduce anxiety, restore order, and promote a sense of self-control and self-worth. *Showing respect* while communicating with patients, families, and communities is extremely important during times when people feel vulnerable. It is important that the way in which GPNs communicate reflects sensitivity to the diversity (including cultural and religious diversity) of the population (ICN & WHO, 2009). GPNs will not use all of these principles in every setting, but knowing and understanding them will allow GPNs to communicate appropriately in whatever setting or capacity they are responding.

Communication must occur within the organization; adequate, accurate, and efficient communication is critical to response operations at all levels. Within each response system, from an organizational level to community, state, and national levels, there will be an organizational structure in place to facilitate efficient command and control and organized communication to effectively and efficiently relay necessary information to enable the decision-making process. Guidance on the reporting structure should be disseminated in advance and include communication-related information on operations, logistics, and the responses required. GPNs should be able to describe and understand the chain of command and their roles within this structure. It is important to note that the way in which communication occurs after an event may vary and that nurses need to remain flexible and adaptable in these situations. Although cell (mobile) phones are convenient, not everyone has a cell (mobile) phone, and those that do may not find them useful or operational during a major event. Cellular (mobile) networks may not be able to handle the sudden influx of calls after a disaster, and cell towers may be affected, thus decreasing signal reach. Other in-house forms of communication such as pagers, agency smartphones, and wearable badges also may not be functional during a crisis situation. It is important to identify alternative modes of communication that the organization may use during a disaster situation and ensure that all personnel are trained in these methods of communication. Other communication options include handheld radios, walkie-talkies, and citizens band radios.

Regardless of the situation, it is important for GPNs to communicate in a calm, clear manner with enough detail to accurately relate information in a timely manner. When communicating with patients, families, and members of the community after a disaster event, it is important that GPNs use therapeutic communication. As with all nurses, GPNs should be attentive and listen actively, focusing on what the patient is saying. In addition, it is vital that GPNs recognize that it is more important to listen than to speak and to seek clarification as necessary. During a disaster it is important to remember to not attempt to placate patients with promises that cannot be kept, to not give unreasonable assurances that a loved one or the patient themselves will be all right. In situations where a GPN does not speak the language of the patient, family, or community, they should be knowledgeable in using available multilingual resources, including ad hoc resources, to provide clear communication with disaster-affected populations (e.g., multilingual staff, family members, community members). Over-the-phone interpretation services, language boards, and phone or tablet apps are some alternatives that may be used. It is incumbent on nurses to determine what multilingual resources are available in the organization and become proficient in using them prior to needing them.

Domain 3: Incident Management Systems

The Incident Management Systems domain provides details on the importance of identifying the actual structure of the disaster or emergency response required by each country, organization, or institution and actions to make them effective and appropriate (ICN, 2019a). To successfully navigate this domain, GPNs should be able to describe their national structure for response to an emergency or disaster. The national structure for response is a guide on how the nation or state will respond in each unique disaster or event. Such plans are typically scalable, flexible, and can be adapted to many types of disasters. For example, the national structure for incident management in the United States is the incident command system (ICS) (Fig. 6.2). Within these plans, the roles and responsibilities of stakeholders are described in each phase of the disaster cycle (mitigation, preparation, response, and recovery). GPNs should be able to identify and know how to use their organization's specific disaster plan. These plans should include details of the chain of command and the GPN's role in an event, exercise, or drill. GPNs should contribute observations and experiences to postevent evaluation, as all information gained is vital to the continuing development of future disaster plans. Finally, GPNs should maintain professional practice within their licensed scope of practice when assigned to an interprofessional team or an unfamiliar location.

Domain 4: Safety and Security

The Safety and Security domain requires assuring and providing education, knowledge, and skills regarding the need for nurses, their colleagues, and patients to maintain safety during a disaster event. It is important to avoid adding to the burden of response through unsafe practices (ICN, 2019a). GPNs should be knowledgeable on how to maintain safety for themselves, their colleagues, patients, families, and members of the community throughout the disaster or emergency event in unusual, austere, or hazardous environments. GPNs must also be knowledgeable and adhere to recognized basic infection control practices and be able to adapt them to the resources available. GPNs should undertake regular assessment of themselves and their colleagues during an event to identify any physical or psychological support needs and know how to provide guidance

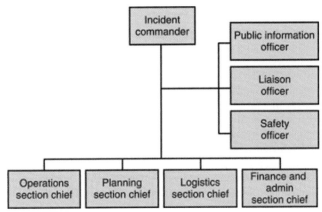

Fig. 6.2 The national structure for incident management in the United States, referred to as the incident command system (ICS). Note that within this incident management structure, there are five major management functions—command, operations, planning, logistics, and finance—and that each function is managed by a single incident commander who coordinates all response efforts. Each of these components has assigned roles that are scalable depending on the size of the event. (From Loesch, M. A., & Giordano, M. J. [2016]. *Ciottone's disaster medicine* [pp. 251–254]. Elsevier.)

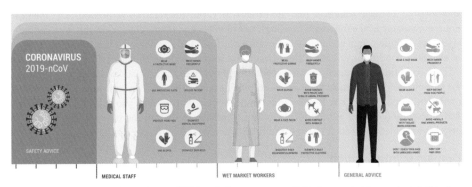

Fig. 6.3 Personal protective equipment (PPE) and other measures of infection control for medical staff, industry workers, and the general population in response to COVID-19. Nurses should be proficient in donning and doffing PPE appropriate to the incident and should educate others on the PPE needed in their working and living environments. (iStock.com\elenabs)

and referral for assistance. To ensure individual safety, all GPNs must be proficient in the use of personal protective equipment (PPE) (Fig. 6.3). Further, GPNs must know how to report possible risks to personnel or others' safety and security and, if possible, voice alternatives that could be considered to address this issue.

The safety and security of the environment in which the GPN is responding can be complicated and hazardous. In particular, when the disaster or event has the potential for sequelae (e.g., earthquake aftershocks) or the working environment has other challenges such as scarce resources, minimal security force support, or people facing uncertainty and hardship, the safety and security of the environment can be at risk. Nurses must realize that those professionals who can secure a dangerous area or building will be in control; and that it is not up to the nurse to attempt dangerous rescues. Understanding and knowing how to provide safety and security for themselves, their colleagues, and affected individuals is paramount to the preparation of GPNs prior to a disaster situation.

Domain 5: Assessment

The Assessment domain requires GPNs to gather data about their assigned patients, families, and communities on which to base subsequent nursing actions (ICN, 2019a). In this domain, GPNs are to report symptoms, clinical results, or events that might indicate the onset of an emergency in their assigned patients, families, and communities. GPNs are to perform rapid physical and mental health assessments of each assigned patient, family, and community based on the principles of triage and the type of emergency or disaster event. A variety of systems are used around the world to triage victims of a disaster, with none being proven superior in terms of patient outcomes, scene management, or allocation of resources (Bazyar, Farrokhi, & Khankeh, 2019). Examples of various triage models include; Simple Triage and Rapid Treatment (START); chemical, biological, radiological, and nuclear (CBRN) triage; Sort, Assess, Life-Saving Interventions, Treatment, and Transport (SALT); military triage; modelo extrahospitalario de triage avanzado (META); medical triage; and Amberg-Schwandorf Algorithm for Primary Triage (ASAV). Fig. 6.4 is one example of a triage tag system used in mass casualty events. It is imperative that GPNs become aware of the triage model used in their country or organization. A more detailed discussion of triage models used in a disaster can be found in Chapter 4. GPNs must maintain ongoing assessment of assigned patients, families, and the community for required changes in care in response to the evolving nature of the disaster event.

Assessments after a disaster require GPNs to be knowledgeable, skilled, and have the ability to perform in potentially difficult or austere conditions for unknown lengths of time. The nurse must appropriately manage resources that are often scarce, provide referrals as needed (e.g., medications, durable medical equipment, housing), and monitor and report changes in the status of individuals to include complications that may arise not from the disaster itself but from the sequelae of events or conditions following the disaster. These may include climatic issues related to heat or cold conditions, increased stress-exacerbating conditions, lack of access to appropriate food for chronic conditions, inadequate access to potable water, the need for critical medications, and myriad other potential hazards that can follow a disaster. Nurses must also collect data on identified illnesses and injuries to monitor them for potential exacerbation and to report communicable diseases to epidemiologists for action and further analysis (ICN & WHO, 2009).

Domain 6: Intervention

The Intervention domain includes any clinical or other actions taken in response to the GPN's assessment of patients, families, and communities within the incident management of the disaster event (ICN, 2019a). To be competent in this domain, GPNs must demonstrate proficiency in implementing basic first aid as needed by individuals in the immediate vicinity of the emergency or disaster event. They also must know when to isolate individuals, families, or clusters of people at risk for spreading communicable conditions to others. GPNs must participate in contamination assessments or assist in the decontamination of individuals when directed by the chain of command and maintain their personal safety while undertaking this duty. GPNs are to engage with patients, their family members, or assigned volunteers within their abilities to extend resources during events. They must also provide patient care based on priority needs and available resources and participate in surge capacity activities as assigned (e.g., mass immunization, mass decontamination). Finally, GPNs are to adhere to their individual organizational protocol for the respectful management of large numbers of deceased. See Chapter 4 for details on response measures.

Domain 7: Recovery

The Recovery domain includes any steps taken to facilitate resumption of pre-event individual, family, community, or organization functioning or moving that functioning to a higher level (ICN, 2019a). GPNs are to assist organizations, within their scope of practice, to maintain or resume

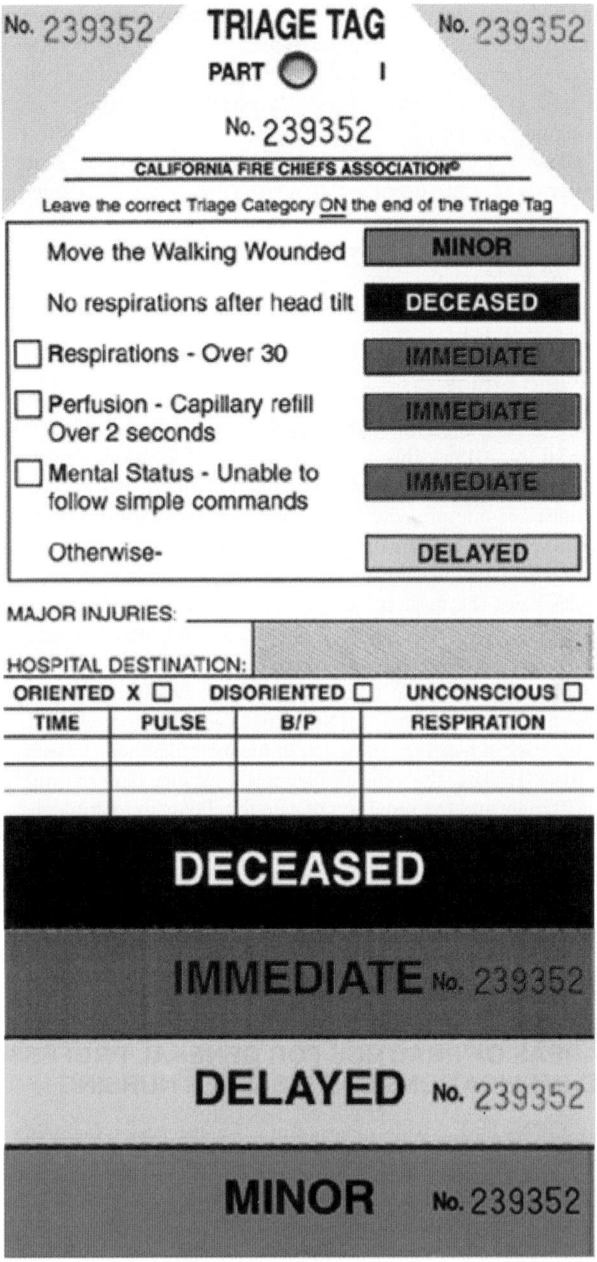

No. 239352   **TRIAGE TAG**   No. 239352

PART ⭕   I

No. 239352

CALIFORNIA FIRE CHIEFS ASSOCIATION©

Leave the correct Triage Category ON the end of the Triage Tag

Move the Walking Wounded	**MINOR**
No respirations after head tilt	**DECEASED**
☐ Respirations - Over 30	**IMMEDIATE**
☐ Perfusion - Capillary refill Over 2 seconds	**IMMEDIATE**
☐ Mental Status - Unable to follow simple commands	**IMMEDIATE**
Otherwise-	**DELAYED**

MAJOR INJURIES: _____

HOSPITAL DESTINATION: _____

ORIENTED X ☐   DISORIENTED ☐   UNCONSCIOUS ☐

TIME	PULSE	B/P	RESPIRATION

DECEASED

IMMEDIATE No. 239352

DELAYED No. 239352

MINOR No. 239352

Fig. 6.4 Triage tag used in mass casualty events. Note the color-coded categorization of victims in green, black, red, or yellow depicting the urgency of the victim's need of medical intervention, with red indicating victims in immediate need and black indicating victims who would no longer benefit from medical intervention. (From Schultz, C. H., & Koenig, K. L. [2018]. Disaster preparedness. In Rosen's emergency medicine: Concepts and clinical practice [x ed., pp. 2406–2417]. Elsevier.)

functioning during and after the event. They are to provide assistance to their assigned patients, families, and communities to maintain or resume functioning during and after the event, including by making referrals for ongoing physical and mental health needs as patients are discharged from care. GPNs are also required to participate in transition debriefing sessions to identify personnel needs for ongoing assistance.

Immediately following a disaster or event, GPNs are to focus on the acute needs of the situation. However, after those acute needs are met, GPNs must begin considering recovery needs. The work in the recovery phase will focus on continued support and assistance for patients, families, and communities affected by a disaster, helping them in recovering from the impacts of the disaster or event. This could involve continued surveillance for communicable diseases, actual or potential mental health issues, and exacerbations of chronic diseases and the recommendation of appropriate referrals as needed.

Domain 8: Law and Ethics

The domain relating to Law and Ethics contains the legal and ethical framework for disaster or emergency nursing (ICN, 2019a). This domain requires GPNs to deliver care within their scope of practice as well as within their applicable nursing and emergency-specific laws, policies, and procedures. They must become proficient in the application of institutional or national disaster nursing ethical frameworks in the care of individuals, families, and communities and demonstrate an understanding of ethical practice during disaster response that is based on utilitarian principles. Utilitarian principles place the highest value on actions that lead to the greatest good for the greatest number of people rather than on actions that are prioritized based on the needs of any one individual.

It is also important for GPNs to consider their perceived duty to provide care and their willingness to respond after a disaster. GPNs must balance the perceived duty to provide care against their potential risk of harm to self to determine their likelihood of responding to a disaster (McNeill et al., 2019). To date, this ethical dilemma, a balance between the health and welfare of oneself and one's family and the provision of care for clients in multiple disaster scenarios, has not achieved consensus (Veenema, 2019). Evidence indicates that a nurse's willingness to respond to a disaster is lower for radiological events and infectious epidemics than it is for mass casualty events and weather-related disasters (Adams & Berry, 2012). However, improvements in the ICN domain of preparedness can result in a higher perceived duty to provide care and subsequent likelihood to respond (McNeill et al., 2019; Nash, 2015). This interconnectedness of domains highlights the need for nurses to be knowledgeable in all domains.

SPECIALTY AREAS OF PRACTICE FOR GENERAL PROFESSIONAL NURSES AND IMPLICATIONS FOR DISASTER NURSING

On any given day, GPNs have a wide range of practice specialties, including hospital or acute care, clinics, health centers, institutions of higher learning, long-term care, students, and volunteers. Each nurse brings a wealth of knowledge from differing perspectives to disaster nursing. Collectively, their expertise in a disaster will provide the tools in each phase of the disaster cycle. Here, we discuss how nurses in various practice settings can contribute to the role of the GPN in a disaster.

Hospital or Acute Care Nurses

GPNs in acute care areas or hospitals may be required to perform in a number of functional capacities after a disaster or event, based on the organizational response plans. This underscores the need for GPNs to review organizational response plans to learn their roles and become proficient in them far in advance of a disaster event. Responsibilities of GPNs working in the emergency department (ED) may include; general assessment, triage of incoming patients, leadership in their clinical area, and emergent psychological care (Alzahrani & Kyratsis, 2017). Overall, disaster response proficiencies for nurses in hospitals and other acute care settings in all departments include patient management to ensure that victims are distributed as evenly as possible to avoid overloading any single area, communication with victims and their families to disseminate information, and making referrals for assistance as needed (Marin & Witt, 2015). GPNs in all areas of hospitals or acute care facilities must be prepared to assess and triage their patients quickly while operating within the incident command system used in their organization. They also should be knowledgeable in donning and doffing PPE, infection control strategies, resource utilization, and the communication needs of victims and their families. It is vital that GPNs understand the consequences of surge capacity due to an influx of patients and how such an influx affects departments throughout the hospital or organization. Technical competencies, including life-saving measures such as airway care, respiratory support, shock management, wound care, infection care, and contaminated patient care, are all vital when a surge of patients is imminent (Noh et al., 2018).

Public Health Nurses

Public health nursing is defined as "the practice of promoting and protecting the health of populations using knowledge from nursing, social, and public health sciences" (APHA, PHN Section, 2013, p.2). As such, the emphasis in public health nursing is prevention, which includes policy, advocacy, planning, and social justice. Public health nurses focus on the needs of the entire population including assessing populations comprehensively and systematically, paying attention to the determinants of health; and apply interventions at all levels to include individual, family, communities, and other systems that might affect health (APHA, PHN Section, 2013). In the disaster continuum (mitigation, preparedness, response, and recovery), the role of a GPN who is a public health nurse includes providing rapid needs assessments of their communities, population-based triage, mass dispensing of prophylaxis or medical countermeasures, education, care or management of shelters for displaced populations, and ongoing essential public health services (Association of Public Health Nurses, Public Health Preparedness Committee, 2014). In addition, a GPN whose practice specialty is public health nursing should participate in response drills, exercises, and training but also possess knowledge to inform disaster policies and plans and be leaders in planning and response efforts. Public health GPNs are uniquely positioned to play a critical role in every phase of the disaster continuum, linking efforts to the nursing process (Jakeway, LaRosa, Cary, Schoenfisch, & Association of State and Territorial Directors of Nursing, 2008). Examples of public health GPN actions in various stages of the disaster continuum includes assessing populations with increased needs after a disaster (e.g., elderly, frail, access and functional needs, cognitive impairment), developing plans to address populations with increased needs, training those populations on preparedness measures as well as conducting drills and exercises related to caring for such populations, and evaluating the feasibility of those plans (Jakeway et al., 2008).

Institutions of Higher Learning

GPNs working in institutions of higher learning have significant opportunity to contribute to positive outcomes after a disaster. Teaching disaster competencies during formal nursing education can create a strong foundation on which to build continued disaster response competency. To date, no single standard for competencies has been developed or tested (Al Thobaity, Plummer, & Williams, 2017; Veenema et al., 2016). However, the ICN (2019a) competencies were derived to serve as a framework for nurses globally as the basis to build knowledge to respond during disasters. To improve and sustain response capacities, the disaster nursing workforce must be developed; a minimum set of competencies should be identified and delivered in nursing schools (Veenema et al., 2016). The eight domains of the ICN *Core Competencies in Disaster Nursing,*

Version 2.0, as depicted in Table 6.1 and discussed throughout this chapter, can be used by nurse educators as the framework to build curricula to ensure that nurses are adequately trained to respond to a wide range of disasters and events (ICN, 2019a).

Nurse educators, many Level I GPNs, can begin efforts to establish didactic and clinical learning opportunities that can be integrated into the curricula at graduate and undergraduate levels (Veenema et al., 2016). Many of the competencies taught in nursing education, such as infection control, epidemiology, and risk assessment, are pertinent in disaster nursing as well. These competencies can be taught in the context of a disaster or other event (Veenema et al., 2016). Knowledge and competencies must also be evaluated using consistent metrics, thus facilitating an evidence-based understanding of the most effective method of delivery of disaster nursing education (e.g., woven throughout the curriculum or provided in a didactic and clinical venue (Veenema et al., 2016).

Schools of nursing have the potential to play significant roles in the disaster plans on their campus and in the larger community and prepare nurses for future disaster events. Nurse educators, thus, need to become familiar with campus-wide emergency plans for internal response to an event and their specific role within the plan. They must also be aware of any institutional connection to the community disaster plan through a memorandum of understanding and be prepared to carry out the nursing role in such plans (e.g., points of distribution activation, supporting the use of campus facilities as alternate care sites).

Student Nurses

Many educational institutions are seeing the need to provide nursing students with appropriate knowledge and skills regarding their future roles in an emergency or disaster event. These individuals are the future of the nursing profession. Proper preparation for nursing roles in the emergency or disaster continuum should be considered just as important as other components of nursing education. The level of education provided to these students will depend on the academic expertise available within the education institution. That said, providing nursing students with curricula based on the ICN competencies will provide the framework for foundational knowledge (ICN, 2019a). Administrators of institutions of higher learning must determine individual response plans for their institution that delineate the roles of nursing students after a disaster.

Academic administrators should also consider the role of the student nurse in disaster response when capacities are overwhelmed. In response to the unprecedented impact of the COVID-19 pandemic, in the United States the National League for Nursing (NLN, 2020) have worked with nursing leaders to propose a model to create academic-practice partnership between health care facilities and institutions providing prelicensure registered nursing and practical/vocational nursing education. Their proposed model calls for the participation of student nurses in response to the pandemic to bolster the capacity of licensed health care providers. The model stipulates that organizations must understand that the participation of student nurses and their faculty is voluntary and must comply with additional requirements mandated in state response plans and federal safety guidelines. It further states that the safety of all front-line providers is paramount and must be safeguarded through prevailing infection control practices. This proposal provides students with a unique opportunity to gain clinical experience while simultaneously learning about population health and emergency management and serving as a resource multiplier at a time when such services are needed most. The proposed model would require careful coordination between health care facilities, nursing programs, and licensing bodies. Using this model, students could serve in a number of capacities depending on the type of disaster. For example, they could assist in clinical facilities with the supervision of their faculty, but they could also augment services in dispensing medical countermeasures after a disaster to increase the throughput and serve all citizens in the community more quickly. Further, they could assist licensed nurses in providing aid in disaster shelters in a number of ways.

Clinic or Outpatient Care and Health Center Nurses

Nurses practice as Level I GPNs in a variety of outpatient care settings, such as health clinics, primary care practices, surgical centers, urgent care centers, home care agencies, and hospice agencies (USDHHS, 2019; (Institute of Medicine) IOM, 2012). Although not consistently well integrated into emergency health care response systems, there is a wide range of available capabilities in these settings. Some of the capabilities include expertise in treating vulnerable populations and low-acuity patients, provision of responder health support or behavioral health support, and the ability to support mass immunizations and dispensing, all valuable assets in a disaster or public health emergency (US Department of Health and Human Services Office of the Assistant Secretary for Preparedness and Response) (US DHSS ASPR, 2019). Such settings may serve as alternative care sites to meet surge capacity needs in the community. Thus, nurses in these outpatient settings should be prepared to provide care for lower acuity hospital overflow patients or those requiring minor trauma care or elective surgery (IOM, 2012). Collaboration with public health Level I GPNs will be important to ensure effective collaboration and coordination of efforts to support community needs.

Long-Term Care

As long-term care facilities are often at capacity during an emergency or disaster event, nurses in these settings likely will not serve in roles to support community surge capacity. Rather, nurses in long-term care should be prepared to support residents who must "shelter in place" during a disaster (IOM, 2012). Of note, residents of long-term care facilities are often at increased risk from the impact of public health emergencies such as influenza or novel viruses (IOM, 2012). Level I GPNs in long-term care facilities thus should be prepared to implement scrupulous infection prevention and control practices based on recommendations described by agencies such as the WHO at https://www.who.int/infection-prevention/en/, the Centers for Disease Control and Prevention at https://www.cdc.gov/infectioncontrol/index.html, or other reputable entities.

Volunteers

Multiple essential service organizations provide disaster services and welcome nurses as volunteers. These organizations conduct emergency or disaster training of their volunteers, preparing them to assist during these events based on the type of services provided and patterns of deployment. The type and frequency of training of volunteers is determined by organizations enlisting the volunteer services, which may include augmenting health care resources in a location affected by a federally declared disaster; providing humanitarian relief such as shelter, food, health assessment and referrals, support for functional needs, mental health services, and supporting local public health organizations during events. Before an event, organizations must clearly articulate the role and scope of practice for their volunteers. It is crucial for the GPN to be aware of the organization's role, protocols, and parameters for disaster service, as they may be more restrictive than the GPN's usual scope of practice. To ensure safe, legal practice, GPNs must maintain awareness not only of the organization's scope of practice and service parameters, but also of whether their license is valid for practice in the location in which they are volunteering.

Working in International Emergency Medical Teams

The number of emergency medical teams (EMTs, formerly foreign medical teams) being sent to low- and middle-income countries affected by a sudden-onset disaster to provide emergency medical care is increasing (Gerdin, Wladis, & von Schreeb, 2013; von Schreeb, Riddez, Samnegård, Samnegård, & Rosling, 2008). Although external assistance provided to countries in a time of need is a sign of global unanimity, such deployments of medical personnel can be challenging and require verification of capacities of such teams to include knowledge, experience, and preparation (Norton, von Schreeb, Aitken, Herard, & Lajolo, 2013). Individuals responding to disasters who are not self-sufficient can add to the burden of the affected country without contributing to the care of the affected population (Camacho et al., 2016). To attempt to overcome this, the WHO (2020c) began its Emergency Medical Teams Initiative to assist member states in building their capacity and strengthening their health systems by coordinating the deployment of medical teams in emergencies with assurances of qualified members (WHO, 2020c). The mission of the WHO Emergency Medical Teams Initiative is to "reduce the loss of lives and prevent disability in sudden-onset disasters and outbreaks through rapid deployment and coordination of quality-assured EMTs" (WHO, 2020c, para 4).

GPNs who wish to become members of international EMT organizations should attend training to appropriately prepare for deployment. Examples of emergency training by relevant EMTs and emergency organizations include: United Nations Disaster Assessment and Coordination (UNDAC), Médecins Sans Frontières (MSF) or Doctors Without Borders, the Red Cross/Red Crescent field-training model, International Search and Rescue Advisory Group (INSARAG), Regional Earthquake Response Exercise, Australian Medical Assistance Teams (AUSMAT), and training initiatives such as those during the Ebola outbreak in West Africa (Camacho et al., 2016). GPNs should inquire about opportunities to attend training and become a part of their international EMT to ensure that they are adequately prepared to respond in this capacity when needed.

There are three steps in the learning process for EMTs (Camacho et al., 2016). Step 1 is *professional competence and license to practice*. Step 2 is *adaptation to context*. Step 3 is *team performance*. These three steps represent the minimum standard for training and education, and no individual should be deployed without completing all three steps. Step 1, *professional competence and license to practice*, is achieved when a GPN is licensed to practice by their respective professional body and has obtained relevant work experience in their home country. Step 2, *adaptation to context*, requires that anyone who is deployed be trained in the context in which they will be deployed, including adapting their professional skills and competencies within the context of limited resources. GPNs must attend EMT training that focuses on critical assessment and analysis of the situation "in order to ensure that priority is given to the most essential health needs of the population and a capacity to triage, based on public health priorities and available resources" (Camacho et al., 2016, p. 10). The following are examples of the training needed to be proficient in Step 2:

- Clinical skills: surgery, wound care, pediatrics, mass casualty
- Public health: disease prevention, health systems, management of epidemics
- Logistics: shelter, water, sanitation

Step 3, *team performance*, is achieved when EMT members are integrated into a multidisciplinary team within the EMT organization and focus their training on teamwork and the organizational values, protocols, communication pathways, security guidelines, teamwork dynamics, personal health and travel, and topics related to the particular deployments and living conditions. While Steps 1 and 2 are individual responsibilities, Step 3 training is the responsibility of the EMT organization.

LESSONS LEARNED

To continue to develop the knowledge and skills required for future emergency or disaster events, nurses must ensure that the lessons learned from previous emergency or disaster events are applied to future event planning and responses. Lessons learned must include the positive and negative events or consequences of particular actions or organizational plans. Continuing to make the same mistakes is costly and can be averted or decreased if organizations appropriately engage in processes centered on learning lessons from each event. Typically, this is a formal process where stakeholders discuss what happened and why, what worked and what did not work, and what should be done differently in the next event. This information needs to be introduced into updated organizational plans in a timely manner.

Case in Point

DISASTER SHELTER MILIEU

Based on weather reports of a hurricane forming in the Atlantic Ocean with movement to the Northeast, state and county emergency management began planning for possible damaging winds and flooding in the state. As more information became available, it was determined that opening shelters would be necessary for the protection of those individuals living in areas at risk for flooding or heavy wind damage. The affected county opened eight shelters. Each shelter was staffed with four to six Level I nurses to provide health services, as necessary, to the shelter population. Guidelines for minimum staffing requirements for general shelters are four Level I nurses per 100 clients for each 24-hour period. If a shelter has a large number of individuals with chronic conditions, additional nurses are requested.

A shelter was set up in a local school with the expectation of 350 clients. Health services initially was staffed with two Level I nurses working days and two Level I nurses working nights. A request was made for additional Level I nurses, though none were immediately available due to the number of shelters open. The nurses on-site selected a room where health services could be set up, providing easy access and privacy. The nurses also conducted a survey of the dormitory area where clients would be staying as well as the kitchen, bathrooms, and feeding area to assure client and staff safety. In addition, the nurses identified an area where clients with special needs, who could not be housed within the general population, could be supported.

When clients arrived at the shelter, they needed to go through a registration process. This was a difficult process due to the number of people trying to register and client concerns that there would not be enough room for everyone. Staff circulated among the clients to let them know that there was room for all and that they would be safe. Once registered, clients were escorted to the dormitory, where they selected a space for their family to sleep. As clients moved through the registration process, a nurse greeted them and spoke with them to determine if they had any health needs or injuries requiring immediate care. For example, the nurse asked clients if they had all their medications, if they were injured, if they had their needed medical equipment, if they had a disability that limited any of their abilities to function, and if special accommodations were required.

Any client who needed immediate assistance (e.g., due to injury, medication loss, or confusion) was taken directly to the health services room, where one of the nurses assessed them and provided care as required. A client who could not be safely managed in a general population was moved to a special needs shelter or other facility, if possible. However, it was important to remember that clients needed to be managed in the general shelter until a special needs shelter became available. The nurse then designated an area for the client and a family member that best met the client need. If a client failed or was unable to bring their medications, it was sometimes possible to send someone back to the home to retrieve the medications. If this was not possible, health services worked to obtain the needed medications from the local pharmacy. Another common issue was clients with in-home health services. Following up with the home health agency was helpful in managing care of the clients in the shelter. Frequently, the agency continued care in the shelter once it was safe to travel. Family members were expected to provide the same support to their family members with health and mobility issues as they did at home. Nurses supported the family by providing any materials they needed to care for their family member or any needed training that helped the family better meet identified needs. One area that was particularly challenging was the need for special beds for clients who could not use the regular cots. For some, this was because of mobility issues or weight. For these clients, it was sometimes necessary to obtain a hospital bed or bariatric bed. There were also times when a client needed special equipment. The nurse worked with the family and local resources to meet these needs.

Once clients were settled in the dormitory area, nurses began the process of interviewing each family to identify any access or functional needs; needs to maintain health and independence; and services, support, and transportation needs. Each family was interviewed, usually in the dormitory area where they chose to sleep. Nurses went to the clients rather than having the clients go to the nurses, as this created a more comfortable dynamic. This was the first time the nurse had the opportunity to establish a relationship with the family and identify health and wellness needs that may not have been identified earlier. For example, needs identified might include that a client did not bring all their medications, a client has dialysis treatment twice a week, a child's wheelchair is lost, a family member is autistic, or a client needs a medical treatment once a week. With this information, the nurse could begin to plan how to meet the client needs. It was important that the nurse had access to resource lists and phone numbers. It was not unusual for clients to come to the shelter without contact information for the resources they needed. The nurses worked with the family to identify the resources and arrange for needs to be met. Most of the health services kits used by the nurses contained resource lists that helped with meeting client needs.

The health room in the shelter, staffed 24 hours a day, was designed to provide care for injured or ill clients and staff. Needs ranged from a situation requiring a Band-Aid to a serious illness or injury. The great majority of the health room visits in any shelter are for minor injuries; clients needing an aspirin for a headache or Band-Aids or clients wanting a blood pressure check. Over-the-counter (OTC) medications were stocked in the health room and managed by the nurses. A health services record was completed for every client treated. For example, a client coming in to request an aspirin would have a health services record completed. It was necessary to complete the health services record, even for a single aspirin, because if the client returned for aspirin multiple times, this may indicate a need for additional assessment. Since nurses changed regularly, documentation was the only way to track care—even with OTC medications.

Nurses in the shelter made periodic rounds of the client and staff areas throughout the day and night. They monitored activities such as feeding to ensure that food was not being left out for too long without proper storage. They reminded workers to wash their hands, talk with clients and staff, and listen to concerns. Nurses also monitored the health of kitchen volunteers and others who were volunteering in the shelter. The importance of the presence of a nurse was illustrated by the following example. Client A mentioned to a nurse that she had seen client B going in and out of the bathroom multiple times that morning. The nurse was concerned and sought out client B. Client B stated that she had not been feeling well but thought it was from the worry and stress of the hurricane. The nurse walked her back to the health room where she assessed client B, determining that the client's blood pressure was high and heart rate was irregular. The nurse immediately arranged for transport to the hospital, where client B remained for several days. Had the nurse not been interacting with clients in the dormitory, client B might have suffered a far worse outcome. Another incident within the shelter occurred with one of the kitchen volunteers who, despite having a cold, continued working as her illness got worse. It was not until several staff also got colds that the nurse realized the volunteer in the kitchen was spreading the virus.

Questions for Discussion

1. Which of the competencies in the ICN *Core Competencies in Disaster Nursing, Version 2.0* are illustrated by the nurses' actions in this case study? Give specific examples.
2. What other elements of care might the nurse working in a disaster shelter need to consider? Give specific examples.

Points to Remember

- The development of the revised ICN disaster nursing competencies provides nurses with a framework for the continuing preparation of individuals for future emergency or disaster events.
- Regardless of the level of the nurse, nurses are usually the first responders. They must assume personal responsibility and accountability for actions taken to ensure that they are competent to respond.
- The domains within the ICN disaster nursing competencies identify the skills needed to show competency. These skills and competencies should be implemented into practice according to nurses' roles.
- GPNs in a variety of practice settings may serve in multiple roles during a disaster or public health emergency. Awareness of these roles is vital to GPNs' ability to prepare for and fulfill these roles.
- Education is a crucial component for nurses to achieve the skills needed within each competency and implement them into their practice roles.

Test Your Knowledge

1. What qualifications are required to be a competent Level I nurse or general professional nurse? *(Choose all that apply.)*
   a. Completion of generalized nursing education
   b. Authorization to practice
   c. Designation on an organization's emergency response team
   d. Prior experience with a deployed emergency response team
2. Which of the following is a principle of crisis and emergency risk communication?
   a. Be first
   b. Be credible
   c. Express empathy
   d. All of the above
3. Proficiency in using PPE is in which competency domain?
   a. Assessment
   b. Safety and Security
   c. Preparation and Planning
   d. Intervention
4. Knowledge of triage models is in which competency domain?
   a. Assessment
   b. Safety and Security
   c. Preparation and Planning
   d. Intervention
5. According to the ICN *Core Competencies in Disaster Nursing, Version 2.0*, what level are military nurses?
   a. Level I
   b. Level II
   c. Level III
   d. None of the above
6. Which of the following statements is true?
   a. The ICN competencies would not be used in schools of nursing.
   b. Student nurses should not consider a role in disaster response.

    c. Preparation for nursing roles in a disaster is not as important as other components of nursing education.

    d. Many of the competencies taught in nursing education are also pertinent in disaster nursing.

7. Nurses in long-term care facilities most frequently serve in which capacity during or after a disaster?

    a. Supporting residents of the facility who must shelter in place during a disaster

    b. Providing care in general shelters for the community after a disaster

    c. Providing care in medical shelters for community members with increased need after a disaster

    d. Deploying on emergency medical teams to provide critical nursing services

8. What are the three steps in the learning process for emergency medical teams?

    a. Professional competence, adaptation to context, team performance

    b. License to practice, adaptation to context, team performance

    c. License to practice and professional competence, adaptation to context, team performance

    d. License to practice and professional competence, adaptation to context and cultural norms, team performance

9. Which of the steps in the learning process for emergency medical teams is an individual responsibility? *(Choose all that apply.)*

    a. Step 1

    b. Step 2

    c. Step 3

    d. Step 4

10. It is important to note that Level I nurses should:

    a. Strive to become experts in a selected area of disaster nursing

    b. Understand that they may develop greater proficiency in one area of disaster nursing based on their area of practice

    c. Wait to use their professional skills until additional responders arrive if they encounter a disaster

    d. Rely on emergency management professionals to understand local risks and hazards

References

Adams LM, Berry D. Who will show up? Estimating ability and willingness of essential hospital personnel to report to work in response to a disaster. *Online Journal of Issues in Nursing.* 2012;17:2.

Al Thobaity A, Plummer V, Williams B. What are the most common domains of the core competencies of disaster nursing? A scoping review. *International Emergency Nursing.* 2017;31:64–71. https://doi.org/10.1016/j.ienj.2016.10.003.

Alzahrani F, Kyratsis Y. Emergency nurse disaster preparedness during mass gatherings: A cross-sectional survey of emergency nurses' perceptions in hospitals in Mecca, Saudi Arabia. *BMJ Open.* 2017;7(4):e013563. https://doi.org/10.1136/bmjopen-2016-013563.

American Public Health Association, Public Health Nursing Section *The definition and practice of public health nursing: A statement of the public health nursing section.* : American Public Health Association; 2013. Retrieved from. https://www.apha.org/-/media/files/pdf/membergroups/phn/nursingdefinition.ashx?la=en&hash=331DBEC4B79E0C0B8C644BF2BEA571249F8717A0.

Association of Public Health Nurses, Public Health Preparedness Committee *The role of the public health nurse in disaster preparedness, response, and recovery: A position paper.* : Association of Public Health Nurses; 2014. Retrieved from. http://nacchopreparedness.org/wp-content/uploads/2014/01/APHN_Role-of-PHN-in-Disaster-PRR_FINALJan14.pdf.

Bazyar J, Farrokhi M, Khankeh H. Triage systems in mass casualty incidents and disasters: A review study with a worldwide approach. *Open Access Macedonian Journal of Medical Sciences.* 2019;7(3):482–494. https://doi.org/10.3889/oamjms.2019.119.

Ben Natan M, Nigel S, Yevdayev I, Qadan M, Dudkiewicz M. Nurse willingness to report for work in the event of an earthquake in Israel. *Journal of Nursing Management*. 2014;22:931–939. https://doi.org/10.1111/jonm.12058.

Camacho NA, Hughes A, Burkle FM, Ingrassia PL, Ragazzoni L, Redmond A, von Schreeb J. Education and training of emergency medical teams: Recommendations for a global operational learning framework. *PLoS Currents*. 2016:8. https://doi.org/10.1371/currents.dis.292033689209611ad5e4a7a3e61520d0.

Errett NA, Barnett DJ, Thompson CB, Tosatto R, Austin B, Schaffzin S, Links JM. Assessment of medical reserve corps volunteers' emergency response willingness using a threat- and efficacy-based model. *Biosecurity and Bioterrorism*. 2013;11(1):29–40. https://doi.org/10.1089/bsp.2012.0047.

Gerdin M, Wladis A, von Schreeb J. Foreign field hospitals after the 2010 Haiti earthquake: How good were we? *Emergency Medicine Journal*. 2013;30(1). https://doi.org/10.1136/emermed-2011-200717.

Institute of Medicine *Crisis standards of care: A systems framework for catastrophic disaster response.* : National Academies Press; 2012.

Intergovernmental Panel on Climate Change. (2018). Summary for policymakers. In V. Masson-Delmotte, P. Zhai, H.-O. Pörtner, D. Roberts, J. Skea, P. R. Shukla, A. Pirani, W. Moufouma-Okia, C. Péan, R. Pidcock, S. Connors, J. B. R. Matthews, Y. Chen, X. Zhou, M. I. Gomis, E. Lonnoy, T. Maycock, M. Tignor, and T. Waterfield (Eds.), *Global warming of 1.5°C: An IPCC Special Report on the impacts of global warming of 1.5°C above pre-industrial levels and related global greenhouse gas emission pathways, in the context of strengthening the global response to the threat of climate change, sustainable development, and efforts to eradicate poverty*. Retrieved from https://www.ipcc.ch/site/assets/uploads/sites/2/2019/05/SR15_SPM_version_report_LR.pdf

International Council of Nurses. (2006). *Disaster nursing: International classification for nursing practice (ICNP) catalogue*. Retrieved from https://www.icn.ch/sites/default/files/inline-files/ICNP_Catalogue_Disaster_Nursing.pdf

International Council of Nurses. (2019a). *Core competencies in disaster nursing, version 2.0*. Retrieved from https://www.icn.ch/sites/default/files/inline-files/ICN_Disaster-Comp-Report_WEB_final.pdf

International Council of Nurses. (2019b). *Position statement: Nurses and disaster risk reduction, response and recovery*. Retrieved from https://www.icn.ch/sites/default/files/inline-files/PS_E_Nurses_and_disaster_risk_reduction_response_and_recovery.pdf

International Council of Nurses & World Health Organization. (2009). *ICN framework of disaster nursing competencies*. Retrieved from http://www.wpro.who.int/hrh/documents/icn_framework.pdf

Jakeway CC, LaRosa G, Cary A, Schoenfisch S, Association of State and Territorial Directors of Nursing The role of public health nurses in emergency preparedness and response: A position paper of the association of state and territorial directors of nursing. *Public Health Nursing*. 2008;25(4):353–361. https://doi.org/10.1111/j.1525-1446.2008.00716.x.

Labrague LJ, Hammad K, Gloe DS, McEnroe-Petitte DM, Fronda DC, Obeidat AA, Mirafuentes EC. Disaster preparedness among nurses: A systematic review of literature. *International Nursing Review*. 2017;65(1):41–53. https://doi.org/10.1111/inr.12369.

Marin SM, Witt RR. Hospital nurses' competencies in disaster situations: A qualitative study in the south of Brazil. *Prehospital and Disaster Medicine*. 2015;30(6). https://doi.org/10.1017/S1049023X1500521X.

Matthews TKR, Wilby RL, Murphy C. Communicating the deadly consequences of global warming for human heat stress. *Proceedings of the National Academy of Sciences of the United States of America*. 2017;114(15):3861–3866. https://doi.org/10.1073/pnas.1617526114.

McNeill C, Alfred D, Nash T, Chilton J, Swanson MS. Characterization of nurses' duty to care and willingness to report. *Nursing Ethics*. 2020;27(2):348–359. https://doi.org/10.1177/0969733019846645.

Melnikov S, Itzhaki M, Kagan I. Israeli nurses' intention to report for work in an emergency or disaster. *Journal of Nursing Scholarship*. 2014;46:134–142. 10.1111.jnu.12056.

Nash T. Unveiling the truth about nurses' personal preparedness for disaster response: A pilot study. *MEDSURG Nursing*. 2015;24(6):425–431.

National League for Nursing. (2020). Policy brief: U.S. nursing leadership supports practice/academic partnerships to assist the nursing workforce during the COVID-19 crisis. Retrieved from http://www.nln.org/

Noh J, Oh EG, Kim SS, Jang YS, Chung HS, Lee O. International nursing: Needs assessment for training in disaster preparedness for hospital nurses: A modified Delphi study. *Nursing Administration Quarterly*. 2018;42(4):373–383. https://doi.org/10.1097/NAQ.0000000000000309.

Norton I, von Schreeb J, Aitken P, Herard P, Lajolo C. *Classification and minimum standards for foreign medical teams in sudden onset disasters.* : World Health Organization; 2013. Retrieved from. https://www.who.int/hac/global_health_cluster/fmt_guidelines_september2013.pdf?ua=1.

Nuclear Threat Initiative. (2018). *Building a framework for assurance, accountability, and action* (4th ed.). https://ntiindex.org/wp-content/uploads/2018/08/NTI_2018-Index_FINAL.pdf

RAND Corporation. (2019, October 28). *Terrorist threat assessment.* Retrieved from https://www.rand.org/topics/terrorism-threat-assessment.html

US Department of Health and Human Services. (2018). *Crisis + Emergency Risk Communication (CERC) introduction.* Retrieved from https://emergency.cdc.gov/cerc/ppt/CERC_Introduction.pdf

US Department of Health and Human Services Office of the Assistant Secretary for Preparedness and Response (ASPR). (2019). *Expanding your partnerships to enhance medical surge: Seven ways to engage outpatient care settings.* ASPR TRACIE. Retrieved from https://www.phe.gov/ASPRBlog/Pages/BlogArticlePage.aspx?PostID=355

Veenema TG, Griffin A, Gable AR, MacIntyre L, Simons RN, Couig MP, Larson E. Nurses as leaders in disaster preparedness and response—A call to action. *Journal of Nursing Scholarship.* 2016;48(2):187–200. https://doi.org/10.1111/jnu.12198.

von Schreeb J, Riddez L, Samnegård H, Samnegård H, Rosling H. Foreign field hospitals in the recent sudden-onset disasters in Iran, Haiti, Indonesia, and Pakistan. *Prehospital and Disaster Medicine.* 2008;23(2):144–151. https://doi.org/10.1017/S1049023X00005768. 153.

Veenema TG. Disaster nursing and emergency preparedness for chemical, biological, and radiological terrorism and other hazards. 4th Ed. New York, NY: Springer Publishing Co; 2019.

World Health Organization. (2020a, January 20). Novel coronavirus (2019-nCoV) situation report – 1.Retrieved from https://www.who.int/docs/default-source/coronaviruse/situation-reports/20200121-sitrep-1-2019-ncov.pdf?sfvrsn=20a99c10_4

World Health Organization. (2020b). *Coronavirus disease (COVID-19) outbreak situation.* Retrieved from https://www.who.int/emergencies/diseases/novel-coronavirus-2019

World Health Organization. (2020c). *Emergency medical teams.* Retrieved from https://www.who.int/emergencies/partners/emergency-medical-teams

Role of the Advanced or Specialized Nurse in Public Health, Advanced Practice, and Military Service[1]

Alice Yuen Loke, RN, PhD, FAAN, FHKAN ▓ Yoomi Jung, RN, PhD ▓ Xiaorong Mao, RN, PhD ▓ Chunlan Guo, PhD

CHAPTER OUTLINE

Introduction 135

Core Competencies of Advanced or Specialized Nurses in Disaster Management 136

Advanced or Specialized Nursing in Public Health Disaster Management 139

A Workshop on Disaster Management for the Community Leaders and Villagers in a Rural Area in Shaanxi, China 140

The Advanced or Specialized Nurses in the Coronavirus Disease 2019 (COVID-19) Epidemic 141

The Response Team at the Fangcang Shelter in Hanyang District, Wuhan, China 142

Korean Armed Forces Nurses as Advanced or Specialized Nurses in Disaster Management 143

The Competencies of Military Nurses in Advanced Disaster Management 143

The Operations of Korean Military Nurses in War and Natural Disasters 144

Continuing Education Courses and Training Offered by KAFNA 146

Case In Point 146

Case Study 1: The Emergency Response of a Head Nurse to an Earthquake 146

Questions for Discussion 146

Case Study 2: Dilemma of a Military Nurse in an Armed Conflict Zone Away from the Home Country 147

Questions for Discussion 147

Points to Remember 147

Test Your Knowledge 148

References 149

---

1 The authors of this chapter would like to acknowledge the contribution of Dr. Sijian Li and Dr. Timothy Sim (The Hong Kong Polytechnic University) to the public health education workshop offered in the Province of Shaanxi, China, in 2018

OBJECTIVES

After reading and studying this chapter, you should be able to:
- Articulate the roles of advanced or specialized nurses in disaster management.
- Recognize differences in the knowledge, skills, and competencies of general professional nurses and advanced or specialized nurses.
- Appreciate the roles of advanced or specialized public health nurses practicing in disaster management as community leaders, using a community program in a rural area of Shaanxi, China, as an example.
- Discuss the roles of advanced or specialized nurses practicing in disaster management, using the COVID-19 outbreak as an example.
- Identify the roles of military nurses in disaster management.
- Describe the unique position of military nurses with regard to their mission and the dilemmas they face in their roles as advanced or specialized nurses.

KEY TERMS

advanced or specialized nurses: Nurses who have achieved knowledge and skill competencies, accumulated a number of years of experience in a specialized area, and/or attained a higher degree.

core competencies: The set of demonstrable abilities and skills that are required in disaster nursing and response that will improve the efficiency and performance of nurses' roles and responsibilities.

COVID-19: A deadly coronavirus pandemic disease. "CO" stands for "corona," "VI" for "virus," and "D" for "disease" and "19" denotes "2019" the year in which the outbreak was first reported to the World Health Organization (WHO, 2020) on December 31.

disaster management: According to the International Council of Nurses (ICN, 2009), disaster management refers to (1) disaster prevention: policy development and planning, risk reduction, disease prevention and health promotion; (2) preparedness: ethical practice, legal practice, and accountability; communication and information sharing, education and preparedness; (3) response: care of the community, care of individuals and families, psychological care, care of vulnerable populations; and (4) recovery or rehabilitation: long-term recovery of individuals, families, and communities.

general professional nurse: Any nurse who has completed a basic general nursing program and is authorized to practice by the regulatory agency of their city, province, or country (ICN, 2019).

military deployment: Refers to service members being sent to a city or country to complete their mission. Deployment is part of the life of military personnel, and an order for deployment is a military order that must be obeyed in accordance with one's place in the chain of command or in accordance with the strategic decision of a higher authority. In some cases, deployment can be voluntary.

military nurses: Nurses who have received a commission in the rank of second lieutenant or higher after graduating from a military or civilian nursing school with a bachelor's degree and receiving authorization to practice as a licensed nurse. These nurses also must complete military training according to their chosen track.

Mobile Army Surgical Hospital (MASH): An army medical unit that originated in the United States Army and was adopted by the Republic of Korea's Army system during the Korean War. After the cessation of the war in 1953, MASH units were retained in the army of the Republic of Korea. The mission of MASH units is to be deployed to the front lines during combat to provide medical services to wounded soldiers.

Introduction

As the largest group of health care providers, nurses shoulder major roles and responsibilities in disaster situations. Nurses possess the knowledge, skills, and ability to support humanitarian efforts in disaster response and management. The primary responsibilities of nurses involve providing direct patient care; giving information; and acting as counselors, communicators, coordinators, and collaborators in managing patients and advocating for the best interest of patients in their daily work. These roles and skills are applicable and significant in all stages of a disaster.

Nurses provide aid in a disaster with the wide range of competencies they possess. The competencies of nurses in the different stages of a disaster can be illuminated by the original framework of disaster nursing competencies put forward by the International Council of Nurses (ICN, 2009). This framework was proposed based on the ICN's views on the competencies of the generalist nurse, as the ICN considers that all nurses, regardless of their area of practice or specialty, should demonstrate the core competencies of disaster nursing. The competencies of generalist nurses in disaster nursing encompass the four stages of disaster: mitigation or prevention, preparedness, response, and recovery or rehabilitation. The core competencies include risk reduction; policy development and planning; ethical practice; communication and information sharing; education and preparedness; care of individuals, families, and community; psychological care; care of vulnerable populations; and long-term recovery (ICN, 2009).

The roles and contributions of nurses in disasters are contingent on the training or education they have received, their clinical experience, and their areas of expertise. For example, in a community prone to hydrological disasters, nurse leaders, managers, or advanced practice nurses are involved in the planning and preparation stages of disaster. They participate in the assessment, planning, development, and modification of the community's disaster mitigation and preparation plans. Their contributions also include the recruitment and allocation of human resources, operation logistics and management, and the provision of training to general nurses to meet local health care needs. When a disaster, such as a huge storm, causes damage to the community or to the health infrastructure, the work of nurses is to protect and provide care to their patients, even when essential medical supplies including medications, water, and food are limited in the response stage of the disaster.

The above scenario clearly illustrates the competencies of nurses in the different stages of a disaster; it also demonstrates the noticeably different levels of competencies among advanced or specialized nurses and general nurses. From 2018 to 2019, the ICN enlisted a panel of international experts in operations and management, research, and academia, representing various organizations involved in disaster nursing around the world. The Steering Committee was established to explore the different levels of core competencies among nurses in dealing with disasters of increasing complexity and to compile the second version of the core competencies in disaster nursing.

In *Core Competencies in Disaster Nursing, Version 2.0* (ICN, 2019) the competencies involved in disaster nursing are classified into three levels. The levels mirror the progression of a novice in disaster care (Level I), to a proficient level with advanced competencies (Level II), to an expert level (Level III). All nurses who have completed a basic education program in general nursing and who are authorized to practice by the regulatory agency in their country should be equipped with the first level of competencies in disaster nursing. The competencies in the next level are demonstrated by nurse leaders, managers, or head nurses who have attained the first level of competencies and are willing to serve in their organizations or professional committees in contributing to emergency planning in the areas of preparation, training, supervision, and management. The third level involves the competencies acquired by frequent responders who deploy to national and international disasters—the military nurses who possess competencies across disaster-associated disciplines. The third level of competencies has not been included in the ICN's recently released publication (ICN, 2019, p. 7).

This chapter focuses on discussing the core competencies of "advanced or specialized nurses" at Level II and on describing their roles in disaster management in the arena of public health, advanced practice, and military nursing. Since there are differences in the job titles of nurses in different countries, the term *advanced* or *specialized nurse* may refer to a nurse supervisor, head nurse, nurse manager, nurse designated for leadership within an organization's emergency plan, or nurse educator preparing for and responding to disaster. The description and discussion of advanced or specialized nurses in disaster management are in accordance with the *Core Competencies in Disaster Nursing, Version 2.0* (ICN, 2019).

In this chapter, the roles and contributions of advanced or specialized nurses in public health are discussed in relation to an effort to strengthen the awareness of community leaders and villagers in a rural village of their disaster risk in the area, to develop an emergency plan, and to hold disaster drills for the villagers. A case study of the COVID-19 outbreak (a case of novel coronavirus that broke out at the end of December 2019 in China) is used to showcase the roles of advanced or specialized nurses in disaster management in relation to an epidemic health emergency. Military nurses have had an impact on global health with their best practices in trauma care, transportation of patients from danger sites, humanitarian medical relief efforts, provision of disaster and emergency training, and diplomatic efforts. The practices of military nurses in the Korean Armed Forces in military deployment, who were advanced or specialized nurses in disaster management, are also discussed.

Core Competencies of Advanced or Specialized Nurses in Disaster Management

For a better understanding of the core competencies of advanced or specialized nurses in disaster management, it is necessary to discuss the differences in the core competencies of advanced or specialized nurses and general professional nurses. For ease of comparison, Table 7.1 lists keywords of the core competencies of advanced or specialized nurses (ASNs) and general professional nurses (GPNs) based on the ICN's (2019) core competencies. The discussion of core competencies is organized according to the eight domains proposed by the ICN.

In Domain 1, Preparedness and Planning, with regard to the competencies of ASNs, the emphasis is on the actions required to collaborate and communicate with people from other disciplines at the institute and community levels in the areas of planning, preparation, response, and recovery, as well as in the evaluation of response actions. These actions include running drills and exercises in one's institution and incorporating basic education and refresher courses for nurses. As for GPNs, the focus is on personal, family, and professional preparation; maintaining up-to-date knowledge of the disaster response policies and procedures of their institution; taking part in drills; and paying special attention to the care of vulnerable populations during a disaster.

In Domain 2, Communication, ASNs are expected to participate in the planning of adaptable emergency or disaster communications systems within their institution or community, convey to nurses in their workplace what is expected of them in a disaster, collaborate with disaster leadership teams on event-specific media messages, and develop guidelines on critical documentation in a disaster or emergency. Meanwhile, the core competencies of GPNs focus on using appropriate terminology in communicating with responders and receivers, providing clear communication with disaster-affected populations, reporting to designated individuals and demonstrating basic skills in crisis communication during emergency or disaster events.

Domain 3, Incident Management, describes how ASNs are expected to develop incident and action plans for nursing practice, participate in exercise or postevent evaluations, and reassign staff and allocate human resources in emergency planning. GPNs are required to have knowledge of the response structure and chain of command, contribute their observations and experiences to

TABLE 7.1 ■ **Comparison of the Core Competencies in Disaster Nursing Between Advanced or Specialized Nurses and General Professional Nurses (ICN, 2019)**

Core Competencies	Advanced or Specialized Nurses Organizational Actions and Guidelines	General Professional Nurses Focus on Personal Skills and Care for Clients
Domain 1: Preparation and Planning		
Preparedness	Work with people from other disciplines at the institution or community level	Be prepared in the personal, family, and professional spheres
Drills or exercises	Evaluate and plan actions for improvement	Participate in exercises with people from other disciplines
Roles and responsibilities	Communicate to others involved in planning, preparation, response, and recovery	Have up-to-date knowledge of policies and procedures
Vulnerable populations	Formulate relevant actions and an emergency plan	Come up with approaches to accommodate
	Incorporate in basic education or refreshment course	
Domain 2: Communication		
Terminology used	Plan for adaptable communication systems	Make appropriate use of responders and receivers
Priority	Communicate expectations of nurses to a workplace	Communicate disaster-related information to designated individuals
Event-specific media messages	Collaborate with disaster leadership teams	Engage in basic crisis communication
Disaster documentation	Develop guidance on critical documentation	Clearly communicate with the disaster-affected population
		Adapt documentation of essential assessments and interventions to the scale of an emergency
Domain 3: Incident Management		
Incident response	Develop an incident plan	Describe the structure for a response
Action plan	Develop action plans for nursing practices	Describe the uses of a specific disaster plan, including a chain of command
Evaluation	Participate in exercise or postevent evaluation	Contribute to observations and experiences to make evaluations
Professional practices	Engage in emergency planning and the reassigning of staff and others	Maintain professional practices
Domain 4: Safety and Security		
Safety	Support nursing decision making that maintains safety	Maintain personal and client safety
Infection control	Provide alternative infection control practices with limited resources	Adapt basic infection control practices
Needed support	Collaborate with others to provide nurses with needed support	Assessment of self or colleagues for physical and psychological needs and support
Personal protective equipment (PPE)	Explain the levels of PPE	Uses of PPE as directed
Possible risks	Create an action plan to correct or eliminate risks to oneself and others	Report possible risks to personnel or others

(continued)

TABLE 7.1 ■ Comparison of the Core Competencies in Disaster Nursing Between Advanced or Specialized Nurses and General Professional Nurses (ICN, 2019)—cont'd

Core Competencies	Advanced or Specialized Nurses Organizational Actions and Guidelines	General Professional Nurses Focus on Personal Skills and Care for Clients
Domain 5: Assessment		
Reporting	Ensure that nurses have up-to-date information on reporting	Report symptoms or events
Triage	Develop guidelines on rapid assessment	Triage: rapid physical and mental assessment
		Ongoing assessment for needed changes
Vulnerable populations	Identify vulnerable populations and the actions needed to help them	—
Domain 6: Intervention		
First aid	Formulate an emergency plan and institutional policy on the administration of first aid	Implement basic first aid as needed
Isolation	Provide guidance on the implementation of isolation	Isolate those at risk of spreading communicable conditions
Decontamination	Describe CBRNE exposure-related decontamination methods	Conduct contamination assessments and decontaminations as directed
Extending resources	Make plans for extending resources	Engage with others to extend resources
Available resources	Implement and reassign nurses within the organization	Provide care based on priority and available resources
Surge activities	Guide nurses in surge activities	Take part in surge capacity activities as assigned
		Adhere to protocol in the management of the deceased in a respectful manner
Domain 7: Recovery		
Responsibility and functioning	Communicate nursing roles and responsibilities in leadership	Assist in maintaining or resuming functioning
		Assist assigned patients, families, or communities to resume functioning
Referral	Maintain referral resources and modifications	Make referrals to address the ongoing physical and mental health needs of clients
		Conduct transition de-briefing to identify personal needs
Domain 8: Law and Ethics		
Emergency-specific laws, policies, and procedures	Provide development and guidance for nurses within the organization or institution	Engage in practices applicable to nursing
Disaster or emergency frameworks for the allocation of resources	Participate in development	Apply when caring for individuals, families, or communities
Utilitarian principles	Develop guidance and support for nurses under utilitarian principles	Engage in ethical practices when responding to a disaster

CBRNE, Chemical, biological, radiological, nuclear, and explosive materials.

postevent evaluations, and maintain the standards of professional practice within the scope of their license.

Domain 4, Safety and Security, involves ensuring the safety of nurses, their colleagues, and victims to avoid increasing the burden on health care workers due to unsafe practices. ASNs are expected to collaborate with others to support nurses in maintaining safety, come up with alternative infection control practices with limited resources, explain the levels of personal protective equipment (PPE), and create action plans to eliminate the risks to themselves and others. GPNs are expected to maintain their own safety and that of their clients, adopt basic infection control practices, assess their own physical and psychological needs and those of their colleagues, use PPE as directed, and report possible dangers and risks.

In Domain 5, Assessment, ASNs are expected to ensure that nurses have up-to-date information and reports, develop event-specific guidelines on making rapid physical and mental assessments, and identify vulnerable populations and the actions needed to treat them. The competencies of GPNs include gathering data; conducting ongoing assessments of assigned patients, families, or communities on which subsequent nursing interventions are to be based; and reporting symptoms or events.

Domain 6, Intervention, involves the clinical actions taken in response to the assessment of patients, families, or communities during a disaster event. ASNs ensure that there is an emergency plan and an institutional policy on the administration of first aid, provide guidance on the implementation of isolation measures, and describe CBRNE (chemical, biological, radiological, nuclear, and explosive materials) exposure-related decontamination methods. They also plan and implement the reassignment of staff within an organization, requisition resources, and guide nurses in surge activities. GPNs implement basic first aid as needed by individuals, isolate those at risk of spreading communicable conditions, carry out decontamination efforts, provide care based on priority, take part in surge capacity activities as assigned, and adhere to protocol.

Domain 7, Recovery, involves taking steps to facilitate the resumption of individual, family, community, or organizational functioning or move it to a higher level than before the event. ASNs communicate nursing roles and responsibilities in leadership and maintain referral resources and make modifications when needed. GPNs assist their assigned clients in maintaining or resuming their ability to function post event and make referrals for the ongoing physical and mental health needs of the clients.

In Domain 8, Law and Ethics, ASNs are expected to contribute to the development of a legal and ethical framework for disaster nursing, contribute to the development and guidance of nurses within their organization, and offer guidance and support to nurses according to utilitarian principles. GPNs are expected to practice within an ethical and legal framework applicable to nursing.

In summary, the core competencies of ASNs focus on organization-related policies and plans and on offering guidance to nursing staff. ASNs are the leaders, planners, managers, and communicators in a disaster-affected health care system, whereas GPNs are the professional practitioners. ASNs are the leaders in developing plans for disasters and emergencies, providing guidance to nurses, and participating in improving disaster nursing responses. They also work with people from other disciplines and organizations to provide professional health care to disaster-affected populations.

Advanced or Specialized Nursing in Public Health Disaster Management

Almost all disasters have an impact on public health. An unanticipated disaster often leads to mass casualties, straining the capacity of health care systems. Regardless of how well government agencies or health care systems have planned and prepared for disasters, people in the community need to be aware of their risk, be prepared, and be able to help themselves when disasters strike.

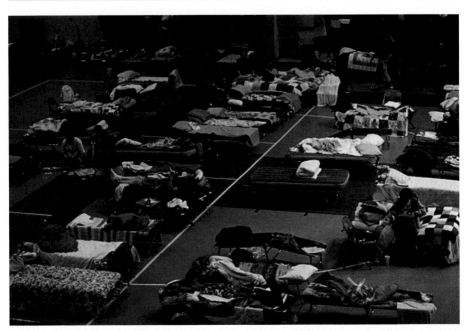

Fig. 7.1   Red Cross shelter in an auditorium that housed flood evacuees in Minot, North Dakota. Burleigh and Ward counties were designated a federal disaster area, opening the way for federal disaster assistance from the Federal Emergency Management Agency (FEMA). (Photo by Andrea Booher/FEMA. Fig. 9.11 from Bullock, J., Haddow, G., & Coppola, D. [2021]. *Introduction to homeland security* [6th ed.]. Elsevier.)

In this regard, community or public health nurses and nurse educators play the essential and vital roles of providing professional services and education to the community at the population level to deal with the full spectrum of disasters.

The public's awareness of and preparedness for the disaster risk in their area is the first step in disaster preparation. This is particularly imperative in remote and resource-poor areas; the public tends to lack awareness of their disaster and health risks, have not made preparations, and have a limited capacity to respond to disasters. This is the case even though these communities may experience frequent and recurrent disasters, such as floods or earthquakes (Fig. 7.1). It has been suggested that, in public health, a bottom-up community-based disaster risk reduction approach is effective at improving the disaster preparedness, response capacity, and overall health outcomes of local individuals, families, and communities.

Public health education using a bottom-up approach can be implemented at minimal cost to empower communities and reduce the public health risks associated with disasters and health emergencies, especially in resource-poor areas. ASNs in public health are responsible for providing education and training to other professionals in community organizations, community leaders, school teachers, and the general public. An example of this approach is illustrated by a public health education workshop offered in a rural area in Shaanxi, China, an area that experiences recurrent earthquakes.

A WORKSHOP ON DISASTER MANAGEMENT FOR THE COMMUNITY LEADERS AND VILLAGERS IN A RURAL AREA IN SHAANXI, CHINA

The public health education workshop was offered in May 2018. It was a two-day disaster management training program conducted by a team consisting of a nurse educator and a social worker specializing in disaster nursing, and four graduates from a master's program on disaster nursing. All of those serving on the disaster response team were ASNs in their respective organizations. The workshop focused on the knowledge, skills, and planning involved in responding to earthquake and fire emergencies, and offered hands-on training and drills to community leaders, officers of community organizations, and villagers.

During the workshop, the team worked closely with the community leaders and officers of organizations to plan and decide on possible escape routes in their rural area during disaster events. A discussion forum was organized, and the participants were divided into several small groups. The team members served as facilitators in leading the discussion on various aspects of disaster response, including the actions to be taken in response to health contingencies. In addition, content included evacuation plans, training in basic first aid skills, identification of vulnerable groups in the community, establishment of a plan for escaping fires or earthquakes, and launching of regular drills in the village. After the discussion forum, a disaster preparation plan for the community was formulated.

The team also led the community leaders in organizing a drill in the event of a fire or earthquake emergency in the rural community. Emergency response teams were organized and assigned among the village officials and community members, with a clear delineation of their roles and responsibilities in different emergency scenarios. The drill provided an opportunity for the villagers and their families to practice their knowledge and skills. The team also taught the villagers basic techniques in first aid to deal with wounds and burns and used interactive games to teach children and their family members. After the workshop, the team together with the community leaders evaluated their plans and actions and discussed possible areas for improvement.

The workshop strengthened the awareness of the community leaders in the rural village of the need to have emergency response plans and hold drills for the villagers. The workshop also provided the villagers with the opportunity to become familiar with potential emergency or disaster situations and equipped them with the skills of self-protection and knowledge of first aid techniques to help others who might require assistance.

These ASNs in public health worked with community leaders in other disciplines to plan and evaluate emergency drills at the community level and offered training in emergency planning for vulnerable populations (people living in resource-poor areas and families with young children). The actions of these ASNs in preparing the village to respond to disasters demonstrated their competencies in Domain 1: Preparation and Planning at Level II, according to the *Core Competencies in Disaster Nursing, Version 2.0* (ICN, 2019).

THE ADVANCED OR SPECIALIZED NURSES IN THE CORONAVIRUS DISEASE 2019 (COVID-19) EPIDEMIC

The health authorities in Wuhan, China, reported the first case of novel coronavirus disease (COVID-19) to the World Health Organization (WHO) on December 31, 2019. On January 30, 2020, the COVID-19 outbreak was declared a public health emergency of international concern by the WHO when human-to-human transmission was confirmed outside of China. The numbers of confirmed cases and deaths were increasing every day. In early March 2020, there were more than 94,209 confirmed cases of COVID-19 worldwide and 3214 deaths, of which the largest majority of both confirmed cases (80,270) and reported deaths (2871) were in China (WHO, 2020). Those who had traveled to Wuhan and come into contact with people confirmed to have COVID-19 were required to quarantine for 14 days. During that time, no one in Wuhan could travel out of the city, and many countries imposed travel restrictions on visitors from China, closed their borders, and suspended flights in an attempt to contain the virus (Francis, 2020). COVID-19 was reported in many countries all over the world and was declared by the WHO to be a pandemic on March 11, 2020.

The large numbers of suspected and confirmed patients far exceeded the normal capacities of Wuhan's health care system, prompting local officials to seek national emergency support. In response to the call for help, the nursing department of a hospital in Sichuan Province quickly activated its volunteer disaster response team, composed of ASNs with specialties in infectious disease and control, critical care, and respiratory care and sent them to Wuhan. The nurses were divided into three emergency response teams. Two teams were sent to Wuhan, and another team was based at the headquarters in the hospital in Sichuan. Next, we discuss the disaster management approach followed by the ASNs in one of the response teams assigned to the Fangcang shelter in Hanyang, Wuhan.

The Response Team at the Fangcang Shelter in Hanyang District, Wuhan, China

The response team deployed to the Fangcang shelter (FCS) in Hanyang District, Wuhan, consisted of 15 nurses, with one nurse manager, five ASNs, and nine experienced nurses. Nurses from other cities also traveled to Wuhan to lend assistance. The FCS was an auditorium that had been hastily renovated into a temporary shelter holding 890 beds for individuals confirmed to have COVID-19 with mild symptoms. Upon arrival, the team took overall leadership and turned the shelter into a "hospital" to receive patients.

The nurse manager and the ASNs quickly arranged the shelter into different zones. Bed units were divided into clean, dirty, and contaminated zones, including staff entrance and exit points from the shelter. All zoning and traffic directions were clearly labeled. The team also established standards and protocols for admitting patients, an identification system, specifications on essential nursing care, the execution of medical instructions and prescriptions, and disinfection and isolation systems.

A three-level operation system was organized to manage human resources. The nurse manager, who was responsible for human resources in the shelter, was responsible for the scheduling of staff and shifts. She also took charge of the registration of medical and nursing staff who arrived at the shelter and the monitoring of their health. Head nurses were responsible for work allocations, and ASNs were team leaders responsible for coordinating and supervising teamwork during a shift. The head nurses or ASNs supervised the disposal of soiled materials, the supply and use of PPE, and the processes for disinfection and isolation in the shelter. They also directed the movement of patients and medical and nursing staff in and out of the shelter.

All nurses received special training on safety and protection in response to the COVID-19 emergency and were given instructions on the standards for the different levels of PPE and on special procedures for disinfection and isolation. All of the GPNs would provide direct patient care and perform ongoing assessments of the condition of the patients. They were instructed to report any changes in a patient's condition to the team leader.

In each team, nurses were assigned special duties and functions, such as being responsible for communicating with external parties on event-specific messages and standing by to provide emergency response. The team leader would reassess the patients and handle the procedure of transferring patients to another medical institution if their condition deteriorated. The head nurse was also responsible for communicating with departments outside of the shelter to deal with problems that could not be solved inside it. The nurse manager was responsible for the daily task of monitoring the body temperature of all staff members and of being alert for symptoms such as coughing.

In summary, at the FCS, the response team took charge of setting up zones in the shelter, establishing standards and protocols, managing human resources and work allocations, providing special training for the safety and protection of the staff, conducting ongoing assessments of the condition of the patients, controlling the spread of infection, and registering and monitoring the health of the medical and nursing staff.

The nurse managers and team leaders assumed vital roles as commanders and executors in responding to the COVID-19 epidemic and demonstrated their core competencies in disaster nursing as specified by the ICN (2019). For example, they demonstrated Domain 3 (Incident Management) competencies by developing standardized action plans for quality nursing practices and providing additional training to staff. They were also concerned about the safety of the staff in the response team, which complied with Domain 4 (Safety and Security). The team first ensured that all nurses provided patient care and performed assessments with up-to-date and event-specific knowledge and skills, which complied with Domain 5 (Assessment). The managers also closely monitored the physical and psychological health of the staff and provided psychological counseling where appropriate. The ASNs worked closely with other nurses to implement clinical care for patients, which illustrates Domain 6 (Intervention).

Korean Armed Forces Nurses as Advanced or Specialized Nurses in Disaster Management

Military health care professionals are the first group of personnel to be deployed to respond to disasters both at home and abroad. In the nature of military service, military nurses are specialized nurses in the areas of trauma nursing and disaster management and have received special training in treating combat casualties. The roles of military nurses in disaster management and response are similar to those of civilian nurses in peacetime. However, as the first group of responders to a disaster, military nurses are always prepared for deployment, have a strong sense of duty, and are equipped with the nursing expertise and leadership skills to respond to disasters.

Wars and disasters share common features in that they are events resulting in mass casualties in an austere environment. However, there are salient differences between wars and other types of disasters. War operations are usually more structured and somewhat predictable, whereas other types of disasters are less predictable as to what, where, and when they occur, making it less likely that people will be prepared and organized to deal with them (Agazio et al., 2016). There is also a difference between the two events in terms of deployment. Military nurses are obligated to respond to an order for deployment during a war, but responding to a call for disaster deployment requires undergoing a process of selection that depends on the type of disaster involved and is sometimes a personal choice not directed by the chain of command. Scenarios of both war and other types of disasters are discussed next in relation to their differences.

THE COMPETENCIES OF MILITARY NURSES IN ADVANCED DISASTER MANAGEMENT

The Korea Armed Forces Nursing Academy (KAFNA) is the only military nursing school in Korea. It trains cadets in the knowledge and skills required in disaster nursing as well as in combat casualty care. Korean military nurses are given special training in trauma and disaster nursing during their 4 years of education and are prepared and ready to be deployed at any time. The majority of Korean military nurses are commissioned at the rank of second lieutenant after they have completed their bachelor's degree in nursing at the KAFNA.

During deployment to disaster scenes, military nurses are expected to work collaboratively with other military and civilian health care professionals. Military nurses are able to set up treatment units. They perform triage on patients (victims) and provide specialized nursing skills in trauma care, intensive care, and life support. They also take the lead in patient or victim registration, transportation or evacuation, documentation, and coordinate work among different health care professionals. Military nurses often pitch in to help in clearing disaster areas, creating space, managing and cleaning equipment and devices, and doing other necessary chores. Their roles vary depending on the disaster situations and conditions. As members of the Korean Armed Forces, they are expected to uphold the positive image of the nation with their humanitarian assistance and cultural activities.

Besides being specialized in trauma nursing and combat casualties, some military nurses are also further specialized in critical care, emergency nursing, perioperative nursing, anesthesia nursing, psychiatric nursing, and artificial kidney nursing. Every year or two, military nurses are selected to go through specialty courses. After they have completed the programs, which last between 4 months and 1 year, they are assigned to work in those areas of specialty. These nurses will be deployed to a specific disaster scene where the specialty is most needed.

The KAFNA also offers advanced disaster nursing and trauma care courses for military nurses to further advance themselves through continuing education and training. In these courses, military nurses are specially trained to take on leadership and coordination roles in disaster management when serving as military officers and disaster commanders. There is a systematic structure of courses for ongoing training and education through which military nurses can advance as leaders in disaster response.

THE OPERATIONS OF KOREAN MILITARY NURSES IN WAR AND NATURAL DISASTERS

Korean military nurses (KMNs) have been dispatched to combat zones and natural and human-made disaster sites to carry out rescue work. KMNs were involved in the Korean War from 1950 to 1953, the Vietnam War from 1964 to 1966, Operation Desert Storm in Iraq in 1991, and peacekeeping operations with the United Nations (UN) Mission for the Referendum in Western Sahara from 1994 to 2006. They were also deployed to Afghanistan from 2001 to 2007, to Iraq from 2003 to 2008, and to Lebanon in 2007.

During the Korean War, which ended in July 1953 with a ceasefire agreement between the United States and North Korea, military nurses took care of more than 397,000 wounded soldiers (Republic of Korea Army Headquarters, 2018). The military nurses were at the front lines to provide care to the wounded. They worked in various settings, including classrooms, halls, doorsteps, and schoolyards. They also helped to evacuate injured patients and civilians from dangerous sites and to escape from the enemy. During the war, under an environment of extreme austerity, military health care teams had to provide services with improvised medical devices, including using fishing line to stitch up wounds and using tin cans as basins.

The Vietnam War was the first international deployment for the Korean military. Upon a request from the United States government, 6 army nurses were selected and deployed in September 1964 with 60 army health care professionals of a Mobile Army Surgical Hospital (MASH) team. The team was made up of army nurses and physicians, interpreters, enlisted soldiers, and trainers of tae kwon do (a Korean martial art). When they arrived, there was no infrastructure that could be used, so they placed the MASH tent beside a stream and made use of whatever they could find as replacements for medical equipment. From October 1964 to October 1965, the military team performed around 850 operations. In the 18 months between October 1964 and March 1966, the team cared for more than 15,300 injured Vietnamese soldiers and civilians (Republic of Korea Army Headquarters, 2018). Delivering humanitarian aid was a big part of their mission, so the team took the risk of taking injured civilians into the MASH tent for needed medical care. When time allowed, the military nurses even performed Korean traditional dances and music to build relationships of trust with the Vietnamese locals, as well as to give a positive image of their country.

In January 1991, when the United States launched Operation Desert Storm in Iraq, the Korean military sent a medical armed force to the conflict zone. Fourteen of the 20 army nurses selected were males, in consideration of the patriarchal culture of the region. Before their deployment, the military medical and nursing personnel were given training in the language, culture, traditions of the local people, and on the characteristics of the desert to prepare them for the environment. The team worked as medical and surgical nurses, scrub nurses, and nurse anesthetists and was also in charge of the central supply room. The military nurses also provided the local enlisted medics and volunteers with training in basic nursing care and first aid.

A total of 143 KMNs responded to the call to join the UN Mission for the Referendum in Western Sahara from 1994 to 2006 and took care of 45,000 UN observers, police officers, and UN civilians as part of the peacekeeping operations (Republic of Korea Army Headquarters, 2018). During the mission, the military nurses also supported reunions of families with refugees. KMNs also went to Afghanistan from 2001 to 2007, Iraq from 2003 to 2008, and Lebanon in 2007 to provide professional nursing care to patients with burns or chronic diseases and offer humanitarian assistance in these conflict zones. In Lebanon, the health care team also traveled to villages to provide general health care services and oversee quarantine efforts.

KMNs have also responded to calls for help in natural disasters at home and abroad. These disasters have included the earthquake in Haiti, the Ebola mission in Sierra Leone, the Middle East Respiratory Syndrome (MERS) pandemic in 2015, and the COVID-19 outbreak in Korea in 2020. The military nurses were deployed to earthquake-struck Haiti from 2010 to 2012. The team cared for an average of 100 patients per day, who mainly suffered from water-borne diseases and skin problems. In a deployment to South Sudan in July 2013, KMNs cared for approximately 22,000 locals (Republic of Korea Army Headquarters, 2018).

One of the highlights in the history of deployment of KMNs is the Ebola mission in Sierra Leone from December 2014 to February 2015. The mission was highly risky, as 42% of patients died from the infection. Nine army, navy, and air force nurses among the team of 25 military and civilian health care physicians and nurses volunteered for the mission, risking their lives to take care of Ebola patients halfway around the globe. The team served for more than 3600 hours and cared for more than 100 patients, according to information provided by the Ministry of Foreign Affairs and the Ministry of Health and Welfare (2015).

Another deployment for a pandemic disease took place in June 2015, when MERS hit Korea. About 40 military nurses volunteered and took care of patients with MERS in 4 civilian hospitals. Despite the chaotic situation, in which health care professionals were at risk of contracting the infectious disease, the military nurses took charge of caring for patients, equipped with the required knowledge, skills, and experience in disaster nursing and a strong sense of duty to serve.

At the time of the writing of this chapter, the COVID-19 outbreak had spread around the world. As fear of the disease intensified among the public, the Korean government asked the Ministry of National Defense to send military nurses and physicians to take charge of quarantine efforts in major ports across the nation. As the situation worsened and the number of patients increased sharply in early March 2020, one-fourth of military nurses willingly volunteered to be deployed to civilian and military hospitals suffering from extreme staffing shortages in Daegu, the city in Korea that was hit hardest by the outbreak. On March 3, 2020, KAFNA commissioned all 75 nursing officers, who were recent graduates of the class of 2020, to join in efforts to contain the outbreak. As the pandemic was expanded and the civilian capacity was overwhelmed, major military hospitals across the country have been designated for civilian as well as military COVID-19 patients since September 2020. As such, almost all nursing officers have been fully or partly contributing to deal with the crisis.

In summary, domestically, KMNs were deployed to the Korean War between 1950 and 1953; to treat survivors of the Sewol ferry disaster in April 2014, which claimed more than 300 lives off the southern coast of Korea; and to care for persons affected by the outbreak of MERS in 2015. Internationally, KMNs have been involved in rescue work and health care operations during the Vietnam War between 1964 and 1966 deployed to Sierra Leone during the Ebola crisis between

2014 and 2015 and sent to conflict zones as part of UN peacekeeping missions, including to Iraq, Afghanistan, Lebanon, and Western Sahara.

CONTINUING EDUCATION COURSES AND TRAINING OFFERED BY KAFNA

KAFNA is also a pioneer in offering disaster health care education in Korea. In 2009, KAFNA began offering a two-week course titled Emergency & Relief Nursing for Disaster. The course was later retitled Disaster Nursing Education Course and has since been offered annually to provide training to both civilian and military nurses. Since 2010 KAFNA has been the only training site in Korea for the Trauma Nursing Course, as designated by the Emergency Nurses Association (ENA) in the United States. Between 2012 and 2015, with funding from the Korean Foundation for International Healthcare, KAFNA also developed and offered a course on advanced disaster health care for the Korean Disaster Relief Team, which included civilian nurses and physicians. The course covered the use of advanced rescue and health care skills at the health station, setting up and delivery of services in the disaster field, and rescuing of victims from confined spaces.

When the Ebola virus broke out in 2014 in West Africa, the Korean government designated KAFNA as the training site for the Korean Disaster Relief Team for Ebola. The team was made up of 25 civilian and military nurses and physicians, who were subsequently deployed to Sierra Leone from December 2014 to February 2015. The team underwent 3 days of intensive training, including in the design and arrangement of the Ebola treatment unit, relevant medical screening and triage, donning and doffing of PPE, disinfection, transfer of patients, and handling of dead bodies. The well-designed training program was considered successful and was highly commended, as all members of the Korean Disaster Relief Team for Ebola accomplished their missions in Sierra Leone and returned home safely.

Case in Point

CASE STUDY 1: THE EMERGENCY RESPONSE OF A HEAD NURSE TO AN EARTHQUAKE

An earthquake with a magnitude of approximately 8 shook County A in the afternoon. There were several strong aftershocks. The earthquake triggered a large number of geohazards, including landslides and quake lakes. It also caused damage to buildings, roads, pipes, railways, and health facilities. Transportation to the nearest provincial capital and to hospitals about 200 kilometers (125 miles) away is not possible, as roads are blocked. Phone lines were damaged.

You are the nurse manager at the only hospital in the county. You have received notifications that thousands of people have been injured, in addition to several hundred fatalities. Most of the injuries involve broken limbs or arms or legs crushed by collapsed buildings and roads. There has also been some damage to the hospital building and facilities. The soon-to-arrive casualties will far exceed the usual capacity of your hospital and human resources.

Questions for Discussion

1. What actions will you take in preparing for the arrival of casualties?
2. What other organizations will you seek assistance from, since there has been damage to the hospital's facilities, blocking your access to equipment?
3. How will you recruit enough nurses or health care workers, knowing that you do not have the human resources needed to help all of the victims?
4. After the event is over, what will you do to prepare for any unforeseeable disasters in the future?

CASE STUDY 2: DILEMMA OF A MILITARY NURSE IN AN ARMED CONFLICT ZONE AWAY FROM THE HOME COUNTRY

You are a military nurse who has been deployed abroad to a clinic in an armed conflict zone. With the collapse of the infrastructure and health facilities in the village due to the conflict between an insurgent group and the government, your clinic has been providing medical services to soldiers as well as locals. Your team has been waiting for the arrival of necessary medical supplies, but it has been delayed by sporadic attacks from the insurgent troops. Your team is worried about the current lack of medical supplies. However, you have received a warning that the base may be attacked tonight.

You are the team leader responsible for triage today, and you predict that wounded soldiers will be coming in if attacks do occur. You surmise that you will need to save the medical supplies that you have on hand. In the afternoon, the insurgent group launches an air attack on the village near your station. Three severely injured local residents are quickly transported to your clinic. A man in his 60s and a woman in her 30s are bleeding severely upon arrival. They will die soon if they do not get immediate treatment and minor surgery. The third victim is a small boy of about 8 years old, who is suffering from multiple trauma injuries and burns; treating him will require the use of a large portion of your limited medical supplies.

Questions for Discussion

1. How would you classify the three victims?
2. Would you treat these victims?
3. How would you balance the role of a nurse with that of a military nurse in charge?

Points to Remember

- ASNs possess the core competencies of disaster nursing as leaders, planners, coordinators, collaborators, supervisors, educators, communicators, and counselors in emergency events or in disaster-affected health care systems. In response to disaster events, nurse leaders and ASNs take charge of situations and assess the environment. They work collaboratively with people from other disciplines and relevant workers in planning, setting up, or rearranging a temporary medical facility if needed, and establishing a standard protocol for all to follow in order to safeguard patients and staff.
- The ICN (2019) core competencies in disaster nursing are a comprehensive list of competencies for the two levels of GPNs and ASNs. The differences between the two levels are outlined in Table 7.1.
- ASNs in public health are community health educators. They function as educators in raising the awareness of community leaders and the general public to strengthen their preparation and planning for disasters and drills. ASNs assist the community in making health contingency plans or evacuation plans. They also are responsible for raising the awareness of families and vulnerable populations to potential emergency or disaster situations, to the importance of being prepared at home, and to the need for self-protection skills and knowledge of first aid techniques. In their emergency plans, ASNs in public health should target the community as their clients, particularly those living in resource-poor areas and members of vulnerable groups.
- ASNs in hospitals or health organizations often work closely with other medical professionals as responders at disaster sites. ASNs lead, plan, coordinate, and manage in the most challenging conditions with limited resources during a disaster. They also formulate specific guidelines on the implementation of protections for medical and nursing professionals in the event of outbreaks of infectious disease and other dangers at various disaster sites.

- Military nurses play the dual role of professional nurse and military personnel. Disaster nursing and management is their specialty in nursing. Military nurses must obey military rules, follow a chain of command, and serve their country by protecting their citizens and country. Military nurses are ready, prepared, and willing to respond to disasters at all times.
- Military nurses have conflicting roles in the provision of nursing care during a deployment because they are nurses who see all patients as equal human beings; however, as members of the military, their priority is to care for their own service members to help them return to their missions as soon as possible. Military nurses often face a dilemma in their triage of victims because they sometimes must decide whether to treat victims in need of urgent trauma care when faced with limited help and a shortage of medical supplies.

Test Your Knowledge

1. What is the best description of the roles of advanced or specialized nurses in disaster management?
   a. Planner
   b. Leader
   c. Communicator
   d. All the above
2. Nurses who have completed a basic education program in general nursing and are authorized to practice by the regulatory agency in their country are:
   a. Equipped with Level II of the core competencies in disaster nursing
   b. Equipped with Level I of the core competencies in disaster nursing
   c. At a basic level and not required to be equipped with the core competencies in disaster nursing
   d. Advanced or specialized nurses in disaster management
3. Nurses who are regarded as being equipped with Level III core competencies in disaster nursing are:
   a. Nurse leaders, managers, or head nurses
   b. Advanced nurses who have attained a higher level of competencies and are willing to be deployed both nationally and internationally to serve in disaster response efforts
   c. Head nurses who volunteered to be deployed to disaster rescue sites
   d. None of the above
4. What are the possible benefits to adopting a bottom-up community-based disaster reduction education program?
   a. Low cost
   b. Increases the public's awareness of disasters
   c. Enhances the public's knowledge and skills in disaster response
   d. All of the above
5. Advanced or specialized nurses in public health are community health educators. Which of the following is not their key responsibility?
   a. Raising the awareness of the general public of the disaster risk in their community
   b. Assisting the community in planning ahead for health contingencies or evacuations
   c. Teaching medical knowledge to the general public
   d. Equipping families and vulnerable populations with self-protection skills and first aid techniques
6. The practice of disaster nursing during an epidemic emergency response includes:
   a. Requisitioning personal protective equipment
   b. Assessing patients for infectious disease
   c. Human resources management
   d. All of the above

7. A specialized disaster nurse description does *not* include:
   a. General professional nurses
   b. Head nurses
   c. Advanced nurses
   d. Nursing managers
8. The zoning in wards for infectious disease does not include:
   a. A contaminated zone
   b. A semicontaminated zone
   c. An office zone
   d. A clean zone
9. Which of the following descriptions of the roles of military nurses in response to a disaster is not true?
   a. Military nurses play similar roles to those of civilian advanced or specialized nurses in daily operations.
   b. Military nurses are deployed to a disaster only by military command.
   c. Military nurses are expected to take part in humanitarian assistance missions as well as in combat casualty care.
   d. Military nurses are the first group of responders to a disaster, therefore, they should be prepared at all times.
10. All of the following statements about the work of advanced or specialized military nurses during triage at a disaster site are true, *except:*
   a. Should prioritize the care of soldiers of their own forces over the needs of civilians when there are shortages in medical supplies
   b. Should exclude prisoners or detainees of war from receiving treatment
   c. Often face ethical dilemmas because of their conflicting roles as nurses and members of the armed forces
   d. The triage system used by the military during a disaster is different from that used by civilian nurses

References

Agazio, J., Goodman, P., Opanubi, O., & McMullen, P. (2016). Ethical issues encountered by military nurses during wartime. *Annu Rev Nurs Res, 34,* 227–246.

Francis, MR. *Just how contagious is COVID-19? This chart puts it in perspective.* Popular Science; 2020, February 20. https://www.popsci.com/story/health/how-diseases-spread/.

International Council of Nurses. *ICN Framework of Disaster Nursing Competencies.* World Health Organization; 2009.

International Council of Nurses. (2019). *ICN core competencies in disaster nursing, version 2.0.* https://www.icn.ch/sites/default/files/inline-files/ICN_Disaster-Comp-Report_WEB_final.pdf

Ministry of Foreign Affairs & Ministry of Health and Welfare *The Korean white paper: Disaster relief for Ebola virus disease in West Africa.* Design Museum; 2015.

Republic of Korea Army Headquarters. *70 Years of history of Republic of Korea Nurse Corps.* ROK Army Publishing Directorate; 2018.

World Health Organization. (2020). *Report of the WHO-China joint mission on coronavirus disease 2019 (COVID-19).* https://www.who.int/emergencies/diseases/novel-coronavirus-2019

Actual Disasters and Public Health Emergencies

CHAPTER 8

Natural Disasters

Joanne C. Langan, PhD, RN, CNE　■　Chrystal R. Glinton, BSW

CHAPTER OUTLINE

Introduction   152

Meteorological Natural Disasters   157
Flooding   157
Drought   157
Climate Change   158
Tornadoes   158
Hurricanes and Tropical Storms   159
Extreme Heat and Cold   160

Geological Natural Disasters   160
Global Earthquakes   160
Tsunamis   162
Landslides   162
Volcanoes   163

School Building Safety   163

Actual Disaster and Public Health
Emergency: The Hurricane Irma
(2017) Experience in the Bahamas   164
Preparedness: A First (Hand) Person
    Account   164
Response   165
Recovery   166
Lessons Learned   167

Case in Point   167
Chemotherapy Patient And Potential Flood   167
Questions for Discussion   168

Points to Remember   168

Test Your Knowledge   168

References   169

OBJECTIVES

After reading and studying this chapter, you should be able to:

- Differentiate biological, geological, and meteorological natural hazards.
- Give two examples of specific types of natural disasters that illustrate geological and meteorological natural hazards.
- List signs and symptoms of heatstroke.
- Discuss the immediate, secondary, and long-lasting effects of disasters.
- Describe at least two devastating circumstances of one of the global disasters described in this chapter.

KEY TERMS

agricultural drought: When the amount of rainfall or moisture cannot meet the needs of a specific crop.

biological natural hazards: Events that occur due to disease of plants, animals, and humans. Examples include pandemic disease and foodborne illnesses.

boil water advisory: A statement to the public advising that tap water must be boiled before drinking.

drought: A period of abnormally dry weather that persists long enough to produce a serious hydrological imbalance.

geological natural hazards: Large-scale, complex natural events that occur on land. Examples include earthquake, tsunami, landslide, subsidence or sinkhole, and volcano.

hydrological drought: When the measurement of surface and subsurface water supplies are below normal.

meteorological drought: When an area gets less precipitation than normal.

meteorological natural hazards: Events that occur due to extreme weather. Examples include climate-related flooding, dam or levee failure, severe thunderstorm (wind, rain, lightning, hail), tornado, windstorm, hurricane and tropical storm, winter storm (snow, ice). Includes droughts and hydrological and climatological events.

mitigation: To reduce the loss of life and property by lessening the impact of a disaster.

natural disasters: Events caused by nature or emerging diseases.

prevention: To avoid, prevent, or stop an imminent threat.

protection: To secure and protect a community against a variety of threats and hazards.

recovery: To assist communities in recovering effectively following a disaster.

response: To save lives, protect property and the environment, and meet the basic needs of a community during a disaster.

tornado warning: A statement to the public issued when a tornado funnel is sighted or indicated by weather radar; it is imminent in the warning area.

tornado watch: A statement to the public issued when weather conditions favor the formation of tornadoes in the watch area.

Introduction

Natural disasters are events caused by nature or emerging diseases. Natural hazards are disasters that have not yet occurred and can be grouped in three broad categories: meteorological, geological, and biological (Box 8.1). Natural disasters can have serious consequences for people and the environment. Fortunately, some natural disasters can be predicted to occur within a range of time, but there is often no definite prevention of loss of life or property. Billions of dollars are spent to restore losses resulting from natural disasters, and billions of dollars are lost to uninsured property (Fig. 8.1). More significantly, natural disasters can cause a large number of deaths (Figs. 8.2 and 8.3). In 2019 there were 292 disaster events. Natural disasters accounted for 193 of those events, and human-made disasters accounted for the remaining 99 events. The monetary loss was $50 billion, and the worldwide loss of life was estimated

---

BOX 8.1 ■ Examples of Natural Disasters

- Epidemic
- Volcanic eruption
- Landslide
- Tsunami
- Mudslide
- Famine
- Avalanche
- Flood

- Earthquake
- Drought
- Wind-driven water
- Tidal wave
- Hurricane
- Tornado
- Storm
- Snowstorm

Dates	Country/Region	Event	Deaths	Overall losses (US$ m)	Insured losses (US$ m)
Oct. 12-13, 2019	Japan	Typhoon Hagibis	90	17,000	10,000
Sept. 9, 2019	Japan	Typhoon Faxai	5	9,100	7,000
Aug. 6-14, 2019	China,Taiwan, Japan, Malaysia	Typhoon Lekima (Hanna)	89	8,100	840
Aug. 1-26, 2019	India	Flood	424	7,000	Minor
June – July 2019	China	Flood	225	6,200	Minor

Fig. 8.1 Top five costliest natural catastrophes by overall losses, 2019. *(From © 2020 Munich Re, Geo Risks Research, NatCatSERVICE. As of January 2020 top_5_world_cost_nat_cats_by_overall_19.gif)* (iStock.com/imaginewithme.)

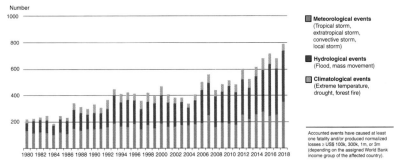

Fig. 8.2 World weather-related natural catastrophes by peril, 1980-2018. (iStock.com\milehightraveler.)

Date	Country/Region	Event	Deaths
Mar. 9-14, 2019	Mozambique, Malawi, Zimbabwe, South Africa	Cyclone Idai	1,014
July 2-29, 2019	Bangladesh, India, Myanmar, Nepal	Flood, landslide	708
Aug. 1-26, 2019	India	Flood, landslide	424
Jan. 25, 2019	Brazil	Flash flood, mudslide	300
June – July 2019	China	Flood, flash flood	225

Fig. 8.3 Top five natural catastrophes by deaths, 2019. *(From © 2020 Munich Re, Geo Risks Research, NatCatSERVICE. As of January 2020. top_5_world_nat_cats_by_fatal_19.gif)*

to be 11,000 including those who died or were missing due to natural and human-made disasters. These numbers and losses were due in large part to tropical cyclones such as Hurricane Dorian in The Bahamas and North Carolina and typhoons Faxai and Hagibis in Japan (Insurance Information Institute, 2020). This chapter focuses on the meteorological and geographical categories of naturally occurring disasters and the global impact of recent disasters on people and the environment (Table 8.1). Biological hazards such as pandemics and foodborne illnesses are addressed in Chapter 11 of this text. When applicable, preventive actions, symptoms, or recognition of the impending natural disaster is presented. The goal of this information is to mitigate the effects of natural disasters and prevent the loss of life and property, when possible. Public service announcements (PSAs) are made to help with mitigation and offer protection of citizens on a global scale as much as possible.

TABLE 8.1 ■ Examples of Major Global Natural Disasters

Event	Year	Estimated Damages (US$ b)	Deaths	Other Damage	Areas Affected
Hurricane Katrina	2005	108 billion	1833 deaths	Loss of life and property damage was heightened by breaks in the levees that separate New Orleans from Lake Pontchartrain. At least 80% of New Orleans was under floodwaters on August 31	Tropical depression formed over the southeastern Bahamas, becoming Tropical Storm Katrina on August 24 as it moved into the central Bahamas. It continued to track west while gradually intensifying and made its initial landfall along the southeast Florida coast, then moved to the US Gulf Coast
Hurricane Sandy	2012	50 billion in United States; 2 billion in Cuba	147 direct deaths	A catastrophic storm surge occurred along the New Jersey and New York coastlines, damaging or destroying at least 650,000 homes	Sandy formed in the central Caribbean on October 22 and intensified to a hurricane as it tracked north across Jamaica, eastern Cuba, and The Bahamas. It moved northeast of the United States until turning west toward the mid-Atlantic coast on October 28. It then transitioned to a post-tropical cyclone just prior to moving onshore near Atlantic City, NJ
Hurricane Florence	2018	24.23 billion	24 direct deaths, 30 indirect deaths	Caused catastrophic damage in the Carolinas, primarily as a result of freshwater flooding due to torrential rain	West Africa, Cape Verde, Bermuda, East Coast of the United States (especially the Carolinas), Atlantic Canada
California wildfires	2019 fire season	Not available	>100 deaths	Fueled by drought, an unprecedented buildup of dry vegetation, and extreme winds, the size and intensity of these wildfires destroyed thousands of homes and exposed millions of urban and rural Californians to unhealthy air	Climate change is considered a key driver of this trend. Warmer spring and summer temperatures, reduced snowpack, and earlier spring snowmelt created longer and more intense dry seasons that increased moisture stress on vegetation and made forests more susceptible to severe wildfire

(continued)

TABLE 8.1 ■ Examples of Major Global Natural Disasters—cont'd

Event	Year	Estimated Damages (US$ b)	Deaths	Other Damage	Areas Affected
Ridgecrest earthquakes	2019	>1 billion	No deaths; emergency crews responded to at least 24 medical and fire incidents	6.4 magnitude	Effects were felt across much of southern California, parts of Arizona and Nevada, as far north as the San Francisco Bay area and Sacramento, and as far south as Baja California, Mexico
Joplin, MO, tornado (United States)	2011	2.8 billion; destroyed 2000 buildings	158 deaths, >1000 injured	Hospital building destroyed	On ground for 22 miles. The injured were taken to 42 hospitals in 4 neighboring states
European heatwave	2019	Not available; wildfires destroyed land, homes, and vehicles and scorched vineyards	8 deaths, 15 firefighters and several police officers injured	The European heat wave was caused by a large dome of high pressure over the continent that was tapping into a hot air mass from northern Africa. An estimated 15,000 heat-related deaths were reported in France following the 2003 heat wave	France, Spain, Italy, and Germany
South Australia blackout	2016	Not available; 850,000 customers affected	None documented	Triggered by severe weather that damaged transmission and distribution assets, which was followed by reduced wind farm output	Statewide power outage in South Australia as a result of storm damage to electricity transmission infrastructure
Indian Ocean earthquake and tsunami	2004	15 billion	227,898 deaths in 14 countries	An undersea megathrust earthquake caused by a rupture along the fault between the Burma Plate and the Indian Plate	Aceh, Indonesia; Sri Lanka; Tamil Nadu, India; and Khao Lak, Thailand
Haiti earthquake	2010	8.7 billion	>300,000 deaths, 3 million affected, >1 million left homeless in the immediate aftermath	7.0 magnitude followed by two aftershocks of 5.9 and 5.5 magnitudes	Haiti, Dominican Republic, and parts of Cuba, Jamaica, and Puerto Rico

(continued)

TABLE 8.1 ■ Examples of Major Global Natural Disasters—cont'd

Event	Year	Estimated Damages (US$ b)	Deaths	Other Damage	Areas Affected
Christchurch earthquake (New Zealand)	2011	30 billion	185 deaths, 1500–2000 injured	6.2 magnitude; buildings and infrastructure were already weakened by the 7.1 magnitude Canterbury earthquake in 2010	The South Island and parts of the lower and central North Island
Nepal earthquake	2015	10 billion	153 deaths, >3200 injured	7.3 magnitude	Nepal, India, Bangladesh, and China

Data from Hurricane Katrina, https://www.weather.gov/mob/katrina; Hurricane Sandy,; Hurricane Florence, https://en.wikipedia.org/wiki/Hurricane_Florence; California wildfires, https://www.fire.ca.gov/incidents/2019/; Ridgecrest earthquakes, https://www.cbsnews.com/live-news/earthquake-california-today-ridgecrest-strikes-near-los-angeles-2019-07-04-live-updates/; Joplin, MO, tornado, https://www.cdc.gov/cpr/readiness/stories/mo.htm; European heat wave, https://weather.com/news/news/2019-06-26-europe-heatwave-germany-france?cm_ven=PS_BI_DSA_09162019_1&par=MK_BING; South Australia blackout, https://www.bing.com/search?q=south+australia+blackout+2016&fo rm=EDGEAR&qs=AS&cvid=565e9a234d084c2e84933897397 4bb44&cc=US&setlang=en-US&elv=AQj93OAhDTt*HzTv1paQdnjs*x3xgOo8qYeWkBu6jZcOhaBYULSln*HaJE xer*UfDWrdbj5b0kXEKjK7JWYK0aLxmI0zhfkFIxo%21YYug8LC&plvar=0; Indian Ocean earthquake and tsunami; https://en.wikipedia.org/wiki/2004_Indian_Ocean_earthquake_ and_tsunami; Haiti earthquake, https://pubs.er.usgs.gov/publication/70042013#:~:text=Additional%20publication%20details%20%20%20%20Publication%20type%20,%20%20 10.1193%2F1.3630129%20%2011%20more%20rows%20, https://en.wikipedia.org/wiki/2011_Christchurch_earthquake#Economic_impact and https://earthquaketrack.com/ nz-e9-christchurch/recent; Nepal earthquake, https://en.wikipedia.org/wiki/List_of_earthquakes_in_Nepal

Meteorological Natural Disasters

Meteorological natural disasters are climate related and include floods, dam or levee failures, severe thunderstorms (wind, rain, lighting, hail), tornadoes, windstorms, hurricanes and tropical storms, and winter storms (snow, ice) (Ready.gov, 2015).

FLOODING

"Turn Around, Don't Drown!" This phrase is one of the most important PSAs that has been shared with communities at high risk of flooding. As little as 6 inches of water can cause a motor vehicle to lose control, stall, or even be completely swept away. Shallow standing water can be dangerous for young children and even deadly in some circumstances due to drowning. In addition, floodwaters or standing water can make citizens susceptible to infectious diseases, chemical hazards, and injuries. These floodwaters may contain human and animal waste; chemical, biological, and radiological waste; and coal ash waste. In addition, downed power lines, lumber, vehicles, debris, wild animals, rodents, and snakes might be in the floodwaters. Besides the physical danger of colliding with or contacting these objects, exposure to contaminants can cause rashes and wound infections, gastrointestinal illness such as diarrheal disease (*Escherichia coli* or *Salmonella* infection), and tetanus (Centers for Disease Control and Prevention [CDC], 2018a).

If a community's water is contaminated, local health authorities are likely to issue a boil water advisory. It is recommended that bottled water be used for drinking and for preparing and cooking food. If bottled water is not available, water should be brought to a full rolling boil for at least 1 minute before consuming it. When water is not safe for consumption, breastfeeding is the best infant feeding option, but ready-to-use formula (which does not require added water) is also approved (Fig. 8.4) (CDC, 2021).

DROUGHT

A drought is a period of abnormally dry weather that persists long enough to result in serious environmental effects such as crop damage, fires, depletion of water resources, deterioration of soil, and loss of plant and animal life (Fig. 8.5). Droughts are defined in three ways. First, meteorological drought occurs when an area gets less precipitation than normal. The severity of a drought depends on the degree of moisture deficiency, duration, and the size of the affected area. A drought area in one part of a country may not be a drought area in another part of the same country. Second, agricultural drought occurs when

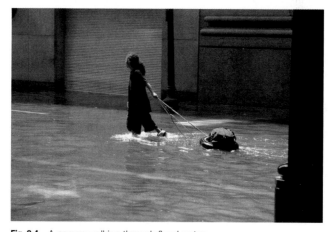

Fig. 8.4 A person walking through flood water

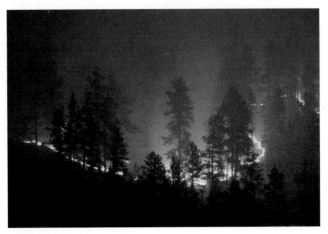

Fig. 8.5   Wild fire

the amount of rainfall or moisture cannot meet the needs of a specific crop. Third, hydrological drought occurs when the measurement of surface and subsurface water supplies are below normal (American Red, 2020). Communities are asked to conserve water when any of these drought conditions exist, and water restrictions both inside and outside of homes are recommended, including prohibiting or limiting watering lawns and washing cars. Although these precautions are crucial during droughts, conserving water is always good for the environment and should be practiced on a regular basis (American Red, 2020).

CLIMATE CHANGE

Climate change, a global systemic risk, increases global warming (rising average temperatures) and the frequency of extreme weather events such as flooding. Heavy rainfalls over short periods of time cause flash floods and necessitate evacuations of communities of people by boat and by air. These weather events also affect wildlife populations, alter habitats, and cause our seas to rise. These extreme weather events due to climate change continue to increase as humans add heat-trapping greenhouse gases such as carbon dioxide from vehicles and methane from agriculture, livestock, natural gas, and mining coal to the atmosphere, which changes the natural rhythms of climate that all living things rely on for survival (Nunez, 2019). The increasing scale of the economic costs of climate change is already forcing financial regulators and the private sector to accelerate the transformation in risk management. The Climate Action Tracker (2019) suggests that without far greater commitment from governments to reduce greenhouse gases, the planet is likely to warm by close to 3°C. To reduce this risk, greenhouse gases must be reduced as rapidly as possible (Glasser, 2019).

TORNADOES

During a severe thunderstorm, a tornado watch might be advised, meaning that weather conditions favor the formation of tornadoes. This level of watch is common during thunderstorms, as tornadoes often accompany thunderstorms. If weather conditions worsen, communities will be asked to prepare to take shelter immediately. A tornado warning means that a tornado funnel has been sighted or is indicated by weather radar. If a tornado warning is issued, all community members should take shelter immediately (Fig. 8.6). Because electrical power often is interrupted during thunderstorms, it is wise to keep fresh batteries and a battery-powered radio or television on hand to be able to receive critical information about weather warnings (CDC, 2012).

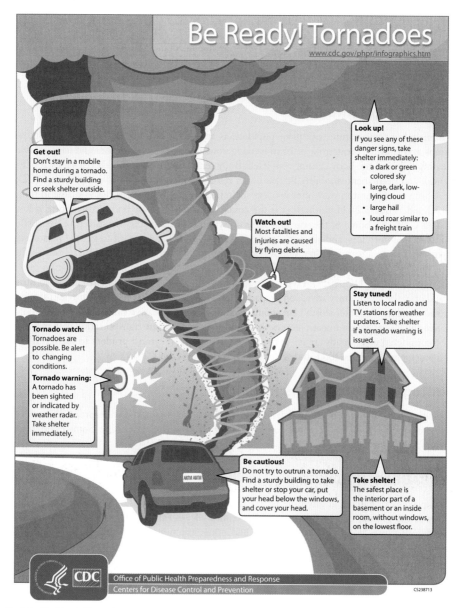

Fig. 8.6   Be Ready Tornadoes

HURRICANES AND TROPICAL STORMS

Hurricanes, also known as cyclones (in the Indian Ocean and South Pacific Ocean) and typhoons (in the Northwestern Pacific Ocean), cause high winds, flooding, heavy rain, and storm surges (CDC, 2020a). Because hurricanes often spawn tornadoes when they make landfall, they cause similar threats to people and the environment as tornadoes. The CDC offers tips to prepare communities for and to cope with a sudden loss of power. Unpowered refrigerators and freezers may lead to spoiled food, which should be thrown away because it may not be safe to eat. At-home generators are useful to restore power to appliances but should be kept a minimum of 20 feet from the home. Also, pressure washers, grills, and other appliances that emit carbon monoxide should be used outdoors only. Depending on the time of year, heat-related illness also may be a concern due to inoperative air conditioning and heating units from loss of power (CDC 2020a).

EXTREME HEAT AND COLD

Extremely hot temperatures can place populations at risk for heat stroke, heat exhaustion, heat cramps, and fainting. Heatstroke is the most dangerous among these conditions and happens when sweating fails and the body cannot cool itself. Body temperature rises quickly (to 41°C/106°F or higher), and permanent disability or death can result if emergency care is not provided (CDC, n.d.). Some communities may offer cooling shelters if air conditioning is not available in homes (CDC, n.d.) (Box 8.2). Hypothermia is the condition when the core body temperature is lower than 35°C (95°F). Some of the warning signs of hypothermia in adults are shivering, exhaustion, confusion, memory loss, and slurred speech (CDC, 2019). It is important to get the person with hypothermia into a warm shelter, remove wet clothing, warm the core areas of the body—chest, neck, head, and groin—and get medical attention quickly. Cardiopulmonary resuscitation may be necessary as well (CDC, 2019). Hypothermia commonly occurs during winter storms, so nurses should offer the community advice on preparing for winter storms and staying warm and safe during snow and ice. A winter storm plan should include a communication plan in the event of power failures and loss of communication services. In addition, an alternate transportation plan may need to be considered when roads are icy. If roads are threatening, it is most prudent to shelter in place with emergency supplies, food, and water readily available (CDC, 2019).

Geological Natural Disasters

Geological natural disasters are land-based events that are complex and widespread. These events have the potential to cause immense damage, loss of property, and loss of life. Some examples are earthquakes, volcanoes, and landslides.

GLOBAL EARTHQUAKES

Earthquakes can happen at any time of day or night across all seasons and all nations. Shaking occurs in the ground due to shifting and breaking rock beneath the Earth's surface along fault lines, which causes buildings, roads, homes, and other structures to crumble. Because fault lines exist throughout the world, early warning systems are being developed to monitor activity globally (University of Washington, 2020). (See Table 8.1 for information on some notable global earthquakes.) Seismic waveforms are being extensively monitored by global, national, and regional networks so that as much information about potential earthquakes can be shared with the affected countries' populations.

Because most natural disasters including earthquakes provide forewarning, preparation, planning, and practice can reduce the health impact and offer the greatest chance of survival. Each family member or individual should consider gathering basic emergency supplies, identifying potential hazards in the home or dwelling, and practicing what to do in advance of an earthquake. For example, tenants of a high-rise building must be aware of the closest emergency exit and identify an alternate exit route if the closest emergency exit is blocked or destroyed. During an actual natural disaster, if debris is falling, seek shelter under a desk or table. Avoid areas near file cabinets, bookshelves, or other structures that may topple and injure people. Also, avoid facing areas with large amounts of windows or glass to prevent being cut by flying shards of

BOX 8.2 ■ Heat-Related Illnesses: What to Look For and What to Do

HEAT-RELATED ILLNESSES

WHAT TO LOOK FOR	WHAT TO DO
HEAT STROKE	
• High body temperature (103°F or higher) • Hot, red, dry, or damp skin • Fast, strong pulse • Headache • Dizziness • Nausea • Confusion • Losing consciousness (passing out)	• Call 911 right away-heat stroke is a medical emergency • Move the person to a cooler place • Help lower the person's temperature with cool cloths or a cool bath • Do not give the person anything to drink
HEAT EXHAUSTION	
• Heavy sweating • Cold, pale, and clammy skin • Fast, weak pulse • Nausea or vomiting • Muscle cramps • Tiredness or weakness • Dizziness • Headache • Fainting (passing out)	• Move to a cool place • Loosen your clothes • Put cool, wet cloths on your body or take a cool bath • Sip water **Get medical help right away if:** • You are throwing up • Your symptoms get worse • Your symptoms last longer than 1 hour
HEAT CRAMPS	
• Heavy sweating during intense exercise • Muscle pain or spasms	• Stop physical activity and move to a cool place • Drink water or a sports drink • Wait for cramps to go away before you do any more physical activity **Get medical help right away if:** • Cramps last longer than 1 hour • You're on a low-sodium diet • You have heart problems
SUNBURN	
• Painful, red, and warm skin • Blisters on the skin	• Stay out of the sun until your sunburn heals • Put cool cloths on sunburned areas or take a cool bath • Put moisturizing lotion on sunburned areas • Do not break blisters
HEAT RASH	
• Red clusters of small blisters that look like pimples on the skin (usually on the neck, chest, groin, or in elbow creases)	• Stay in a cool, dry place • Keep the rash dry • Use powder (like baby powder) to soothe the rash

(From Centers for Disease Control and Prevention (n.d.). *Warning signs and symptoms of heat-related illness.* https://www.cdc.gov/disasters/extremeheat/warning.html)

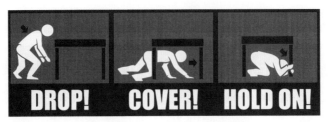

Fig. 8.7 Staying safe during an earthquake. (From Centers for Disease Control and Prevention. (2017). *Earthquakes*. https://www.cdc.gov/disasters/earthquakes/index.html)

glass. Similarly, distance yourself from exterior walls that may crumble or be destroyed. Locate a battery-powered radio or television so that you can listen to the news and emergency directions, which will alert you to whether you should vacate the building or shelter in place. Once a decision has been made to leave the building, do not use the elevators. As you descend the stairs, stay to the right side so that you do not hinder emergency workers from ascending, and carry your emergency supply kit with you.

Learning what actions to take can help you and your family to remain safe and healthy in the event of an earthquake. In most situations, you will reduce your chance of injury from falling objects (and even building collapse) if you immediately follow the CDC's recommendations (Fig. 8.7) (CDC, 2020b).

TSUNAMIS

Tsunamis, also known as seismic sea waves, exist deep below the ocean's surface. Unfortunately, this depth shields them from satellite signal for detection, and the movement of the sea floor faults can unleash a deadly intensity in the form of earthquakes, landslides, or volcanic eruption (CDC, 2013; University of Washington, 2020). Nurses and other rescue personnel are encouraged to consider immediate, secondary, and long-term effects of tsunamis. Immediate concerns include providing clean drinking water, food, shelter, and medical care in order to stabilize injuries. Environmental hazards such as insect exposure and heat are likely as well because some victims may lose shelter. Drownings are associated with tsunamis, but traumatic injuries are a primary concern. Injuries occur when people are washed into debris of all kinds; as the water recedes, the associated strong suction can cause further injuries (CDC, 2013). Although decaying bodies create little risk of major disease outbreaks, those who handle the bodies to prepare them for burial are most at risk (CDC, 2013). The effects of a disaster are long-lasting. The affected area must be surveyed for infectious and water- or insect-transmitted diseases. Health care, financial, and material assistance are needed for months or even years after a disaster, and personnel and supplies in nonaffected areas must be diverted to affected areas. Restoring health care services, water systems, shelter or housing, and employment are critical in helping the community to recover some semblance of normalcy, and mental and social aspects of life must be considered when the crisis is resolved (CDC, 2013).

LANDSLIDES

Landslides may be caused by earthquake activity, heavy rains, and mining or construction on steep degrees of sloping land. Landslides result in the downward and outward movement of materials such as rock, soil, and debris. In March 2014, a deadly landslide occurred in Oso, Washington, that killed 43 people and destroyed the community (University of Washington, 2020). Landslides and mudflows create health hazards due to a number of conditions they cause. Rapidly moving water and debris and broken electrical, water, gas, and sewage lines can all lead to injury and illness. Roadways and railways are disrupted, and motorists cannot drive to safety or use railways to access health care (CDC, 2018b).

VOLCANOES

Volcanic eruptions occur when magma rises through cracks or weaknesses in the Earth's crust and are considered one of the most dramatic and violent natural hazards. Lava, dangerous gases, and mud destroy forests, agricultural lands, and entire communities. The most common cause of death from a volcano is suffocation. The 1980 explosion of Mount St. Helens in Washington state was one of the deadliest volcanic events in US history and led to 57 deaths. Communities that are forewarned and have sufficient time can implement mitigation measures to decrease the negative consequences of the volcanic eruption. Mitigation activities include moving away from rivers and streams that might carry mud or debris, being prepared to stay indoors, avoiding downwind areas if ashfall is expected, and moving toward higher ground by following evacuation instructions and road signs if mudflows are approaching (University of Washington, 2020). Although many mitigation measures are targeted to adults, children and other vulnerable populations must be considered in all that we do in disaster preparedness, response, and recovery.

School Building Safety

One common aspect of children around the globe is the education endeavor and the buildings where children are taught. These buildings need special consideration. Regardless of the country, state, region, or tribal nation, children are sent to school with the expectation that they will be safe from natural hazards. In many instances, however, school buildings are susceptible to severe damage or collapse from natural disasters such as earthquakes, tornadoes, hurricanes, floods, tsunamis, or windstorms. Some school structures are at risk due to poor construction or are located in tsunami hazard zones without access to safe ground within the expected warning time. After school hours, school buildings are frequently used for community events such as social and sporting events and as polling stations, but they also may be repurposed as designated shelters for displaced families after disasters or public health emergencies (Federal Emergency Management, 2017). Because of the various uses for schools, school buildings must be inspected for structural integrity and heating, ventilation, and air conditioning (HVAC) if the community is able to support the additional maintenance costs.

Nurses provide professional health care relief in all areas of the world. They must be ready to contribute to the preparedness, response, and recovery efforts in the regions in which they work. Knowledge of the communities' available assets will aid the nurse in helping citizens cope with the social, economic, and environmental effects of natural disasters. Natural disasters have a range of devastating effects on communities, depending on the severity, location, duration, and length of exposure to its citizens. As has been discussed in other chapters in this text, the nation's most vulnerable persons must be considered. Nurses can teach valuable safety and preparedness measures to help mitigate disaster effects on their populations' physical, emotional, spiritual, and mental well-being.

Actual Disaster and Public Health Emergency: The Hurricane Irma (2017) Experience in the Bahamas

The Bahamas is an archipelagic nation with a population of 393,244. It is described as a beautiful country of 700 islands, cays, and islets in the Atlantic Ocean, located north of Cuba and Hispaniola Island, northwest of the Turks and Caicos Islands, southeast of the US state of Florida, and east of the Florida Keys. The 700-island chain comprises 2000 rocks and cays spread over 100,000 square miles of ocean, and only 30 of the islands are inhabited. The capital of The Bahamas is Nassau, which is located on the island of New Providence, with a population of 274,400. Hurricanes, tropical storms, and weather systems generally traverse The Bahamas during June through November.

The Hurricane Desk and other such entities have been around in the Bahamas since the 1960s but by an Act of Parliament, February 6, 2006, The Disaster Preparedness and Response Act gave the National Emergency Management Agency (NEMA) the authority to focus on Comprehensive Disaster Management (CDM) that is coordinating preparedness, mitigation, response and recovery to natural, human-made, technological and biological hazards and disasters. The National Emergency Operations Center (NEOC) is housed at NEMA, which is located on New Providence (Nassau) and headed by a director, Captain Stephen M. Russell, formerly of the Royal Bahamas Defense Force. For many years NEMA has ensured that all inhabited Family Islands have personnel who are trained in the areas of shelter management, initial damage assessment, damage assessment and needs analysis, community emergency response training (CERT), swift water rescue, and firefighting, with the assistance of local trainers and international organizations, namely the Office of Foreign Disaster Assistance (OFDA) and the Northern Command (NC).

One of NEMA's roles is to ensure that teams are identified at each Family Island and trained in disaster response and how to be self-sufficient for 5 to 7 days until the national response team can arrive from New Providence. NEMA's primary role is to coordinate with the 14 Emergency Support Function (ESF) groups: Transportation, Communications, Public Works and Engineering, International Assistance, Planning and Information, Shelter Services, Relief Supplies and Distribution, Health and Medical Services, Search and Rescue (Urban and Maritime), Hazardous Materials (Land and Marine) and Bioterrorism, Food, Tourism, Volunteers, and Veterinarian Services and Animal Care. The functions are performed by government agencies, nongovernment agencies, and faith-based organizations and through private partnerships.

PREPAREDNESS: A FIRST (HAND) PERSON ACCOUNT

As the next senior person to the Director of NEMA, one of my many responsibilities is that of preparedness. Prior to the impact of Hurricane Irma, my team and I had mounted an aggressive preparedness program throughout The Bahamas. The month of May 2017, activities started with a national church service. NEMA staged a media blitz in which we included the majority of the agencies represented in the ESF groups and speaking engagements at schools, churches, civic groups, and community-based organizations. We distributed thousands of preparedness brochures throughout the country and went door to door in the communities affected by Hurricane Matthew in 2016, including other communities that were considered vulnerable. Due to The Bahamas being an archipelagic country, programs executed in New Providence are duplicated in the Family Islands.

The media played a significant role as they worked closely with NEMA to promote the importance of preparedness. "NEMA's Tech Squad," the students at the University of The Bahamas, formerly the College of The Bahamas, was crucial to our team as they managed social media, Facebook, WhatsApp, and Twitter.

The Bahamas was encouraged to prepare for the 2017 hurricane season because Acklins, Long Island, San Salvador, and Cat Island had been affected by Hurricane Joaquin in 2015 and New

Providence had been affected by Hurricane Matthew in 2016. As a people, we were beginning to experience the full wrath of Category 4 and greater superstorms.

Hurricane Irma affected The Bahamas from September 7 to 11, 2017. Each inhabited island has a senior manager or managers known as Island Administrators who are responsible for the administration and coordination of central government financial and administrative matters. The Administrators are also responsible for the coordination of disaster management for their districts. Local government was introduced to the Family Islands over 20 years ago to bridge the gap between central government and the community. Island Administrators were alerted as usual once the Director of Meteorology informed the Director of NEMA that Hurricane Irma was a threat to The Bahamas. Acklins, Bimini, Crooked Island, Inagua, Mayaguana, and Ragged Island were immediately contacted and a Cabinet decision was made to evacuate these islands within 2 days, as all commercial aircraft and large vessels including the Royal Bahamas Defence Force vessels were scheduled to leave The Bahamas within 3 days to secure them from the anticipated impact.

According to Arnold King's report on Hurricane Irma from the Department of Meteorology, the storm became an extremely dangerous Category 5 hurricane with winds of 175 miles per hour at 7:45 a.m. Eastern Standard Time on September 5, 2017. The eye of the hurricane passed over Little Inagua and south of Acklins during the early hours of September 8th. Hurricane Irma passed directly over Duncan Town, Ragged Island, on the afternoon of September 8th as a Category 4 storm, with winds of 150 miles per hour. Bimini sustained hurricane-force winds on September 10th.

RESPONSE

NEMA mounted a multi-island volunteer evacuation exercise, which had never occurred in the Caribbean or Atlantic. Aircrafts were dispatched to Acklins, Bimini, Crooked Island, Inagua, Mayaguana, and Ragged Island, and people were airlifted to New Providence to live with relatives and friends. However, New Providence Community Church (NPCC) was selected as a shelter for the 155 people from Acklins who had nowhere to live (Tables 8.2 and 8.3).

TABLE 8.2 ■ Population, Households, and Number of Persons Evacuated by Island Affected by Hurricane Irma, 2017

Island	Capital	Population	Males	Females	Households	Number Evacuated by NEMA
Acklins	Colonel Hill	428	227	201	134	318
Crooked Island	Colonel Hill	350	172	178	132	106
Bimini	Alice Town	1988	1063	925	751	365
Inagua	Matthew Town	969	476	493	302	487
Mayaguana	Abraham's Bay	259	129	130	96	163
Ragged Island	Duncan Town	72	44	28	26	40

NEMA, National Emergency Management Agency.

TABLE 8.3 ▪ **Number of Persons Who Were in Shelters by Island During the Passage of Hurricane Irma**

Abaco	105	The Exumas	249
Andros and the Berry Islands	591	Grand Bahama	392
Bimini	1	Inagua	1
Cat Island	103	Long Island	172
Crooked Island	36	New Providence	1024
Eleuthera	461	Rum Cay	98

It is to be noted that NEMA was informed that many persons left the islands prior to the evacuation orders. To ensure the total well-being of the evacuees at NPCC, the members of the church, hotels, and the community at large provided additional food, toys, games, and clothing.

Social workers and members of the Royal Bahamas Defense Force manned the shelter 24 hours a day. In addition, nurses and doctors as well as a psychological team were assigned to the shelter. NEMA coordinated all of these efforts. The Department of Social Services reported that 3233 persons were in emergency shelters throughout The Bahamas.

Once the "all clear" was given on September 11, 2017, NEMA organized a flyover that included the Prime Minister and selected members of his Cabinet. The following day, initial damage assessments teams were deployed to the affected areas. NEMA has a Memoranda of Understanding with the major supermarket (Super Value) and a major bottled water company (AquaPure) in The Bahamas. Aircraft were dispatched with emergency lifelines consisting of water, food, and requested medication due to contractural agreements.

RECOVERY

The Bahamas government wanted to ensure that persons who were affected by Hurricane Irma would begin rebuilding their lives quickly. The Prime Minister, who at that time was also the Minister of Finance, issued an Exigency Order (which is usually executed in the aftermath of a disaster in The Bahamas) on September 11, 2017, to last for 180 days initially. The order stipulated that persons from the affected islands of Acklins, Bimini, Crooked Island, Grand Bahama, Inagua, Long Cay, Mayaguana, Ragged Island, and South Andros could purchase locally or import items such as building materials; electrical fixtures and materials; household furniture, furnishings, and appliances; generators; and vehicles in New Providence or the United States free from duty and value-added tax (VAT).

Two retired permanent secretaries and a former director from the Ministry of Works and her team had been retained after Hurricane Matthew to ensure that building inspection and assessments were executed in a timely fashion and that the building code was enforced. These persons were also responsible for assisting NEMA with the coordination of recovery efforts in the aftermath of Hurricane Irma. One of the permanent secretaries was assigned to work with the island of Andros, and the other worked directly with the National Recovery and Reconstruction Unit (NRRU) and NEMA. The Bahamas received financial assistance as well as goods and services, including tarpaulins, blankets, water, and generators from volunteer groups, the Office of US Foreign Disaster Assistance (OFDA), international businesses, several countries, local businesses, and the community at large.

The Ministry of Works and the Department of Social Services performed door-to-door assessments at all affected islands. In the past, the Bahamian government rebuilt homes for senior citizens, disabled persons, and unemployed persons with children that were owner-occupied during the passage of hurricanes dating back to Hurricane Floyd in 1999 without cost to the homeowner. I found a senior citizen at Cupid's Cay in Eleuthera who stated that the government at that time rebuilt his home after it was destroyed by Hurricane Betsy in 1965. However, after Hurricane Irma, a decision was made by the government to give each household a one-time payment to assist homeowners whose houses had been destroyed and to give material and labor to homeowners whose homes had sustained minor damage, based upon the assessment report from the Ministry of Works and the Department of Social Services.

LESSONS LEARNED

The people of The Bahamas remember with sorrow Hurricane Dorian that devastated the Abacos and Grand Bahama in 2019, even though Hurricane Irma in 2017 is the focus of this discourse. However, many lessons have been learned and changes continue to be made such as:

1. One can never be overprepared for natural disasters.
2. Governments should issue mandatory evacuation orders rather than volunteer evacuation orders.
3. Provisions should be made so that every child over the age of 5 years can learn how to swim.
4. Mandatory first aid training should be taught in schools.
5. Each government ministry and department must allocate a percentage of its budget for disaster preparedness and response.
6. Ministries and departments must submit preparedness and response multicomplex disaster plans.
7. Families should be encouraged to prepare go-kits with special provisions for children, the elderly, and those with special needs.
8. Important documents should be kept in secure waterproof and fireproof packages.
9. Photographs of your house (inside and outside), vehicle(s) and special items, documents (passports, driver's licences), or heirlooms should be emailed to yourself for insurance purposes and to have documents readily available, such as a government-issued identification cards.
10. Cash should be secured ahead of an anticipated event.

NEMA reported directly to the Prime Minister of The Bahamas up to the onslaught of Hurricane Dorian. The Ministry of Disaster Preparedness, Management and Reconstruction headed by a minister was created on October 3, 2019, and the Disaster Reconstruction Authority, headed by a chairperson, was created on December 1, 2019. These two significant changes have been legislated in The Bahamas in recent times to assist in the execution of disaster management, response, and recovery activities.

I would be remiss if I did not mention the role that nurses have played since 1999 in the aftermath of all natural disasters that have affected The Bahamas. The majority of nurses requested to remain in their post, particularly at the Family Islands, even when nurses were deployed to the impacted areas to offer relief assistance. Those who left the islands returned shortly thereafter, and all gave the same response: "My people, my community need me; my patients are depending on me. No one knows or understands my patients like I do. They would feel as though I abandoned them. I must return." And they all returned to their assigned communities.

NEMA reported directly to the Prime Minister of The Bahamas. In the aftermath of Hurricane Dorian, the Ministry of Preparedness was created on October 3, 2019, and the Disaster Reconstruction Authority, headed by a chairperson, was created on December 1, 2019.

Case in Point

CHEMOTHERAPY PATIENT AND POTENTIAL FLOOD

The home health nurse is visiting a 59-year-old married, male client who was discharged from the hospital yesterday. The purpose of the visit today is to review the care and dressing change instructions for his new central line catheter through which he will receive chemotherapy. While driving to the home, the nurse notices the couple's close proximity to the town's main river. They have a dock at the back of their home. It has been raining off and on for the past 3 days and the forecast calls for several more days of heavy rainstorms.

QUESTIONS FOR DISCUSSION

1. What types of questions will the nurse ask this client and his wife regarding their proximity to the water?
2. What will the nurse assess regarding their preparations for emergencies?
3. What types of items should the couple keep with them at all times, especially if swift evacuation is required?
4. What will the nurse teach about foods and water if they should lose power to their home?
5. What other types of information will the nurse be sharing to prepare them for emergencies?

Points to Remember

- Natural disasters often result in human pain and suffering, injury, and loss of life.
- Social and economic disruptions occur with the physical destruction of dwellings, schools, churches, businesses, and other significant structures.
- Natural hazards may be clustered in geographical areas and be predictable or sudden in onset; all have long-term effects.
- Advanced warning systems can mitigate the devastating effects of natural disasters.
- Nurses should be familiar with the natural disasters that occur frequently in their regions and mitigation activities and be ready to participate in the preparedness, response, and recovery activities in their communities.

Test Your Knowledge

1. Which of the following are examples of meteorological natural disasters? *(Choose all that apply.)*
   a. Tornadoes
   b. Hurricanes
   c. COVID-19
   d. *Salmonella* poisoning
2. Which of the following are examples of biological natural disasters? *(Choose all that apply.)*
   a. Tornadoes
   b. Hurricanes
   c. COVID-19
   d. *Salmonella* poisoning
3. Which of the following are examples of geological natural disasters? *(Choose all that apply.)*
   a. Earthquakes
   b. Volcanoes
   c. Hurricanes
   d. Tornadoes
4. A patient suspected of having heatstroke is brought to the emergency department. Which of the following is true?
   a. Pale skin
   b. Normal core body temperature

    c. Core body temperature of at least 41°C (106 °F)

    d. Not in need of emergency care

5. A person who is diagnosed with hypothermia would likely exhibit which of the following symptoms? *(Choose all that apply.)*

    a. Shivering

    b. Exhaustion

    c. Alert and oriented

    d. Slurred speech

6. Appropriate treatment for persons diagnosed with hypothermia would include: *(Choose all that apply.)*

    a. Warm the core areas of the body

    b. Seek medical attention quickly

    c. Cardiopulmonary resuscitation

    d. Remove wet clothing

7. Nurses should be aware of the immediate health needs after disasters, such as: *(Choose all that apply.)*

    a. Clean drinking water

    b. Nutritious food

    c. Shelter

    d. Medical care for injuries

8. Nurses are in a position to teach the general public about secondary health effects of disasters. Which of the following statements are true? *(Choose all that apply.)*

    a. Decaying bodies create a substantial risk to major disease outbreaks.

    b. Those most at risk are those who handle bodies and prepare them for burial.

    c. Natural disasters will cause an increase in infectious disease outbreaks.

    d. Contaminated food and water may cause worsening illnesses that already exist in the affected region.

9. The long-term duties of public health officials and others engaging in disaster relief and recovery include: *(Choose all that apply.)*

    a. Monitoring for infectious water or disease-transmitted diseases

    b. Restoring primary health services, water systems, and housing

    c. Diverting medical supplies from nonaffected areas to meet the needs of the affected regions

    d. Assisting community members to recover mentally and socially when the crisis has subsided

10. Massive heat waves such as the European heat wave of 2019 can cause which of the following effects? *(Choose all that apply.)*

    a. An extensive number of deaths

    b. Wildfires that destroy land, homes, and vehicles

    c. Deaths and injuries among first responders, police, and firefighters

    d. An increase in the number of wild animals

References

American Red Cross. (2020). Drought preparedness. https://www.redcross.org/get-help/how-to-prepare-for-emergencies/types-of-emergencies/drought.html

Centers for Disease Control and Prevention. (2012). *Preparing for a tornado.* https://www.cdc.gov/disasters/tornadoes/prepared.html

Centers for Disease Control and Prevention. (2013). Tsunamis. https://www.cdc.gov/disasters/tsunamis/

Centers for Disease Control and Prevention. (2018a). Floods. https://www.cdc.gov/disasters/floods/index.html

Centers for Disease Control and Prevention. (n.d.). Heat related illnesses. https://www.cdc.gov/disasters/extremeheat/pdf/Heat_Related_Illness.pdf

Centers for Disease Control and Prevention. (2018b). Landslides and mudslides. https://www.cdc.gov/disasters/landslides.html

Centers for Disease Control and Prevention. (2019). Winter storms (snow and ice). https://www.cdc.gov/disasters/winter/index.html

Centers for Disease Control and Prevention. (2020a). Hurricanes and other tropical storms. https://www.cdc.gov/disasters/hurricanes/index.html

Centers for Disease Control and Prevention. (2020b). Natural disasters and severe weather: Earthquakes. https://www.cdc.gov/disasters/earthquakes/index.html

Centers for Disease Control and Prevention. (2021). Water, sanitation, & hygiene (WASH)–related emergencies & outbreaks. https://www.cdc.gov/healthywater/emergency/drinking/drinking-water-advisories/boil-water-advisory.html

Climate Action Tracker. (2019). Dec 2019 update. https://climateactiontracker.org/global/temperatures

Federal Emergency Management Agency. (2017). Safer, stronger, smarter: A guide to improving school natural hazard safety. https://www.fema.gov/media-library-data/1503660451124-33b33bb90d4a6fe-62c89e6de2b11dd78/FEMA_p1000_Aug2017_508.pdf

Glasser. R. (2019). *Special report: Preparing for the era of disasters*. Australian Strategic Policy Institute.

Insurance Information Institute. (2020). World natural catastrophes 2019. https://www.iii.org/fact-statistic/facts-statistics-global-catastrophes

Nunez. C. (2019). *Causes and effects of climate change. National Geographic*. https://www.nationalgeographic.com/environment/global-warming/global-warming-overview/.

Ready.gov. (2015). Risk assessment. https://www.ready.gov/risk-assessment

University of Washington. (2020). Natural hazards. https://hazards.uw.edu/geology/

CHAPTER 9

Preparedness and Response to Radiological Emergencies

Roberta P. Lavin, PhD, FNP-BC, FAAN ▪ Laura Mangano, MSN, RN ▪ Tener Goodwin Veenema, PhD, MPH, MS, RN, FAAN ▪ Sandy J. Cobb, MSN, FNP-C, RN, REEG

CHAPTER OUTLINE

Introduction	172	Use Of Potassium Iodide (KI)	180
Radiation Emergencies	173	Preparedness, Shelter, and Evacuation	183
Nuclear Weapons	174	Short-Term Health Concerns Of Radiation	183
Radiological Dispersal Device	175	Long-Term Health Concerns Of Radiation	184
Radiological Exposure Device	175	**Radiation Emergency Response**	**184**
Nuclear Power Plant Accidents	175	The Role Of Nurses	185
Transportation Accidents	176	**Legal Issues**	**187**
Occupational Accidents	176	**Ethical Considerations**	**187**
Sentinel Nuclear Events	176	**Conclusion**	**189**
Three Mile Island (1979)	176	**Points to Remember**	**189**
Chernobyl (1986)	178	Resources for a Radiation or Nuclear	
Fukushima Daiichi (2011)	178	Public Health Emergency of	
Radiation Exposure	**179**	International Concern	189
Instantaneous And Near-Immediate		**References**	**190**
Health Concerns Of Radiation	180		

OBJECTIVES

After reading and studying this chapter, you should be able to:

- Describe the major radiation emergencies that may occur.
- Identify the health impacts of radiation exposure and contamination.
- Understand the burden on health care systems that would result from a large-scale radiation event.
- Appreciate the role of the nurse in radiation response.

KEY TERMS

acute radiation syndrome: Also known as radiation sickness, is a condition caused by irradiation of the entire body by a substantial dose of penetrating radiation in a short window of time.

ionizing radiation: A type of energy emitted by radioactive materials, is of most concern after a nuclear event.

nuclear weapon: Create massive explosions by rapidly releasing energy through nuclear fission or fusion.

potassium iodide: (KI) may protect a person's thyroid from ionizing radiation damage by saturating the thyroid with KI, thus blocking the thyroid gland's uptake of radioiodine.

radiological dispersal device: (RDD), also known as a "dirty bomb," combines conventional explosives, such as dynamite, with radioactive material to create an explosion.

radiation emergency: A nuclear event.

radiological exposure device: (RED) exposes people to radiation without spreading radioactive material.

Introduction

Our capacity as a health care system to respond to a large-scale radiation emergency or nuclear event will depend on the preparedness and capabilities of the health care workforce. As the largest group of health care professionals in the world, nurses are expected to respond and must prepare for these emergencies to minimize harm in a nuclear-threatened world (Veenema, Burkle, & Dallas, 2019). This chapter presents an overview of radiological emergencies and discusses the importance of preparedness and response activities for nurses across the globe in order to reduce mortality and optimize population outcomes.

Much of what we know about radiation comes from medical and other legitimate uses. There are many beneficial uses of radiation, such as x-rays and medical treatment (World Health Organization [WHO], 2016a, 2016b); however, in large doses such as those emitted by nuclear disasters, this type of radiation can cause an array of short- and long-term health issues in humans (Agency for Toxic Substances and Disease Registry [ATSDR], 1999). As early as 1896, only 4 months after the first use of x-rays, adverse biomedical effects were reported (Walker & Cerveny, 1989). Radiation went from being a potentially helpful medical tool to an instrument of war with the beginning of the Manhattan Project, which led to the creation of the first nuclear weapons used in World War II against Japan. The detonation of the first nuclear bomb on Hiroshima on August 6, 1945, destroyed most of the city, killed more than 80,000 people, and set off the nuclear arms race, continuing the fear of nuclear war and terrorism (Fig. 9.1). The fear has been realized with increasing frequency.

As people have become more aware of major radiological and nuclear events, it has caused an increase in fear of the unknown in civilian populations (Berger Ziauddin & Marti, 2020). An examination of the number of nuclear accidents that have occurred since the Manhattan Project makes clear that the rate of accidents has decreased with increasing safety standards. For example, in the 1950s there were 14 publicly reported accidents, and in the 2010s the number had declined to 4 (Fig. 9.2) (The Guardian, 2016). Ionizing radiation, a type of energy emitted by radioactive materials, is of most concern after a nuclear event (U.S. Environmental Protection Agency, 2012).

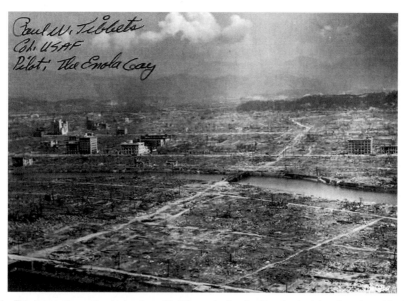

Fig. 9.1   This image shows the destruction of buildings shortly after the atomic detonation above Hiroshima, Japan, in 1945. (From U.S. Navy Public Affairs Resources. https://upload.wikimedia.org/wikipedia/commons/a/a0/Hiroshima_aftermath.jpg.)

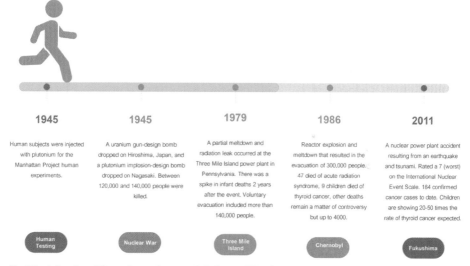

1945	1945	1979	1986	2011
Human subjects were injected with plutonium for the Manhattan Project human experiments.	A uranium gun-design bomb dropped on Hiroshima, Japan, and a plutonium implosion-design bomb dropped on Nagasaki. Between 120,000 and 140,000 people were killed.	A partial meltdown and radiation leak occurred at the Three Mile Island power plant in Pennsylvania. There was a spike in infant deaths 2 years after the event. Voluntary evacuation included more than 140,000 people.	Reactor explosion and meltdown that resulted in the evacuation of 300,000 people. 47 died of acute radiation syndrome, 9 children died of thyroid cancer, other deaths remain a matter of controversy but up to 4000.	A nuclear power plant accident resulting from an earthquake and tsunami. Rated a 7 (worst) on the International Nuclear Event Scale. 184 confirmed cancer cases to date. Children are showing 20-50 times the rate of thyroid cancer expected.
Human Testing	Nuclear War	Three Mile Island	Chernobyl	Fukushima

Fig. 9.2   A timeline of the major nuclear events in the world to date.

Radiation Emergencies

Radiation emergencies occur when large amounts of radiation are released through an accident or a deliberate attack. These events can cause immediate injury or death but may also produce delayed or long-term health effects. Nuclear disasters can place significant strain on emergency responders, health care systems, public health administrators, and government officials

(Ohtsuru et al., 2015). Disaster plans for radiation emergencies must be made at federal, state, and local levels. Health care workers must be knowledgeable of these plans in radiation emergencies in order to provide appropriate care to victims.

NUCLEAR WEAPONS

Nuclear energy, such as energy harvested within power plants, is an efficient way to produce energy. Though the management of nuclear wastes follows strict regulations set by the United States Nuclear Regulatory Commission (NRC), its use comes with many risks for our health and environment (U.S. Environmental Protection Agency, 2012). In addition, the use of nuclear energy, fueled by political power, has caused a great shift in our history of weapons in war. Fears regarding the possibility of nuclear war diminished when the Cold War ended with the signing of the Intermediate-Range Nuclear Forces Treaty (INF Treaty); however, the manufacturing of nuclear weapons has not ended (Berger Ziauddin & Marti, 2020). In fact, nuclear weapons capabilities have advanced to the point that mutually assured destruction is a possibility. Because of the proliferation of nuclear weapons and nuclear reactors, nurses must remain vigilant and prepare for large-scale humanitarian aid in the event of a radiological emergency (Berger Ziauddin & Marti, 2020).

Nuclear weapons create massive explosions by rapidly releasing energy through nuclear fission or fusion. The Manhattan Project's atomic bombs that were detonated over Hiroshima and Nagasaki, Japan, in World War II are examples of nuclear weapons (Reed, 2017). The fireball produced by a nuclear detonation expands and vaporizes everything inside it, and carries it upward to create a mushroom cloud (Radiation Emergency Medical Management, 2019). The explosion instantaneously compresses the surrounding air and increases pressure to above atmospheric pressure (overpressure), causing a blast wave that exerts tremendous force outward from the detonation site (Blast Injury Research Coordinating, 2019). The blast wave is followed by a superheated blast wind, a wave of negative pressure that pulls debris back toward the detonation site. As vaporized radioactive material in the mushroom cloud cools, it condenses into solid particles and falls back to earth, known as "fallout" (The National Academies, 2005). Damage from the initial radiation, thermal energy, and blast waves can stretch for miles and is distributed evenly around the blast site. Radioactive fallout travels in a unidirectional path determined by wind direction and extends far beyond the blast zone.

According to the National Security Staff, Interagency Policy Coordination Subcommittee for Preparedness and Response to Radiological and Nuclear Threats, 2010, nuclear weapon detonation causes significant damage to infrastructure. The blast creates a large crater at the detonation site. Blast waves and blast wind cause structural damage to buildings, automobiles, roadways, and utility lines. The intense heat generated by the explosion produces widespread fires. Fallout can travel for hundreds of miles and contaminate water and crops. The ionization of the atmosphere can generate an electromagnetic pulse that damages electronics and communications equipment.

Injuries to humans occur secondary to physical trauma or radiation exposure. Casualties are highest at the detonation site, where the potent thermal energy is 100% lethal. The intensely bright light, or thermal flash, causes temporary "flash blindness," macular retinal burns, or permanent blindness. According to Blast Injury Research Coordinating, 2019, blast injuries result from physical trauma from the explosion. Primary blast injuries result from the blast overpressure and include blast lung (pulmonary barotrauma), tympanic membrane rupture, abdominal hemorrhage and perforation, globe (eye) rupture, and mild traumatic brain injury (TBI). Secondary blast injuries are caused by flying debris, resulting in penetrating ballistic or blunt injuries, eye penetration, and open or closed TBI. Tertiary blast injuries occur when a person is thrown by blast wind, causing bone fractures, traumatic amputations, blunt and crush injuries, and open or closed TBI. Quaternary blast injuries are caused by heat, light, or exposure to toxic substances with resulting burns or breathing problems from inhalation of toxins. Quinary blast injuries include problems related to postdetonation exposure to contaminants, such as chemical burns, radiation exposure, and viral or bacterial infections.

The Centers for Disease Control and Prevention (CDC, 2018d) warns that humans closest to the blast site are immediately exposed to high levels of radiation, causing radiation sickness. Other effects from acute exposure may take weeks or years to manifest. Nuclear fallout can travel for hundreds of miles and expose people to radioactive material. External exposure occurs when skin comes into direct contact with fallout particles. Internal exposure occurs through inhaling radioactive particles, eating contaminated food, or drinking contaminated water. A study by the CDC (2014) on weapons testing fallout found that most people received their highest doses of radiation through drinking contaminated milk from cows that ingested contaminated vegetation.

RADIOLOGICAL DISPERSAL DEVICE

According to the CDC (2018e), a radiological dispersal device (RDD), also known as a "dirty bomb," combines conventional explosives, such as dynamite, with radioactive material to create an explosion. The radioactive material may be in the form of pellets or powder. RDDs do not produce atomic blasts or mushroom clouds as nuclear weapons do (Pichtel, 2011). The main danger of an RDD is injury from the explosion, as most RDDs do not release enough radiation to cause immediate illness. However, people who are very close to the blast site may be exposed to high levels of radiation, causing serious illness. After the blast, radioactive dust and smoke may disperse to areas outside the immediate blast zone. This places people at risk of inhaling radioactive dust, drinking contaminated water, and eating contaminated food (CDC, n.d.). People may not realize they have been exposed to radiation since it is odorless, colorless, and tasteless (Federal Emergency Management Agency, 2007). The size of the RDD, amount of radioactive material, method of dispersal, and weather conditions affect the extent of local radiation contamination (NRC, 2020a). The magnitude of deleterious health effects is proportional to the radiation dose. Health effects are determined by the amount of radiation absorbed, type of radiation, distance from the blast site, means of exposure, and length of exposure time.

RADIOLOGICAL EXPOSURE DEVICE

A radiological exposure device (RED) exposes people to radiation without spreading radioactive material (FEMA, 2014). An example of an RED is unshielded radioactive material placed in a container and location in which people are exposed to leaking radiation. Touching the container does not cause contamination, but close proximity to an RED for extended periods results in high levels of radiation exposure. These devices are often used to target specific individuals, and a perpetrator may plant an RED in the victim's home, office, or vehicle (Bland et al., 2018). REDs also may be hidden by terrorists in public places, such as shopping malls, or on public transportation vehicles. However, terrorists are less likely to use REDs since extended exposure time to the device is needed to cause harm. Acute symptoms of exposure include radiation sickness and radiation burns (CDC, 2018e). Other health effects occur in days or weeks and may lead to cancer or death.

NUCLEAR POWER PLANT ACCIDENTS

Nearly 20% of the United States' electricity was produced by nuclear energy in 2019 (United States Energy Information Administration, 2020). The United States has 96 of the world's 442 nuclear reactors and generates more nuclear power than any other country (World Nuclear Association, 2020). Nuclear power plants generate electricity by creating controlled nuclear reactions (Murray & Holbert, 2015). Atoms of uranium, a radioactive element, are split (nuclear fission) to produce heat. The heat creates steam, which flows through a turbine connected to an electric generator that produces electricity and disperses it through power grids.

Despite heavy regulation, nuclear power plant accidents still occur. Mukhopadhyay et al. (2016) found that accidents are caused by faulty system design, equipment failure, and human error. If the reactor core cooling system fails, the core begins to melt and release massive amounts of radiation into the air and ground. Plumes from the melted core spread fallout over vast areas and contaminate the environment. The fallout from the Chernobyl nuclear plant disaster in Ukraine in 1986 was detected in nearly all of Europe, parts of Russia (De Cort et al., 2009), and the United States (EPA, 2019a). The Chernobyl fallout permanently contaminated the area with radioactive material, and an 18-mile "exclusion zone" around the reactor is still in place today (U.S. Nuclear Regulatory Commission, 2018). External and internal exposure to radioactive materials can cause long-term health effects, including cancer.

TRANSPORTATION ACCIDENTS

Radioactive materials are transported globally via trucks, trains, planes, and ships (EPA, 2019b). The United States Department of Transportation and the U.S. Nuclear Regulatory Commission, 2003 regulate the shipping and transportation of radioactive materials. All radioactive material must be packaged in special protective containers that can withstand damage. Packaging is based on the type of radioactive material being transported and the risk of contamination if the package ruptures. Transportation accidents can put people at risk of contamination if the radioactive cargo leaks or escapes its container. Since 1971 there have been more than 500 reported transportation accidents that caused radioactive spills, fires, explosions, or gas dispersions (Pipeline and Hazardous Materials Safety Administration, 2020). Many of these incidents involved improper packaging of radioactive material. Injury or death were reported in only three incidents.

OCCUPATIONAL ACCIDENTS

Occupational exposure to radiation can occur in many settings, including nuclear power plants, medical facilities, research laboratories, mining sites, industrial plants, and radioactive materials transportation. The NRC (2020b) regulates occupational radiation dose limits. The Occupational Safety and Health Administration (2004) sets standards for occupational protection against radiation exposure. Workers may be exposed to radiation if radioactive materials are stored improperly, safety controls malfunction, or safety procedures are not followed (CDC, 2018e). Occupational accidents can expose workers to DNA-damaging alpha particles, beta particles, x-rays, and gamma rays (Fig. 9.3).

SENTINEL NUCLEAR EVENTS

Over the past century, sentinel nuclear disasters such as those that have occurred in Chernobyl, Ukraine, and Fukushima, Japan, have elicited devastating health effects for those involved directly as well as for generations following these events (Dallas, 2012). Although the chemical composition of nuclear power reactor destruction and nuclear weapon detonation is not an exact match, the effects seen in the damage zones can be quite similar (Adams et al., 2019). Three Mile Island, Chernobyl, and Fukushima Daiichi are the most well-known examples of nuclear accidents (see Fig. 9.2).

Three Mile Island (1979)

On March 28, 1979, the United States experienced its only major nuclear disaster. The water pumps at the Three Mile Island Nuclear Generating Station stopped working and combined with a series of equipment and management failures, led to a partial meltdown of the nuclear reactor (Charles River Editors, 2014). The accident quickly made clear that the local hospitals

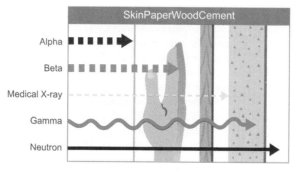

Fig. 9.3 An illustration of alpha particles, beta rays, gamma, or x-rays, and neutrons penetrating through matter. (From U. S. Nuclear Regulatory Commission. https://www.nrc.gov/reading-rm/doc-collections/nuregs/brochures/br0322/r1/br0322r1.pdf.)

and nursing homes were not prepared for a nuclear disaster and that their disaster plans were not adequate for a nuclear incident (Maxwell, 1982). Within the 5-mile evacuation zone were three nursing homes; when the evacuation zone was expanded to 20 miles, it contained 14 hospitals and 62 nursing homes (Maxwell, 1982). Planning began with an assumption that 1308 short-term care patients, 2400 nursing home patients, and 30 outpatients requiring renal dialysis would need to be evacuated (Smith & Fisher, 1981).

Because there were hospitals in the potential evacuation zone, these hospitals needed to assess measures to reduce the hospital census and prepare for an evacuation, if ordered. The first step was to discharge stable patients to their families, resulting in the freeing of 30% of the beds. Next, they cancelled all nonemergency surgeries and restricted admissions to life-threatening conditions (Maxwell, 1982). Finally, the hospitals worked with surrounding communities to take patients if the government ordered an evacuation. Ultimately, only one nursing home and three neonates were evacuated. The government did not institute an evacuation order but recommended that pregnant women and preschool children leave the 5-mile evacuation zone (Maxwell, 1982).

ACTIONS TO REDUCE HOSPITAL CENSUS DURING A NUCLEAR ACCIDENT

- Rapid discharge of emergency department (ED) ambulatory patients
- Cancellation of elective procedures and admissions
- Reduction of the routine use of ancillary services (e.g., x-rays, laboratory testing)
- Acceptance of admitted patients from the ED into "hallway" beds
- Early discharge of stable inpatients
- Expansion of critical care capacity (moving stable patients requiring ventilator support to monitored or stepdown beds)
- Conversion of private rooms to double occupancy
- Use of nonpatient care areas (e.g., lobbies, classrooms) for patient care

(From Pekarev, M., Singh, K., Lavin, R. P., Hsu, S., & Broyles, T. (2010). Hospital impact: Long-term issues. In R. Powers & E. Daily (Eds.), *International disaster nursing.* (pp. 119–138). Cambridge University Press)

Chernobyl (1986)

On April 26, 1986, the power plant in Chernobyl, Ukraine, was scheduled for experimental testing when a series of explosions in one of the nuclear reactors occurred, killing more than 30 people. It released more than 100 times the amount of radioactivity of the bombs dropped on Hiroshima and Nagasaki (Dallas, 2012). Radiation spread over what was then the Soviet Union, much of Europe, and eventually to other continents. The Chernobyl power plant explosion resulted in food, plants, animals, surfaces, water, and soil contamination. Radiation was transferred from plants to the cows that ate them, to milk and the people who drank the milk, resulting in significant thyroid disease, especially in children (International Atomic Energy Agency, Vienna Austria, 2005) (Fig. 9.4). It was critical to be able to instruct community members on what was safe to eat and drink and on cleaning procedures for food and utensils. In addition, the public in the Soviet Union and across Europe needed information about the future risk of developing cancer (Cardis et al., 2006).

FOOD SAFETY AFTER A NUCLEAR ACCIDENT

- Food in sealed containers is safest (bottles, cans, boxes, etc.).
- Food that was in the refrigerator is safe.
- Food stored in a pantry or drawer that was closed is safe.
- Bottled water, juices, or milks should be from a sealed container.
- DO NOT pick or eat food from outside until emergency management personnel declare it safe to eat.
- Water from the toilet or water heater is also safe.

CARE IN PREPARING FOOD

- Wipe containers with a damp or clean towel.
- Wipe counters and all cooking equipment.
- Take the cloth used for cleaning and put it in a sealed container or plastic bag away from people or pets.
- Tap water is safe for cleaning containers or oneself, as any contamination will be very diluted.

(From CDC, 2018b, 2018c.)

Fukushima Daiichi (2011)

On March 11, 2011, the Fukushima Daiichi Nuclear Power Plant failed in the aftermath of an earthquake and the resulting tsunami that destroyed the power supply. Because of the meltdown and explosions, ^{131}I, ^{134}Ce, and ^{137}Ce were released. In comparison to Chernobyl, which had 600 emergency workers and more than 500,000 recovery workers, Fukushima had 20,000 workers during the immediate response and the following 9 months (Shimura et al., 2015). In addition, there was a 20-kilometer (12.42-mile) evacuation zone that affected approximately 154,000 residents.

Occupational health personnel played a significant role in helping to monitor and minimize the exposure of workers. Both occupational health physicians and nurses were needed to assist with worker safety and mental health checks (Shimura et al., 2015). The occupational health personnel monitored 31,383 workers, among which 173 exceeded the 100 mSv recommended maximum levels, and found an average worker level of 12.5 mSv (Shimura et al., 2015). In addition, the workers were able to address other emergency response–related injuries of workers.

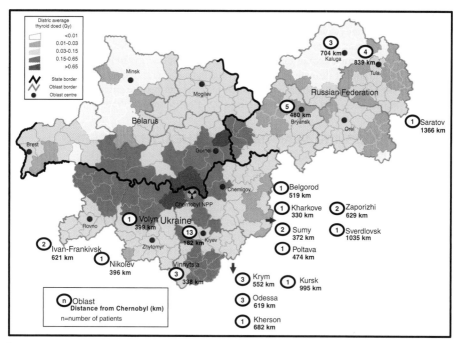

Fig. 9.4 A map depicting the prevalence of thyroid disease in Chernobyl, Ukraine, and the surrounding areas following the Chernobyl nuclear event. (From Fisher SB, Cote GJ, Bui-Griffith JH, et. al. Genetic characterization of medullary thyroid cancer in childhood survivors of the Chernobyl accident. Surgery. 2019; 165(1):58–63. doi: 10.1016/j.surg.2018.08.029. Epub 2018 Nov 2. PMID: 30392857.)

ROLE OF OCCUPATIONAL HEALTH IN NUCLEAR ACCIDENT PREPAREDNESS AND RESPONSE

- Maintaining an occupational health exposure tracking system
- Improving radiation dosimetry
- Administering iodine
- Providing occupational medicine and preventative care
- Ensuring that guidelines are in place prior to a disaster
- Ensuring that sufficient occupational health measures and systematic preparation for radiation exposure are in place
- Assisting with decontamination after the initial measurement of exposure

(From Shimura et al., 2015.)

Radiation Exposure

When people encounter radioactive materials, they are exposed to ionizing radiation, a type of energy that is given off during radioactive decay as alpha particles, beta particles, and gamma rays. Once exposed, the radioactive particles quickly begin to disrupt electrons in molecules within DNA and proteins that make up tissues of the human body (U.S. Environmental Protection Agency, 2012). Exposure to ionizing radiation, whether through contaminated clothing or ingestion of radioactive food, can lead to extreme health conditions in people of all ages. For this reason, it is important to intervene quickly and begin treatment when an individual has been exposed to prevent further damage (Coleman et al., 2009).

When a nuclear reactor combusts or a nuclear weapon is detonated, a chain reaction of combustion occurs within milliseconds in the nuclear material. The energy from the explosion is transferred to our environment through a flash of thermal radiation, and nuclear radiation is deposited into the air. The effects of a nuclear explosion on humans can be categorized as either instantaneous, near-immediate, short term, or long term (U.S. Environmental Protection Agency, 2012).

INSTANTANEOUS AND NEAR-IMMEDIATE HEALTH CONCERNS OF RADIATION

When the explosion first occurs, a blinding flash is seen instantaneously. The intense light emitted by the flash can damage cells in the retina of the human eye, causing temporary or permanent blindness (Dallas, 2012). After the flash, a large blast of thermal radiation is emitted from the center of the explosion (U.S. Department of Homeland Security, 2019). Temperatures well over several million degrees generate winds traveling thousands of kilometers an hour, propelling the scalding heat waves out from the center to the perimeter of the explosion. This envelops the core in fire and causes mass destruction to structures in the immediate area. This heat instantly vaporizes any flammable materials in its path, including human flesh, and can cause immediate death or severe injury depending on proximity. If humans are exposed to the blast or are not properly protected, there is a chance that they will suffer from burn injuries and other types of trauma involving building destruction. In addition, the electromagnetic pulse emitted from the explosion can destroy electrical power lines, causing a power outage for several miles (U.S. Department of Homeland Security, 2019).

After the blast, the explosion creates a large mushroom cloud that erupts over the top of the center. This pulls in debris from the environment (i.e., soil, building particles, concrete, dust, etc.) that will be laced with radioactive materials and displaced into the environment over the next few days. This fallout debris is known to contaminate the air people inhale, exposing the body to radiation internally. Fallout debris also contaminates skin and clothes, exposing humans to radiation externally (CDC, 2018e). Furthermore, the large fires at the explosion core will continue to burn and emit toxins into the environment as building remains collapse, contributing to the fallout debris and increasing human exposure to radiation. Furthermore, fallout debris is known to travel several miles from the center of an explosion due to strong winds, mixing radioactive materials with air in the atmosphere to be deposited later to the ground and water sources (ATSDR, 1999). Nuclear materials can interfere directly with human health; however, the radioactivity of fallout debris decreases over time due to the short half-life of ionizing radiation and other radionucleotides embedded in it (Adams et al., 2019).

USE OF POTASSIUM IODIDE (KI)

The ongoing fear of terrorist events has Americans and others concerned about the possibility of terrorists using radioactive materials in an attack. This fear led the US Congress to extend the 10-mile radius described in 10 CFR 50.47(b)(10) to 20 miles in the Public Health Security and Bioterrorism Preparedness and Response Act of 2002, Section 127, Public Law 107–188. The American Association of Clinical Endocrinology (AACE) and the American Thyroid Association support the use of potassium iodide (KI) as a protective measure for radioactive iodine exposure (AACE, 2004). As indicated in the Federal Guidelines for Requesting, Stockpiling, Distributing Potassium Iodide (KI) From the Strategic National Stockpile (SNS) (Office of Public Health Emergency Preparedness, 2005), the law requires that KI be made available through the SNS in quantities sufficient for the vulnerable population within a 20-mile radius of commercial nuclear power plants and that guidelines be developed for "stockpiling, distribution, and utilization of KI" (p. 2).

This law leads to many individual tasks, including (1) identifying the extent of the vulnerable population, (2) identifying the level of threat, (3) identifying the countermeasures, (4) identifying available distribution systems, (5) evaluating existing plans for state and federal roles and responsibilities, (6) evaluating the appropriateness of the existing KI messaging for health education, (7) proposing plan modifications to address gaps, and (8) identifying an appropriate conceptual model by which to best address the identified tasks. Addressing all of these tasks is outside the scope of this chapter. However, the key issues related to KI are discussed in order to give a broad perspective of the problem.

The WHO (2006) reported that there remains a finite risk of a nuclear power plant accident, despite the extensive safety measures that are in place. Based on its evaluation of epidemiological cancer data after the Chernobyl accident, the WHO concluded that the possibility of significant doses of radioactive iodine exposure can occur more than 100 kilometers (60 miles) from the accident site.

Within the United States, extensive measures are in place to prevent accidents. However, in a worst-case scenario, the design of nuclear power plants should be able to contain the radioiodine for several days. However, there are other sources of radioactive iodine, including nuclear weapons and dirty bombs as well as research and medical facilities.

If KI is taken within 3 to 4 hours after exposure to radioactive iodine and continued every 24 hours while exposure continues, it may protect a person's thyroid from ionizing radiation damage by saturating the thyroid with KI, thus blocking the thyroid gland's uptake of radioiodine (U.S. Department of Health and Human Services, 2001). This dosage is most effective for children and lactating women. There is no apparent effect for persons over age 40 unless they have been subjected to long periods of internal exposure (e.g., drinking contaminated milk or water or eating contaminated food) to radiation doses that may put them at risk of hypothyroidism. However, it does not protect the thyroid from direct exposure to radiation. The safety and effectiveness of the short-term use of KI was demonstrated after the Chernobyl accident, with generally mild side effects (U.S. Department of Health and Human Services, 2001).

The National Research Council found that KI is a reasonable, prudent, and inexpensive supplement to evacuation and sheltering for specific local conditions. The National Research Council (2004) reported that KI is an important protection against the health effects of exposure to radioiodine and should be available to everyone at risk. This means that KI should be available to all persons under the age of 40 within a 20-mile radius of a nuclear power facility. The National Research Council established two emergency planning zones. The first zone is within a 10-mile radius of ground zero and includes persons who did not evacuate, came in contact with the plume, and received the highest radiation exposure. Additional exposure may come from airborne particles, ground surface particles, and inhalation. In the first zone there can be sufficient exposure, within a short period, to cause acute radiation effects. The second zone is between 10 and 50 miles from ground zero. Because the primary route of exposure tends to come from contaminated food, milk, and water, the best method of protection is to avoid contaminated products. The Federal Guidelines for Requesting, Stockpiling, Distributing Potassium Iodide (KI) From the Strategic National Stockpile (SNS) (Office of Public Health Emergency Preparedness, 2005) note that public education is the most important component in the success of any KI plan. Education is especially important because the public is its own major source of protection when it comes to avoiding contamination. Radioiodine has a short half-life of 8 hours, so avoiding contamination should be a priority until there has been sufficient decay of the radioactive source. In other words, if canned food and grains are stored for several months after an accident, they should not pose a risk of contamination.

TABLE 9.1 ■ U.S. Food and Drug Administration Recommendations for the Administration of Potassium Iodide (KI)

Threshold Thyroid Radioactive Exposures and Recommended Doses of KI for Different Risk Groups				
	Predicted Thyroid Exposure (cGy)	KI Dose (mg)	Number of 130 mg Tablets	Number of 65 mg Tablets
Adults over 40 years	>500	130	1	2
Adults over 18 through 40 years	>10	–	–	–
Pregnant or lactating women	–	–	–	–
Adolescents over 12 through 18 years*	>5	–	–	–
Children over 3 through 12 years	–	65	½	1
Over 1 month through 3 years	–	32	¼	½
Birth through 1 month	–	16	⅛	¼

*Adolescents approaching adult size (>70 kg) should receive the full adult dose (130 mg).
(Modified from U.S. Department of Health and Human Services. (2001, December). *Guidance potassium iodide as a thyroid-blocking agent in radiation emergencies*. Food and Drug Administration. https://www.fda.gov/media/72510/download.)

KI is approved by the U.S. Food and Drug Administration (FDA) as a nonprescription drug for use as a blocking agent to prevent the human thyroid gland from absorbing radioactive iodine. In addition, on January 12, 2005, the FDA approved ThyroShield, a 65 mg/mL oral solution for children (ThyroShield, 2005). The current dosages (Table 9.1) are based on the FDA's evaluation of the dose exposure and cancer risk after the Chernobyl accident (U.S. Department of Health and Human Services, 2001). The WHO recommended doses different from those suggested in FDA guidelines. The FDA attempted to reduce the variation in the doses in order to simplify administration regimes.

It should be noted that KI does not offer any protection to organs other than the thyroid but is protective of the thyroid for children, young adults, and pregnant or lactating women and is relatively inexpensive. Since the Chernobyl accident in 1986 there have been extensive epidemiological studies documenting the benefit of KI in children (Moysich et al., 2002). Shakhtarin et al. (2003) supported the link between exposure to iodine 131 (^{131}I) and thyroid cancer in children and adolescents but added the factor of iodine deficiency as influencing the rate of cancer. The National Research Council (2004) did an extensive review of the evidence linking thyroid cancer to nuclear events and concluded that there is a dose-dependent link to cancer; young children are at greater risk for cancer after exposure, and the risk of thyroid cancer in exposed adults is very low.

While the benefits of KI vary with age, so too do the associated risks. There are negligible risks of side effects of KI for those younger than 40 years old. Individuals over age 40 and persons with iodine deficiencies have an increased incidence of thyroid disease (WHO, 1999). Even with minimal risks of side effects over age 40, there is very little risk of severe side effects and few contraindications (WHO, 1999). The contraindications include thyroid disease, iodine hypersensitivity, dermatitis herpetiformis, and hypocomplementemic vasculitis (WHO, 1999). Due to the minimal risk of KI prophylaxis, the major decisions become economic.

The need to take KI within 3 to 4 hours drives the distribution plans. The KI must be readily available, and recipients must know when and how to take it. The Final Rule for the Nuclear

Regulatory Commission, 2001 does not specify whether particular plans are necessary but does require a plan for a range of protective measures for workers and the public based on zones. The protective measures must include shelter, evacuation, and the use of KI. If a state confirms that it has a plan, that state can petition the NRC for funding to maintain a KI stockpile.

In the United States, public health is a state responsibility, and therefore each state that chooses to distribute KI has its own plan. Some states have chosen to have stockpiles in schools and hospitals, whereas others have chosen to give KI to each household or make the drug available for pickup at the local health department. It is evident that the success of any program depends on the mechanism and success of public education. State pickup programs were generally unsuccessful, and the National Research Council (2004) reported that the average pickup rate in the community was approximately 5%.

PREPAREDNESS, SHELTER, AND EVACUATION

For humans to increase their likelihood of survival and decrease their exposure to radioactive materials, they must plan to take appropriate shelter inside their homes or the nearest building. The CDC guidelines for a nuclear event are *Get Inside, Stay Inside, Stay Tuned* (CDC, 2020). Ideally shelters should be free of windows, underground, or in the center of a building, with several layers of opaque concrete or brick walls (U.S. Department of Homeland Security, 2019). If possible, there should be an adequate amount of prepackaged food, water, medications, and other essentials to last at least 2 days (Berger Ziauddin & Marti, 2020). If there is no basement in the home or apartment complex, an alternative is to evacuate from inadequate shelter and travel to a nearby public shelter for safety. Due to limited time between notification and the arrival of a nuclear attack, families who require public shelter should identify themselves in advance to increase their chances of survival (Yoshimura & Brandt, 2011). For this reason, it is important for families to discuss the possibilities of a nuclear attack and develop an action plan so that they can take necessary precautions for sheltering (U.S. Department of Homeland Security, 2019).

In the postexplosion period, the evacuation of sheltered populations affected by nuclear contamination can be time-consuming depending on the route and proximity to health care facilities. Some buildings may be difficult to evacuate due to destruction and may require assistance from search and rescue teams for evacuation. Prolonged evacuation can affect the dose of radiation that individuals receive due to an increase in time between initial exposure and the decontamination process of skin and clothing (Adams et al., 2019). If individuals are able to exit their shelters independently, they may feel inclined to seek immediate medical attention, contributing to a mass influx of patients to nearby hospitals. According to Coleman et al. (2009), most of the affected population will be transported to hospitals and designated treatment sites via local and regional resources or personal vehicles. For this reason, it is important for injured individuals to receive information about available safe routes and sites where they can seek treatment.

SHORT-TERM HEALTH CONCERNS OF RADIATION

Those who have been exposed to radioactive fallout will be affected in the days following exposure, but the multitude of illnesses varies with the dose and type of radiation. Thermal radiation exposure most likely will lead to cutaneous radiation syndrome, affecting the basal layer of the skin via burns, inflammation, and erythema, whereas ionizing radiation exposure can lead to acute radiation syndrome (Coleman et al., 2009).

Acute radiation syndrome, also known as "radiation sickness," is a condition caused by irradiation of the entire body by a substantial dose of penetrating radiation in a short window of time (CDC, 2018a). It manifests in three phases: prodromal, latency, and clinical manifestations (Coleman et al., 2009). In the prodromal phase, symptoms include nausea, vomiting, diarrhea, fever, and chills. These symptoms are followed by a dormant period, or latency phase, of several weeks during which the individual may appear healthy and unaffected (Coleman et al., 2009). After the latency phase, the individual's bone marrow is unable to regenerate essential components of the immune system, causing the individual to become immunocompromised. In addition, the individual may develop gastrointestinal syndrome or cardiovascular and central nervous system syndrome, both of which are irreversible and serious conditions that lead to death. Although it is rare, recovery from acute radiation syndrome is possible (CDC, 2018a).

LONG-TERM HEALTH CONCERNS OF RADIATION

According to Coleman et al. (2009), long-term epidemiological studies after the Chernobyl accident have identified a clear increase in radiation-induced cancers and organ dysfunction in the surrounding populations. Furthermore, radiation exposure has a deleterious effect on developing fetuses. According to the U.S. Environmental Protection Agency, 2012, pregnant women who are exposed to radiation have an increased chance of experiencing spontaneous abortion or having a child born with genetic defects. In addition, ionizing radiation exposure can damage reproductive cells, causing birth defects in children born years after the event (U.S. Environmental Protection Agency, 2012).

Radiation Emergency Response

To reduce the rate of mortality following a radiological event, medical response teams must be prepared to address the population's health needs. It is critical for nurses and physicians to receive special training to obtain the knowledge and skills necessary for the nuclear response (Adams et al., 2019). In population-dense cities, hospitals may be responsible for the care of thousands of victims who have experienced burns and contamination and are suffering from acute radiation sickness (Berger Ziauddin & Marti, 2020). The DHHS, in conjunction with the Department of Energy, has designated radiation emergency training sites where health care and emergency responders can gain further knowledge on the appropriate medical response in a nuclear event. Furthermore, online training modules and pocket guides have been developed for clinical staff to refer to during radiological emergencies (CDC, 2020).

It is essential for medical staff to understand the mechanism of radiation injury, organ physiology, inflammation processes, immune system function, and tissue repair mechanisms before implementing treatment and managing victims of nuclear crisis (Coleman et al., 2009). Nurses play a critical role in the assessment, triage, and treatment of individuals affected by radiological disasters. For effective treatment, nurses must recognize the signs and symptoms of various conditions after a nuclear crisis and begin the decontamination process as soon as possible (Coleman et al., 2009). Nurses are responsible for treating and decontaminating patients, but they must first protect themselves from radioactive materials via personal protective devices. Protective measures include the use of disposable gowns, gloves, masks, and a radiation meter (Fig. 9.5) before exiting the contaminated area (CDC, 2018d).

The triage of affected individuals begins with maintenance of the airway and treating major trauma. It is also important for the nurse to obtain blood samples for monitoring complete blood counts, specifically analyzing lymphocyte counts, and human leukocyte antigen (HLA) typing (CDC, 2018d). After initial triage, nurses should assess and treat major burns by following the burn protocol of their facility. An example of the flow of health care triage is shown in Fig. 9.6. Due to an insufficient number of burn care nurses required to treat large populations affected by cutaneous radiation injuries, the DHHS has implemented additional training for nurses to prepare for burn care mass-casualty events (Coleman et al., 2009).

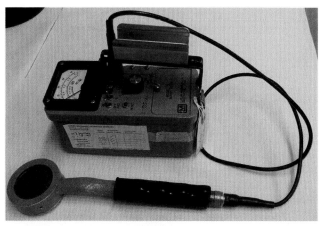

Fig. 9.5 An image of a Geiger-Mueller (GM) survey meter that can be used in emergency settings to detect small amounts of radioactive contamination. (Courtesy of Tim Vickers. http://fathersonpreppers.com/top-7-geiger-counters-how-they-work/.)

After triage, the decontamination process must occur to remove any radioactive material from the body. This process includes removal of all clothing, rinsing all skin with water, washing hair with shampoo, and treating additional surface injuries underneath clothing (WHO, 2016a, 2016b). Advancements in the decontamination process have been made. These advancements include the ability to measure the dose of radiation absorbed by the body via blood samples and removing internally deposited radionucleotides via pharmaceutical intervention (Dallas, 2012).

According to the CDC (2018a), physical injuries will account for most of the immediate health concerns in the triage process after a nuclear disaster. However, nurses also must be prepared to manage large quantities of people suffering from psychological trauma, as these events can trigger memories of previous traumatic events. According to Dallas (2012), mental health concerns were discovered to be the greatest health impact following the Chernobyl accident due to fear and the stressful conditions of both the general public and health care workers.

Nurses and physicians also need to consider the long-term effects of radiological disasters (Coleman et al., 2009). After the initial wave of acute health treatment, health care workers should anticipate large numbers of people suffering from cancer, birth defects, central nervous system abnormalities, immunosuppression, mental illnesses, and more during the recovery phase. Additional training for these types of effects is necessary for hospitals to prepare for the intense need for medical interventions and corresponding supplies in these circumstances (Dallas, 2012).

THE ROLE OF NURSES

Nurses play a critical role in the effective and timely response to any radiation emergency. They provide triage, provide clinical and palliative care, provide care to and address the unique needs of infants and children, and coordinate health systems response efforts (Veenema & Thornton, 2015). However, nurses may not possess the knowledge, skills, and abilities they need to respond during large-scale radiological emergencies (Veenema et al., 2018; Veenema, Lavin, et al., 2019). Calls to schools of nursing to extend education and to integrate training into their curricula to address radiation and nuclear disaster response have been made (Veenema et al., 2017).

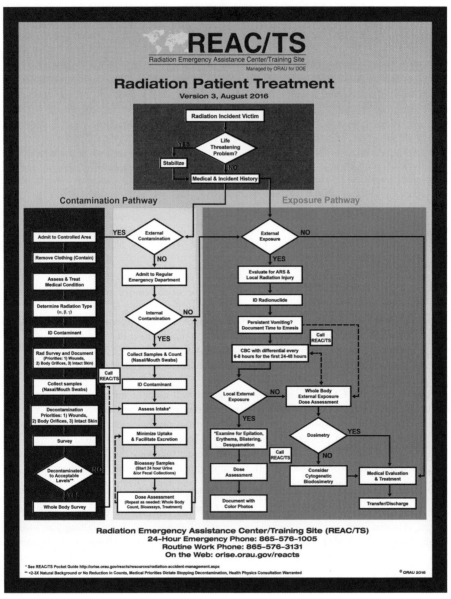

Fig. 9.6 An example of the flow of triage steps for emergency health care providers immediately after a radiological disaster.

During disaster response, the role of the nurse changes drastically from that of day-to-day bedside nurse. Proper training and preparation through nursing schools and hospitals should be implemented to ensure effective communication, strong leadership skills, and knowledge about radiological emergencies from nurses during the response (Veenema, Lavin, et al., 2019). Nurses assist in evacuating survivors to safe shelters, triaging those who have been injured or exposed to radiation, allocating resources, and filling in many other gaps to create an efficient health care environment. This also includes the administration of appropriate medications, such as 131 and assisting in the decontamination of those who have been affected by ionizing radiation in the environment (Kako et al., 2014). Furthermore, nurses may be required to address the mental health needs of those who have been affected by the disaster, which can subsequently affect their own mental health during the response efforts (Veenema, Lavin, et al., 2019). For this reason, nurses must be flexible, resilient, and strongly committed to assisting those in need during radiological emergencies (Kako et al., 2014).

Legal Issues

Nurses may confront difficult ethical and legal issues during large-scale public emergencies. They may feel conflicting obligations of caring for patients, their families, and themselves during times of crisis. A provision of the American Nurses Association (ANA, 2015) *Code of Ethics* states that nurses primarily should be committed to patient. However, another provision states that nurses must take care of themselves as they do for others. It also acknowledges the nurse's struggle to protect human rights in the face of extreme emergencies. During disasters, nurses may be worried about the liability of triaging, allocating resources, and practicing in a different setting with less supervision (Aliakbari et al., 2015). Nurses must be aware of local disaster response plans and current emergency laws covering health care workers.

There are many federal and state laws regarding disasters, emergency response, and recovery. The Public Readiness and Emergency Preparedness (PREP) Act allows the Secretary of the DHHS to issue a declaration that provides immunity to licensed health professionals involved in prescribing, distributing, and administering medical countermeasures against radiological and nuclear agents (Office of the Assistant Secretary for Preparedness and Response, 2019). Some Health Insurance Portability and Accountability Act (HIPAA) provisions may be waived if the US President declares an emergency and the DHHS Secretary declares a public health emergency (U.S. Department of Health and Human Services, 2013).

The Emergency Management Assistance Compact allows states to share assets, including volunteer health professionals, across state lines during a governor-declared emergency (Lopez et al., 2013). It was ratified by the US Congress in 1996 and has been adopted in all 50 states. Health care workers licensed in their home states are considered licensed in the receiving state while providing disaster relief. While assisting with the emergency response, visiting health care workers cannot be held liable for any act or omission made in good faith. However, these provisions apply only to health care workers who are government employees of their home states. To help fill this coverage gap, the Uniform Law Commission (ULC) drafted the Uniform Emergency Volunteer Health Practitioners Act (UEVHPA). This model legislation allows licensed health care workers from the private sector to practice across state lines during an emergency without having to seek licensure in the receiving state. The health care worker must be registered as a volunteer in a public or private registration system to be covered. Since 2007, 17 states and 2 territories have enacted the UEVHPA (ULC, 2020).

Policies on a leave of absence or work release during a disaster vary by employer. The ANA (2002) recommends that if a nurse requests a work release to help in disaster recovery, the employer should make every effort to honor the request. It is the nurse's responsibility to keep the employer up-to-date on plans for length of absence. Nurses should speak to their employers about the possibility of participating in disaster recovery at the time of employment or when emergency preparedness education or certification is obtained.

Ethical Considerations

There are always extremes in ethical considerations in nursing. At one end of the continuum is injecting human beings with plutonium, such as done in the Manhattan Project in 1945. At the other end of the continuum is determining how to allocate scarce resources. Somewhere in between is the individual decision of whether to report to work during a nuclear disaster or evacuate with family. All of these are issues that nurses should consider seriously. The most common ethical issues discussed in relation to nuclear disasters are (1) duty to care, (2) resource allocation, and (3) mandatory evacuation (Khaji et al., 2018).

Philosophers like Jeremy Bentham, John Stuart Mill, and David Hume have long pondered the big questions. How do we decide between good and bad, and how do we enhance the happiness and well-being of society and weigh it against the happiness and well-being of an individual? The early writers on utility conceptualized it as the maximization of happiness. While it might seem odd to think of nursing ethics in terms of happiness: is good health not consistent with happiness? Have you ever seen a parent who is happy when their child is denied health? Or, is it acceptable to support risk communication that is not based on evidence, such as was the case in Japan of insisting that 100 mSv radiation exposure resulted in no or insignificant increased risk of cancer (Westacott, 2020)?

When a disaster occurs, it is expected that triage will respond and assist in caring for those affected. From the ethical nursing standpoint, the nurse's main responsibility is to the health and well-being of patients and those in need of nursing care (ANA, 2017). This is known as the nurse's duty to care and considers the moral and ethical obligation of nurses. However, the ethical paradigm makes a drastic shift during a disaster; the goal of disaster response is to save as many lives as possible. For nurses, this conflicts with the ethical principles of beneficence and nonmaleficence that guide traditional nursing practices, as not all patients in emergency settings can be saved due to limited resources and time (Leider et al., 2017).

Another factor that influences the nurse's duty to care in disaster settings is the refusal to work due to perceived risks of harm associated with providing care during the disaster. Nurses spend the highest amount of time with patients and therefore are at increased risk of disease transmission in the event of a pandemic emergency or transfer of biocontaminants during patient care. The decision to care for patients during radiological events requires moral commitment and acceptance of possible environmental risks (Holt, 2008). However, the duty to provide care may conflict with one's duty to self and family or the commitment to always provide the highest quality care rather than providing triage that ultimately may lead to withdrawal of care for those with poor prognoses (Leider et al., 2017).

The allocation of a scarce resource depends on the moral evaluation of those who have control of the resource. Nurses and other health care workers in emergency response settings must be accountable for assessing patients and distributing resources as needed. These difficult decisions are based on prioritizing treatment for those who have the highest chance of survival and/or those who require palliative care measures (Holt, 2008). Unlike in traditional health care settings, the ethical principle of justice takes higher precedence over autonomous decision making of both the patient and the provider when it comes to treatment in disasters. Allocation decisions are based on the fair distribution of health care goods and services among large populations of affected people, ensuring that no one resource is depleted on one individual or subgroup of people (Satkoske et al., 2019). Similarly, utilitarianism, the philosophy that an action is deemed ethical if it produces the greatest benefit for the greatest number of people, is often used in disaster response to guide the distribution of resources. These principles shift the focus of caregivers toward saving as many individuals as the available resources will allow (Leider et al., 2017).

With the allocation of scarce resources, often a great deal of moral distress can arise. For example, moral distress may occur when the health care worker experiences inner conflict between what is ethically right and what is necessary in that circumstance to provide efficient, effective, and equitable health care (Leider et al., 2017; Satkoske et al., 2019). Caregivers also may experience the loss of trust as patients feel they are being abandoned in their most vulnerable states, which can further perpetuate their moral and psychological distress (Satkoske et al., 2019. For this reason, prior training and discussion of expected roles and altered standards of care is necessary to minimize moral distress and psychological trauma experienced by caregivers in disaster settings when following ethical protocols (Holt, 2008; Leider et al., 2017).

The mandatory evacuation of individuals who live in the affected area of a disaster has posed many ethical concerns in the past. Requiring residents to leave their homes violates their privacy, freedom, and rights. However, evacuation is critical to ensure safety, medical treatment, and the distribution of necessary resources such as food, water, and medications (Khaji et al., 2018). Once evacuated, the affected populations can be taken to hospitals to receive care or to shelters where they can remain safe (Holt, 2008). Although requiring evacuation is among one of the most difficult ethical decisions for disaster response teams to make, it is important to ensure the safety of all who have been affected by the event.

Conclusion

Despite international treaties and regulations set for nuclear energy use, the possibility of a major radiological emergency occurring in the United States has not been completely eradicated (Berger Ziauddin & Marti, 2020; U.S. Environmental Protection Agency, 2012), and the global threat remains ubiquitous. After Chernobyl, Alvin Weinberg was reported to say "A nuclear accident anywhere is a nuclear accident everywhere," and nurses must be prepared. Medical response teams need to prepare for such events to decrease mortality based on our current knowledge. For the public, it is critical for families to ensure access to adequate shelter and resources for the immediate impact and to develop a safe evacuation route for necessary medical treatment (Berger Ziauddin & Marti, 2020; Yoshimura & Brandt, 2011). In addition, it is important to know the potential health hazards after exposure to nuclear fallout and act accordingly to mitigate risks. For health care workers, proper training for nuclear events is essential for the care of cutaneous radiation injury and acute radiation syndrome in large populations (Coleman et al., 2009). Nurses are at the forefront of response and must follow efficient treatment protocols and acquire training before radiological emergencies. For this reason, there are available training courses, via emergency training centers or online modules, that can provide adequate knowledge and skills for medical staff (CDC, 2018e). In conclusion, with proper preparation and response, it is possible to decrease the rate of mortality following a radiological emergency.

Points to Remember

1. Radiation emergencies occur when large amounts of radiation are released through an accident or a deliberate attack.
2. Following a radiation event, nurses conduct triage, provide clinical and palliative care, and coordinate health systems response efforts.
3. Nurses must be aware of local disaster response plans and current emergency laws covering health care workers.
4. The most common ethical issues discussed in relation to nuclear disasters are (1) duty to care, (2) resource allocation, and (3) shelter-in-place and mandatory evacuation.

RESOURCES FOR A RADIATION OR NUCLEAR PUBLIC HEALTH EMERGENCY OF INTERNATIONAL CONCERN

Centers for Disease Control and Prevention (CDC), Clinician Outreach and Communication Activity (COCA)
https://emergency.cdc.gov/coca/index.asp

Centers for Disease Control and Prevention (CDC), Emergency Preparedness and Response/ Radiation Emergencies
https://www.cdc.gov/nceh/radiation/emergencies/clinicians.htm

Centers for Disease Control and Prevention (CDC), Environmental Health Training in Emergency Response (EHTER)
https://www.cdc.gov/nceh/ehs/elearn/ehter.htm

Centers for Disease Control and Prevention (CDC), Health Information for Disaster Relief Volunteers
https://www.cdc.gov/disasters/volunteers.html

Radiation Emergency Assistance Center/Training Site (REAC/TS)
https://orise.orau.gov/reacts/

Radiation Injury Treatment Network
https://ritn.net/

The Guardian. (2016). *Nuclear power plant accidents: listed and ranked since 1952.*
https://www.theguardian.com/news/datablog/2011/mar/14/nuclear-power-plant-accidents-list-rank

US Department of Health and Human Services (DHHS), Radiation Emergency Medical Management (REMM)
https://remm.hhs.gov/index.html

US Nuclear Regulatory Commission (NRC), Emergency Preparedness in Response to Terrorism
https://www.nrc.gov/about-nrc/emerg-preparedness/respond-to-emerg/response-terrorism.html

References

Adams, T. G., Yeddanapudi, N., Clay, M., Asher, J., Appler, J., & Casagrande, R. (2019). Modeling cutaneous radiation injury from fallout. *Disaster Medicine and Public Health Preparedness*, *13*(3), 463–469. https://doi.org/10.1017/dmp.2018.74.

Agency for Toxic Substances and Disease Registry. (1999, September). *Public health statement: Ionizing radiation.* https://www.atsdr.cdc.gov/ToxProfiles/tp149-c1-b.pdf

Aliakbari, F., Hammad, K., Bahrami, M., & Aein, F. (2015). Ethical and legal challenges associated with disaster nursing. *Nursing Ethics*, *22*(4), 493–503. https://doi.org/10.1177/0969733014534877.

American Association of Clinical Endocrinology. (2004). http://www.aace.com/members/leg/ki.php

American Nurses Association. (2002, June). https://www.nursingworld.org/~4af83e/globalassets/practiceand-policy/work-environment/health--safety/wrkrel.pdf

American Nurses Association. (2015, January). *Code of ethics for nurses with interpretive statements.* https://www.nursingworld.org/practice-policy/nursing-excellence/ethics/code-of-ethics-for-nurses/

American Nurses Association. (2017). *Who will be there? Ethics, the law, and a nurse's duty to respond in a disaster 2017.* https://www.nursingworld.org/~4af058/globalassets/docs/ana/ethics/who-will-be-there_disaster-preparedness_2017.pdf

Berger Ziauddin, S., & Marti, S. (2020). Life after the bomb: Nuclear fear, science, and security politics in Switzerland in the 1980s. *Cold War History*, *20*(1), 95–113. https://doi.org/10.1080/14682745.2018.1536121.

Bland, J., Potter, C., & Homann, S. (2018). *Radiological exposure devices (RED) technical basis for threat profile.* Sandia National Laboratories. https://prod-ng.sandia.gov/techlib-noauth/access-control.cgi/2018/186003.pdf.

Blast Injury Research Coordinating, Office. (2019, June). https://blastinjuryresearch.amedd.army.mil/index.cfm/blast_injury_101/science_of_blast

Cardis, E., Krewski, D., Boniol, M., Drozdovitch, V., Darby, S. C., Gilbert, E. S., … Boyle, P. (2006). Estimates of the cancer burden in Europe from radioactive fallout from the Chernobyl accident. *International Journal of Cancer*, *119*(6), 1224–1235. https://doi.org/10.1002/ijc.22037.

Centers for Disease Control and Prevention. (n.d.). *Dirty bomb or radiological dispersal device.* https://www.cdc.gov/nceh/radiation/emergencies/pdf/infographic_radiological_dispersal_device.pdf

Centers for Disease Control and Prevention. (2014). https://www.cdc.gov/nceh/radiation/fallout/rf-gwt_home.htm

Centers for Disease Control and Prevention. (2018a, April 4). *Acute radiation syndrome: A fact sheet for clinicians.* https://www.cdc.gov/nceh/radiation/emergencies/arsphysicianfactsheet.htm

Centers for Disease Control and Prevention. (2018b, April 4). *Drinking water safety.* https://www.cdc.gov/nceh/radiation/emergencies/watersafety.htm

Centers for Disease Control and Prevention. (2018c, April 4). *Food safety.* https://www.cdc.gov/nceh/radiation/emergencies/foodsafety.htm

Centers for Disease Control and Prevention. (2018d, April 4). *Frequently asked questions about a nuclear blast.* https://www.cdc.gov/nceh/radiation/emergencies/nuclearfaq.htm

Centers for Disease Control and Prevention. (2018e, April 4). *More information on types of radiation emergencies.* https://www.cdc.gov/nceh/radiation/emergencies/moretypes.htm

Centers for Disease Control and Prevention. (2020, March). https://www.cdc.gov/nceh/radiation/emergencies/stayinside.htm

Charles Rivers Editors. (2014). *Chernobyl and Three Mile Island: The history and legacy of the world's most notorious nuclear accidents.* CreateSpace Independent Publishing Platform.

Coleman, C. N., Hrdina, C., Bader, J. L., Norwood, A., Hayhurst, R., Forsha, J., … Knebel, A. (2009). Medical response to a radiologic/nuclear event: Integrated plan from the Office of the Assistant Secretary for Preparedness and Response, Department of Health and Human Services. *Annals of Emergency Medicine, 53*(2), 213–222. https://doi.org/10.1016/j.annemergmed.2007.12.021.

Dallas, C. E. (2012). Medical lessons learned from Chernobyl relative to nuclear detonations and failed nuclear reactors. *Disaster Medicine and Public Health Preparedness, 6*(4), 330–334. https://doi.org/10.1001/dmp.2012.72.

De Cort, M., Dubois, G., Fridman, S. D., Germenchuk, M. G., Izrael, Y. A., Janssens, A., & Avdyushin, S. I. (2009, July). https://op.europa.eu/en/publication-detail/-/publication/110b15f7-4df8-49a0-856f-be8f681ae9fd

Federal Emergency Management Agency. (2007, June). *Fact sheet: Dirty bomb.* U.S. Department of Homeland Security. https://www.fema.gov/media-library-data/20130726-1621-20490-3999/dirtybombfactsheet_final.pdf.

Federal Emergency Management Agency. (2014). *WMD definitions for use in the DHS/FEMA course materials developed by CTOS.* U.S. Department of Homeland Security. http://www.ctosnnsa.org/docs/CTOS_WMD_Definitions.pdf.

Final Rule for the Nuclear Regulatory Commission. (2001, January). *Federal Register, 66*(13). (to be codified at 10 C.F.R. pt. 50). https://www.govinfo.gov/content/pkg/FR-2016-07-29/pdf/2016-17766.pdf

Holt, G. R. (2008). Making difficult ethical decisions in patient care during natural disasters and other mass casualty events. *Otolaryngology-Head and Neck Surgery, 139*(2), 181–186. https://doi.org/10.1016/j.otohns.2008.04.027.

International Atomic Energy Agency, Vienna Austria. (2005). *Environmental consequences of the Chernobyl accident and their remediation: Twenty years of experience. Report of the UN Chernobyl Forum Expert Group "Environment"(EGE) Working material (INIS-XA–793).* International Atomic Energy Agency (IAEA).

Kako, M., Ranse, J., Yamamoto, A., & Arbon, P. (2014). What was the role of nurses during the 2011 great east earthquake of Japan? An integrative review of the Japanese literature. *Prehospital and Disaster Medicine, 29*(3), 275–279. https://doi.org/10.1017/S1049023X14000405.

Khaji, A., Larijani, B., Ghodsi, S. M., Mohagheghi, M. A., Khankeh, H. R., Saadat, S., … Khorasani-Zavareh, D. (2018). Ethical issues in technological disaster: A systematic review of literature. *Archives of Bone and Joint Surgery, 6*(4), 269–276.

Leider, J. P., DeBruin, D., Reynolds, N., Koch, A., & Seaberg, J. (2017). Ethical guidance for disaster response, specifically around crisis standards of care: A systematic review. *American Journal of Public Health, 107*(9), e1–e9. https://doi.org/10.2105/AJPH.2017.303882.

Lopez, W., Kershner, S. P., & Penn, M. S. (2013). EMAC volunteers: Liability and workers' compensation. *Biosecurity and Bioterrorism: Biodefense Strategy, Practice, and Science, 11*(3), 217–225. https://doi.org/10.1089/bsp.2013.0040.

Maxwell, C. (1982). Hospital organizational response to the nuclear accident at Three Mile Island: Implications for future-oriented disaster planning. *American Journal of Public Health, 72*(3), 275–279. https://doi.org/10.2105/AJPH.72.3.275.

Moysich, K. B., Menezes, R. J., & Michalek, A. M. (2002). Chernobyl-related ionizing radiation exposure and cancer risk: An epidemiological review. *The Lancet Oncology, 3*(5), 269–279. https://doi.org/10.1016/S1470-2045(02)00727-1.

Mukhopadhyay, S., Halligan, J., & Hastak, M. (2016). Assessment of major causes: Nuclear power plant disasters since 1950. *International Journal of Disaster Resilience in the Built Environment, 7*(5), 521–543. https://doi.org/10.1108/IJDRBE-11-2015-0056.

Murray, R., & Holbert, K. (2015). *Nuclear energy: An introduction to the concepts, systems, and applications of nuclear processes* (7th ed.). Elsevier/Butterworth-Heinemann.

National Research Council. (2004). *Distribution and administration of potassium iodide in the event of a nuclear incident.* The National Academies Press.

National Security Staff, Interagency Policy Coordination Subcommittee for Preparedness and Response to Radiological and Nuclear Threats (2010). *Planning guidance for response to a nuclear detonation.* Federal Emergency Management Agency. https://asprtracie.hhs.gov/technical-resources/resource/1432/planning-guidance-for-response-to-a-nuclear-detonation-second-edition.

Occupational Safety and Health Administration. (2004). *Ionizing radiation control and prevention.* https://www.osha.gov/SLTC/radiationionizing/prevention.html

Office of Public Health Emergency Preparedness. (2005, August 29). *Federal guidelines for requesting, stockpiling, distributing potassium iodide (KI) from the Strategic National Stockpile (SNS).* U.S. Department of Health and Human Services. https://www.federalregister.gov/documents/2005/08/29/05-17223/federal-guidelines-for-requesting-stockpiling-distributing-potassium-iodide-ki-from-the-strategic.

Office of the Assistant Secretary for Preparedness and Response. (2019). *PREP Act Q&As.* U.S. Department of Health and Human Services. https://www.phe.gov/Preparedness/legal/prepact/Pages/prepqa.aspx.

Ohtsuru, A., Tanigawa, K., Kumagai, A., Niwa, O., Takamura, N., Midorikawa, S., … Clarke, M. (2015). Nuclear disasters and health: Lessons learned, challenges, and proposals. *The Lancet, 386*, 489–497. https://doi.org/10.1016/S0140-6736(15)60994-1.

Pekarev, M., Singh, K., Lavin, R. P., Hsu, S., & Broyles, T. (2010). Hospital impact: Long-term issues. In R. Powers & E. Daily (Eds.), *International Disaster Nursing* (pp. 119–138). Cambridge University Press.

Pichtel, J. (2011). *Terrorism and WMDs: Awareness and response.* CRC Press.

Pipeline and Hazardous Materials Safety Administration. (2020). *HAZMAT incident report search tool.* https://portal.phmsa.dot.gov/analytics/saw.dll?Portalpages

Radiation Emergency Medical Management. (2019, November). *Nuclear detonation: Weapons, improvised nuclear devices.* U.S. Department of Health and Human Services. https://www.remm.nlm.gov/nuclearexplosion.htm#fireball.

Reed, B. C. (2017). *The Manhattan Project: A very brief introduction to the physics of nuclear weapons.* Morgan & Claypool Publishers. https://doi.org/10.1088/978-1-6817-4605-0.

Satkoske, V. B., Kappel, D. A., & DeVita, M. A. (2019). Disaster ethics: Shifting priorities in an unstable and dangerous environment. *Critical Care Clinics, 35*(4), 717–725.

Shakhtarin, V. V., Tsyb, A. F., Stepanenko, V. F., Orlov, M. Y., Kopecky, K. J., & Davis, S. (2003). Iodine deficiency, radiation dose, and the risk of thyroid cancer among children and adolescents in the Bryansk region of Russia following the Chernobyl power station accident. *International Journal of Epidemiology, 32*, 584–591. https://doi.org/10.1093/ije/dyg205.

Shimura, T., Yamaguchi, I., Terada, H., Okuda, K., Svendsen, E. R., & Kunugita, N. (2015). Radiation occupational health interventions offered to radiation workers in response to the complex catastrophic disaster at the Fukushima Daiichi Nuclear Power Plant. *Journal of Radiation Research, 56*(3), 413–421. https://doi.org/10.1093/jrr/rru110.

Smith, J. S., & Fisher, J. H. (1981). Three Mile Island: The silent disaster. *JAMA, 245*(16), 1656–1659. https://doi.org/10.1001/jama.1981.03310410034023.

The Guardian. (2016). *Nuclear weapons and accidents waiting to happen.* https://www.theguardian.com/world/2013/sep/14/nuclear-weapons-accident-waiting-to-happen

The National Academies. (2005). *Nuclear attack.* U.S. Department of Homeland Security. https://www.dhs.gov/xlibrary/assets/prep_nuclear_fact_sheet.pdf.

ThyroShield. (2005). ThyroShield. http://www.thyroid.org/professionals/publications/documents/ThyroShieldinsert.pdf

Uniform Law Commission. (2020). *Emergency Volunteer Health Practitioners Act.* https://www.uniformlaws.org/committees/community-home?CommunityKey=565933ce-965f-4d3c-9c90-b00246f30f2d

U.S. Department of Health and Human Services (2001, December). *Guidance potassium iodide as a thyroid-blocking agent in radiation emergencies.* U.S. Food and Drug Administration. https://www.fda.gov/media/72510/download.

U.S. Department of Health and Human Services. (2013). https://www.hhs.gov/hipaa/for-professionals/faq/1068/is-hipaa-suspended-during-a-national-or-public-health-emergency/index.html

U.S. Department of Homeland Security. (2019, September). https://www.ready.gov/nuclear-explosion

U.S. Energy Information Administration. (2020). https://www.eia.gov/tools/faqs/faq.php?id=427&t=3

U.S. Environmental Protection Agency. (2012, April). *Radiation: Facts, risks, and realities.* https://www.epa.gov/sites/production/files/2015-05/documents/402-k-10-008.pdf

U.S. Environmental Protection Agency. (2019a). *Historical radiological event monitoring.* https://www.epa.gov/radnet/historical-radiological-event-monitoring

U.S. Environmental Protection Agency. (2019b). *Transportation of radioactive material.* https://www.epa.gov/radtown/transportation-radioactive-material

U.S. Nuclear Regulatory Commission. (2003). https://www.remm.nlm.gov/NRC_for-educators_11.pdf

U.S. Nuclear Regulatory Commission. (2018, August). *Backgrounder on Chernobyl nuclear power plant accident.* https://www.nrc.gov/docs/ML0511/ML051160016.pdf

U.S. Nuclear Regulatory Commission. (2020a, February). *Backgrounder on dirty bombs.* https://www.nrc.gov/docs/ML1814/ML18143B254.pdf

U.S. Nuclear Regulatory Commission. (2020b, February 21). *Part 20—Standards for protection against radiation.* https://www.nrc.gov/reading-rm/doc-collections/cfr/part020/full-text.html#part020-1201

Veenema, T. G., Burkle, F. M., Jr., & Dallas, C. E. (2019). The nursing profession: A critical component of the growing need for a nuclear global health workforce. *Conflict and Health, 13*(9), e1–e8. https://doi.org/10.1186/s13031-019-0197-x.

Veenema, T. G., Lavin, R. P., Bender, A., Thornton, C. P., & Schneider-Firestone, S. (2018). National nurse readiness for radiation emergencies and nuclear events: A systematic review of the literature. *Nursing Outlook, 67*(1), 54–88. https://doi.org/10.1016/j.outlook.2018.10.005.

Veenema, T. G., Lavin, R. P., Griffin, A., Gable, A. R., Couig, M. P., & Dobalian, A. (2017). Call to action: The case for advancing disaster nursing education in the United States. *Journal of Nursing Scholarship, 49*(6), 688–696. https://doi.org/10.1111/jnu.12338.

Veenema, T. G., Lavin, R. P., Schneider-Firestone, S., Couig, M. P., Langan, J. C., Qureshi, K., … Sasnett, L. (2019). National assessment of nursing schools and nurse educators readiness for radiation emergencies and nuclear events. *Disaster Medicine and Public Health Preparedness, 13*(5–6), 936–945. https://doi.org/10.1017/dmp.2019.17.

Veenema, T. G., & Thornton, C. P. (2015). Understanding nursing's role in health systems response to large scale radiologic disasters. *Journal of Radiology Nursing, 34*(2), 63–72. https://doi.org/10.1016/j.jradnu.2014.11.005.

Walker, R. I., & Cerveny, T. J. (Eds.). (1989). *Textbook of military medicine: Part I—Warfare, weaponry, and the casualty: Vol 1—Medical consequences of nuclear warfare.* Office of the Surgeon General.

Westacott. E. (2020, February). *Three basic principles of utilitarianism, briefly explained.* ThoughtCo. http://thoughtco.com/basic-principles-of-utilitarianism-3862064.

World Health Organization. (1999). *Guidelines for Iodine Prophylaxis following Nuclear Accidents.* https://www.who.int/ionizing_radiation/pub_meet/Iodine_Prophylaxis_guide.pdf

World Health Organization. (2006). *Health effects of the Chernobyl accident: An overview.* https://www.who.int/ionizing_radiation/chernobyl/backgrounder/en/

World Health Organization. (2016a, April). *1986–2016: Chernobyl at 30: An update.* https://www.who.int/ionizing_radiation/chernobyl/Chernobyl-update.pdf?ua=1&ua=1

World Health Organization. (2016b, April). *Ionizing radiation, health effects, and protective measures.* https://www.who.int/news-room/fact-sheets/detail/ionizing-radiation-health-effects-and-protective-measures

World Nuclear Association. (2020, February). *Nuclear power in the world today.* https://www.world-nuclear.org/information-library/current-and-future-generation/nuclear-power-in-the-world-today.aspx

Yoshimura, A. S., & Brandt, L. D. (2011). *Analysis of sheltering and evacuation strategies for a national capital region nuclear detonation scenario.* Sandia National Libraries. https://doi.org/10.2172/1031881.

Chemical Disasters

Karen Hammad, RN, PhD

CHAPTER OUTLINE

Introduction 195

Chemicals That Cause Disasters 195

Bhopal Disaster 198

Tokyo Subway Attacks 199

Preparedness 199

Risk Assessment 199

Plans 200

Health Care Facility and Staff Readiness 200

Response 200

Indicators of a Chemical Release 201

Personal Protective Equipment (PPE) 202

Decontamination 203

Life-Saving Treatment and Triage 204

Identifying the Chemical 205

Medical Management 205

Psychological Impacts 206

Recovery 206

Legal Considerations 207

Ethical Considerations 207

Special Considerations 208

Points to Remember 208

Test Your Knowledge 209

References 210

OBJECTIVES

After reading and studying this chapter, you should be able to:

- Classify the main groups of chemical compounds and broadly describe their effects on humans.
- Provide examples of past chemical disasters and discuss their effects on the local community.
- Discuss the roles, responsibilities, and key considerations for nurses across different phases of the disaster cycle in relation to chemical disasters.
- List indicators that a chemical disaster has occurred.
- Identify the type of agent responsible for an exposure.
- Discuss the principles of responding to a chemical disaster, including decontamination, triage, and medical management.

KEY TERMS

antidote: A medication that counteracts the effects of a chemical agent.

chemical disaster: An incident in which existing resources are overwhelmed due to the release of toxic chemicals that are hazardous to public health and the environment.

chemical weapon: Toxic chemicals used to cause intentional death or harm, including munitions, devices, and other equipment specifically designed to weaponize toxic chemicals.

decontamination: The removal or inactivation of a chemical compound and its toxic abilities.

deliberate release: Occurs when chemical agents are intentionally released with the aim to cause harm.

off-gassing: Secondary chemical exposure from the clothing and bodies of people exposed to chemicals, particularly among first responders and health professionals treating casualties without wearing appropriate protection.

Introduction

A chemical disaster is an incident in which existing resources are overwhelmed due to the release of one or more toxic chemicals that are hazardous to public health and the environment. The release of hazardous chemicals can be accidental or deliberate. An accidental release might occur when critical infrastructure such as chemical installations, pipelines, storage sites, transportation links, waste sites, and mines are damaged or weakened due to human error, equipment or technological malfunction, transportation incidents, or a natural disaster such as an earthquake or flooding. A deliberate release occurs when chemical agents are intentionally released with the aim to cause harm (World Health Organization [WHO], 2020). Perpetrators might be terrorists or military organizations.

Although there are many examples of chemical incidents, full-blown chemical disasters are relatively infrequent compared to other types of disasters. Despite this, the potential for chemical disasters remains high because chemical compounds are a mainstay of modern society. Chemicals are manufactured, stored, and transported across the globe and are used domestically around the home for cleaning, in agricultural ventures as pesticides and fertilizers, and in industrial manufacturing. Chemical disasters can have devastating long-term and wide-reaching consequences for individuals, communities, and health systems. Nurses, particularly those working in frontline roles, should know what chemical hazards exist in their region as well as how to identify and respond to a chemical release in a safe and effective manner. This level of readiness can mitigate the harsh consequences of a chemical disaster on themselves, their colleagues, the individuals directly affected by the event, the wider community, and the health care facility.

This chapter discusses different types of chemicals, the effect they have on humans, and the role of nurses across the disaster spectrum from preparedness through to response and recovery. The focus of this chapter is predominately the roles and responsibilities of nurses working in health care facilities. Two cases—the Bhopal disaster in India in 1985 and the Tokyo subway attacks in Japan in 1995—are woven throughout the chapter to illustrate the real-life consequences of chemical disasters. Useful lessons can be learned from both events, particularly in regards to preparedness. Bhopal is often referred to as one of the world's worst chemical disasters and despite significant conjecture over the exact cause, it is largely agreed that the Bhopal disaster was accidental. By contrast, the Tokyo subway attacks were a well-publicized, well-documented deliberately caused event.

Chemicals That Cause Disasters

A large array of chemicals can cause disasters. A chemical weapon is a toxic chemical used to cause intentional harm or death. These weapons include "munitions, devices and other equipment specifically designed to weaponise toxic chemicals" (Organisation for the Prohibition of Chemical Weapons [OPCW], 2020, p. 1). Table 10.1 lists a sample of common groups of

TABLE 10.1 ■ Chemical Agents, Characteristics, Symptoms, and Treatment

Classification and Examples	Characteristics	Mode of Transmission and Symptoms	Treatment
Lung irritants (choking or pulmonary agents) Ammonia, bromine, chlorine, hydrogen chloride, phosgene, phosphine	Colorless; chlorine is a greenish-white gas or clear amber liquid	Inhalation Coughing; chest constriction; wheezing; respiratory distress; burning of eyes, nose, and throat; blurred vision; skin irritation; chemical burns; decreased cardiac output; blistering; vomiting Asymptomatic for 20 min After 24 h, fluid leakage into lungs followed by tight chest, shortness of breath, dyspnea, pulmonary edema	N-acetylcysteine (NAC) for chlorine or phosgene exposure Supportive therapies of humidified oxygen bronchodilators, inhalatory sodium bicarbonate, corticosteroids, mechanical ventilation, suction, fluid replacement, diuretics; heparin, antibiotics, extracorporeal membrane oxygenation (ECMO) for acute respiratory distress syndrome (ARDS)
Nerve agents (organophosphorus chemical compounds) G agents: sarin, soman, tabun; V agents (VX)	Odorless, colorless, or yellow-brown liquids	G agents: inhalation VX: penetration of skin Rhinorrhea, pinpoint pupils, miosis, blurred vision, hypersecretions, bronchoconstriction, respiratory distress, increased sweating, muscular fasciculation, nausea, vomiting, diarrhea, generalized weakness, rapid loss of consciousness, convulsions, flaccid muscle paralysis, respiratory and circulatory failure Can be fatal within several minutes	Anticholinergic drugs such as atropine Oximes such as pralidoxime (2-PAM) Benzodiazepines such as diazepam Supportive therapies such as airway management, suctioning, tropicamide 0.5% ophthalmic solution or atropine eye drops for eye pain
Blister agents (vesicants) Lewisite, mustards, phosgene oxime	Oily, colorless, may have mustard or garlic odor; Lewisite has an odor like geraniums	Inhalation or direct contact with skin, eyes Pain and blistering to skin, eyes, and respiratory tract; intense eye pain; swelling; lacrimation; photophobia; corneal edema, perforation; blindness; skin erythema, blistering, itching Inhalation: burning nasal pain, epistaxis, sinus pain, laryngitis, loss of taste and smell, cough, wheezing, dyspnea, airway obstruction Ingestion: burns to gastrointestinal (GI) tract, nausea, vomiting; abdominal pain Systemic: insomnia, tremors, convulsions, bone marrow suppression, fatal complicating infection, hemorrhage, anemia	Antidote for Lewisite is dimercaprol (British anti-lewisite [BAL]) Supportive therapies such as NAC, inhaled bronchodilators, corticosteroids, local emollients, systemic antihistamines, topical corticosteroids, topical antibiotics and steroids for ocular exposures Replacement of fluids, electrolytes in hypovolemic shock after severe exposure Some burns may need surgical treatment

Classification and Examples	Characteristics	Mode of Transmission and Symptoms	Treatment
Blood agents (cyanogenic or systemic agents) Arsine, carbon monoxide, cyanide	Bitter almond smell	Inhalation or skin absorption Affects central nervous system, heart; headache; nausea, vomiting; anxiety; confusion; drowsiness; tachycardia; hypertension; dyspnea; tachypnea; faint pale-red hue to skin Death occurs within minutes	Antidotes for cyanide include amyl nitrite perles, sodium thiosulphate, sodium nitrate, hydroxocobalamin Aggressive oxygenation, airway management Acidosis treated with sodium bicarbonate Seizures treated with benzodiazepines Hypotension treated with vasopressors Supportive care for arsine exposure includes blood transfusions, renal dialysis
Incapacitating agents (psychomimetic agents) Opioids (fentanyl, etorphine), lysergic acid diethylamide (LSD), marijuana derivative, glycolate anticholinergics, 3-quinuclidinyl benzilate (BZ)	Fentanyl released as fine particles, aerosol; can contaminate water, food, agricultural products	Inhalation; ingestion through skin, eyes, intravenous (IV), intramuscular (IM), transdermal Restlessness, dizziness, failure to obey orders, confusion, erratic behavior, stumbling or staggering, vomiting, dryness of mouth, tachycardia at rest, elevated temperature, blurred vision, pupillary dilation, slurred speech, hallucinations, disrobing, altered conscious state, inappropriate smiling or laughing, irrational fear, distractibility, perceptual distortions, pinpoint pupils, depressed breathing	Opioid intoxication: naloxone (Narcan) Treatment depends on substance ingested
Riot control agents (RCAs) (lacrimators or tear gas) Chlorobenzylidene malononitrile (CS), chloroacetophenone (CN), dibenzoxazepine (CR), chloropicrin (PS), oleoresin capsicum (pepper spray)	Liquids or solids (powder). Low toxicity, rapid onset, short duration of action	Aerosolized or dispersed via a spraying solution Eye pain or burning, conjunctivitis, erythema of eyelids, blepharospasm, lachrymation, photophobia, burning in throat or nose, rhinorrhea, erythema of nasal membrane, epistaxis, sneezing, coughing, vomiting, skin burning	Remove to fresh air, change clothes, eye wash solution, naloxone or physostigmine might be used to counteract effects of agent, bronchodilators, steroids Burns are treated like other burn injuries
Biotoxins Botulinum toxin, digitalis, nicotine, staphylococcal enterotoxin, snake poisons, insect venoms, plant alkaloids, ricin, marine toxins, strychnine, colchicine	—	Inhalation (most toxic), ingestion, injection Pain or weakness, headache, joint or back pain, dry mouth, nausea, fever, cough, sore throat, dizziness, drowsiness, anxiety	As with incapacitating agents, treatment is symptomatic and depends on biotoxin exposure Wash with soap and water, use eye wash solution

Data from Anderson, P. D. (2012). Emergency management of chemical weapons injuries. *Journal of Pharmacy Practice*, 25(1), 61–68; Centers for Disease Control and Prevention. (2018). *Emergency preparedness and response: Chemical categories*. https://emergency.cdc.gov/agent/agentlistchem-category.asp; Organisation for the Prohibition of Chemical Weapons. (2016). *Practical guide for medical management of chemical warfare casualties*. https://www.opcw.org/sites/default/files/documents/ICA/APB/Practical_Guide_for_Medical_Management_of_Chemical_Warfare_Casualties_-_web.pdf chemicals, including lung irritants, nerve agents, blister agents, blood agents, incapacitating agents, riot control agents, and biotoxins. These groups are so named primarily due to the effects they have on humans. The effect of chemical exposure on humans relies on many different variables, such as the physical state of the agent. Chemicals come in three physical states: solid, gas, and liquid. An exposure of a chemical in gas form likely will be through inhalation and will affect parts of the body that the gas comes into contact with, such as the skin, facial mucous membranes, and respiratory tract. In contrast, exposure to a liquid likely will affect the skin or the gastrointestinal tract through ingestion. The different physical states also behave in different ways. For example, a gas might settle into low-lying areas, meaning that movement to a higher point or well-ventilated area would limit exposure, whereas a liquid might soak through clothing, causing direct exposure to the skin. The mode of delivery of the chemical plays a role in how a human is affected. A chemical release might be associated with an explosion and release of a toxic gas, or it might be delivered via weaponry such as bombs and missiles, in a spray mechanism, through water and sanitation systems, or within food. Terrorists might mix different chemicals to cause multifaceted effects and make it difficult to initially identify what chemical exposure has occurred. Off-gassing of chemicals from the clothing and bodies of people exposed to chemicals also can occur, resulting in secondary exposure particularly to first responders and health professionals who are not using appropriate protection when treating casualties. A person whose clothes are soaked in a chemical compound might experience leakage through to the skin and would continue to experience chemical exposure until the clothes have been removed and the skin has been washed. This process is referred to as decontamination and is addressed later in this chapter.

Bhopal Disaster

The Bhopal disaster occurred on December 3, 1984, at the Union Carbide India Limited pesticide plant in Bhopal, Madhya Pradesh, India, when more than 40 tons of toxic gas used in the production of pesticides leaked from the plant during the night. Methyl isocyanate (MIC), a lung irritant, was the primary chemical involved in the Bhopal disaster, which killed up to 5000 people. Inhabitants of Bhopal were awakened from sleep with breathlessness, cough, throat irritation or choking, chest pain, hemoptysis, eye irritations such as severe watering of the eyes, photophobia, profuse lid edema, corneal ulcerations, vomiting, and a feeling of suffocation (Eckerman & Børsen, 2018; Mehta et al., 1990). Other acute effects reportedly included gastrointestinal symptoms such as diarrhea and abdominal pain; impaired audio, visual, and psychomotor function; and psychological effects such as neuroses and anxiety (Broughton, 2005; Dhara & Dhara, 2002; Mehta et al., 1990). Although there are many differing opinions on the exact cause of the disaster and the numbers of dead and injured, there is agreement that the suboptimal safety standards at the plant were a major causative factor in the disaster (Broughton, 2005; Chernov & Sornette, 2016; Eckerman & Børsen, 2018; Mehta et al., 1990). It is also commonly agreed that as a result of safety failings, water infiltrated the tank containing MIC, causing an exothermic reaction and the release of toxic gas containing a mix of MIC, hydrogen cyanide, nitrogen oxides, carbon dioxide, carbon monoxide, phosgene, and monomethylamine (Broughton, 2005; Dhara & Dhara, 2002; Eckerman & Børsen, 2018; Mehta et al., 1990). The plant was built in an area that had been zoned for light industry and commercial use. However, it is reported that at least 100,000 people were living within a 1 kilometer (0.6 mile) radius of the plant (Mehta et al., 1990). Within the first 24 hours, approximately 90,000 to 100,000 sought medical treatment at the four major hospitals as well as at smaller health clinics in the region (Mehta et al., 1990). Exact numbers of those killed and injured as a result of the incident remain unknown due to poor record keeping, deliberate misinformation, and people leaving the city immediately after the event. However, it is suggested that between 3800 and 5000 people were killed immediately, a further 200,000 to 500,000 were injured, and 100,000 to 200,000 were left with permanent injuries (Broughton, 2005; Dhara & Dhara, 2002; Eckerman & Børsen, 2018; Mehta et al., 1990).

Tokyo Subway Attacks

The Tokyo subway attacks occurred in Tokyo, Japan, on the morning of March 20, 1995. The attacks were carried out by members of the Aum Shinrikyo cult to distract police from carrying out a raid at the cult's headquarters (Okumura et al., 2005). The terrorists put a sarin mixture in nylon and polyethylene bags wrapped in newspaper and punctured the bags with the tips of their umbrellas before leaving the subway (Okumura et al., 1998, 2005; Taki et al., 2009). The sarin was released in 5 carriages of Tokyo's subway transportation system, and 15 subway stations were affected by the incident (Okumura et al., 1998). Tokyo citizens experienced burns, inhalation injuries, eye pain, dim vision, miosis, decreased visual acuity, weakness, difficulty breathing, fasciculation, convulsions, and cardiopulmonary arrest (Okumura et al., 1996). Overall, 12 people died and approximately 5000 were affected. It is suggested that this passive way of dispersing sarin is one reason why there were few deaths from the incident (Okumura et al., 2005). Evidence on the Tokyo subway attacks largely focuses on St. Luke's Hospital, which received 640 patients as a result of the event (Okumura et al., 1996, 2005). The first call to the emergency department reported that there had been a gas explosion at a subway station, so preparations began for an influx of burn and carbon monoxide poisoning casualties. Around 8 minutes later, the first casualty arrived on foot from a subway station, and in that first hour St. Luke's received 500 patients. The hospital had no specific plan in place to manage mass casualties and as a result the response was described as chaotic (Okumura et al., 1998).

Preparedness

Chemical disasters require a different management approach to that used in response to other types of disasters. Factors to consider in the preparedness phase from a health care facility perspective include risk assessments, plans, facility readiness, and staff readiness. From an individual standpoint, nurses also should be able to identify that a chemical release has occurred and understand how to safely and effectively manage a response. Unfortunately, due to the relative infrequency of chemical disasters, the preparedness phase is often overlooked. Both the Bhopal disaster and the Tokyo subway attacks provide examples of inadequate preparation and planning. Health care facilities in Bhopal were unprepared for a large influx of patients, and clinicians had not been trained in chemical exposure management (Chernov & Sornette, 2016). Whereas Bhopal did not have previous experience with a chemical incident, Japan did yet it is still reported that the response was chaotic and hospitals were overwhelmed (Okumura et al., 1996).

RISK ASSESSMENT

Performing a risk assessment is an essential part of the preparedness phase. Health facilities must determine the potential for hazardous chemical exposure in the region and develop an understanding of facilities and industries that operate in the region, the type of chemicals they use or store, and the antidotes for exposure to those chemicals. Prior to the disaster in Bhopal, neither the pesticide plant nor the health care facilities had undertaken an appropriate risk assessment. As a result, the health care facilities were unaware of the risk posed by the plant, the chemicals that could have been released, and the stock of antidotes (medications that counteract the effects of the chemical agent) (Chernov & Sornette, 2016).

PLANS

A key consideration in the preparedness phase is to have mass casualty plans in place. It was reported that four major hospitals in the Bhopal region did not have mass casualty response plans at the time of the incident (Broughton, 2005). Existing mass casualty plans should provide instruction for the management of mass casualties with chemical exposure because this requires specific management. These plans are dynamic and should respond to any changes or new information that could make a response more effective. Plans should be practiced regularly to ensure that they are relevant, and staff should understand the plan and be aware of their roles within it. Where emergency response plans are inadequate or outdated, nurses can demonstrate leadership and influence safe practice by encouraging management of the facility to update and practice plans. Because chemical disasters are so complex, an effective response relies on strong collaboration across sectors at the local, state/regional, or national levels in the preparedness phase. This collaboration ensures that emergency response plans are coordinated and efficient and mitigate the effects of a chemical release. Emergency services such as ambulance, fire, and police must be aware of the capabilities of the health care facility. Effective communication between the incident site and the health care facility is essential. Multisector exercises are especially important in planning for chemical disaster response, as they can generate knowledge and understanding of the response capabilities across sectors, key players, their roles and responsibilities, decontamination capabilities in the region, and availability and access to antidotes and treatments.

HEALTH CARE FACILITY AND STAFF READINESS

Health facilities must have adequate infrastructure, capacity, and resources in place to decontaminate and treat an influx of people who have been exposed to a chemical hazard. For example, decontamination showers should be easily accessible outside of the facility and, if possible, remotely accessed to promote staff safety. Waiting areas should be separated from the general population and well ventilated but under cover to protect patients from inclement weather. Health care facilities need to calculate supply requirements and stockpile personal protective equipment (PPE) or install remote-controlled lockdown systems to prevent access to the health care facility prior to decontamination. A prepared workforce can produce a more effective response, which might reduce mortality and morbidity in the affected population, reduce mental health impacts on hospital staff, and help ensure human resource and facility protection. Limited knowledge among clinicians in past events has been cited as a possible cause of disorganization, ineffective response, or higher mortality and morbidity rates (Chernov & Sornette, 2016; Firouzkouhi et al., 2017; Okumura et al., 1996). Nurses should give some thought to whether they are prepared to respond to a chemical disaster. Factors that reduce willingness to respond include fear of the unknown. If health care facilities' plans for a chemical response are inadequate, nurses should encourage their employers to address this. If a barrier to response is limited understanding of chemical disasters, nurses can address this by enhancing their own knowledge.

Response

The initial management of a mass casualty incident differs from the management of other disasters and mass casualty incidents due to the potency of the chemical exposure and the potential for secondary contamination. Decontamination and contamination controls must take precedence over the provision of medical care to ensure that staff and the health care facility are protected from secondary exposure. This section explores the factors that nurses need to consider during the response phase, including indicators of a chemical disaster, protection, decontamination, triage,

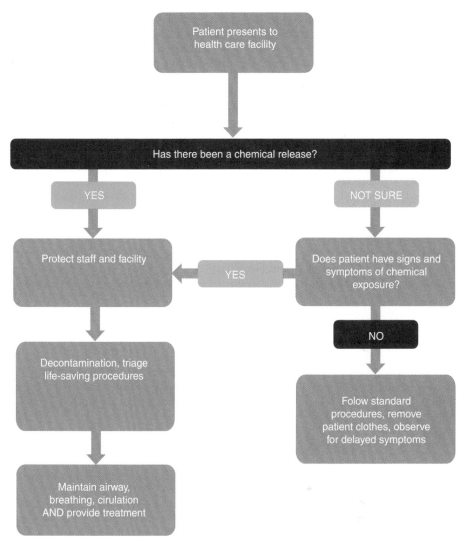

Fig. 10.1 Initial management of chemical exposure.

medical management, and psychological impacts. The flowchart shown in Fig. 10.1 provides clear guidance on the initial management steps for people with chemical exposure.

INDICATORS OF A CHEMICAL RELEASE

One of the first indictors of a chemical release often occurs when people begin presenting to the hospital. Nurses, particularly those in the emergency department, need to be astute to the signs and symptoms that indicate a chemical release. A cluster of people from the same area displaying similar signs and symptoms should ring alarm bells and prompt the implementation of the chemical response plan. Notification of a chemical release might come through the media, which have been informed directly by the perpetrators, or in the case of an accident by the company associated with the storage or transportation of chemicals. Other indicators might include an explosion followed by a strange odor or a colored mist. Chlorine is linked to a greenish-yellow gas and has a very strong odor similar to bleach. The odor associated with sulfur mustard is that of mustard or garlic, Lewisite is said to smell of geraniums, and tabun and cyanide smell like almonds. Chemical agents are almost all heavier than air, so a fog or mist might be visible in low-lying areas and casualties might be found on lower levels of buildings or on the ground. The presence of canisters or weaponry that may have contained chemicals could indicate that a deliberate event has occurred. The presence of injured or dead animals in a particular area also can indicate a chemical exposure. The clothes of people directly affected might provide clues of an exposure if they are wet, covered in a fine powder or dust, discolored, or burnt. People affected might have a distinctive odor, or the people around them might show signs and symptoms signifying that they were involved in the same event or have secondary exposure. If a person is displaying signs and symptoms of respiratory distress that do not fit with any other etiology and has no history of respiratory disease, a chemical exposure is suspected. Obtaining a good history from people who have been exposed can help determine that their symptoms are likely the result of a chemical exposure, the cause (accidental or deliberate), and the type of chemical involved. Questions a nurse might ask someone to generate this information could include: Where were you when you started feeling unwell? Did you notice anyone else around you experiencing the same symptoms? Did you notice anything unusual, such as a strange odor or taste or a colored mist?

PERSONAL PROTECTIVE EQUIPMENT (PPE)

If chemical exposure is suspected, an appropriate code or alert should be sent out so that hospital staff are aware of the exposure and contaminated people are prevented from entering the facility. Communication strategies need to be considered in the preparedness phase to ensure that nonaffected people do not present to the health care facility and potentially become exposed. To protect staff, PPE is the first line of defense in a chemically contaminated environment (OPCW, 2016). Exposure will occur through direct contact with a contaminated person or object or by inhaling fumes from affected people (off-gassing). Nurses who are working outside the health care facility in the predecontamination environment must wear PPE that includes a respirator, protective clothing, gloves, and boots. Respirators are especially important in this environment because many chemical agents affect the respiratory system (OPCW, 2016). There are many issues associated with nurses working in a predecontamination environment. First and foremost, staff who are likely to leave the health care facility to treat contaminated patients must be trained to use high-level PPE, must practice working in PPE regularly under the conditions that they might be exposed to in an actual event, and must be physically fit. It is incredibly difficult to work in high-level PPE and function effectively due to poor vision, decreased dexterity and mobility, limitations to communication, and the potential for heat stress (OPCW, 2016). The following transcript (Hammad, 2017) is a first-hand experience from a nurse of how difficult it is to work in PPE and what it feels like to wear it:

> We had never worked in an actual event. We had trained in it. I can tell you that the suits are very hot. This event happened in August, so summer. It was 96 degrees [Fahrenheit] outside—hot. Humid, hot. There was 90 percent humidity and we were standing outside on a black coal parking lot wearing nonpermeable suits that don't breathe and a hood. Of the five people that were actually working that day, the first person passed out in the tent after about 10 minutes from the heat. And then, the second person dropped after about 20 minutes which left us with three … They have sealed joints. There's really no breathability to them…. Before the first patients arrived, I had people dressed in suits for 20 minutes already, just kind of standing around in the hot sun, baking. At the time that the actual incident started when the bus rolled up, these people were already 20, 25 minutes into that 30 minutes in the suit. As

they started to do things, and they started to super heat, after 10 or 15 minutes, they were done. They were baked (Participant 8—chemical spill).

The health care facility should stock a range of high-level PPE so that all staff responders have the appropriate size available to them. In addition, PPE needs to be checked regularly to ensure that it is functional and replaced if necessary. Once decontamination has occurred, standard precautions apply.

DECONTAMINATION

The aim of decontamination is to remove or inactivate the chemical compound and its toxic abilities. The decontamination process limits the duration and continuation of exposure to the patient, minimizes the potential for off-gassing (which causes secondary exposure), and prevents contamination of the health care facility and its staff. Ideally decontamination should occur as soon as possible after exposure for the patient's protection and to prevent the spread of contaminants. The first step of the decontamination process is to remove all clothes, shoes, jewelry, and accessories, as they can trap and hold liquid agents and vapors (OPCW, 2016). It is estimated that the removal of clothes alone decreases the contaminant by 80% (OPCW, 2016). When removing clothes, it is best to cut them off or slowly remove them, paying special attention not to transfer contaminants to noncontaminated areas. The act of pulling a shirt off over the head might transfer contaminants from the shirt across the patient's face and into the eyes and mouth. Decontamination can be continued by washing with copious amounts of water and soap using the "rinse-wipe-rinse" technique (OPCW, 2016). Contact lenses must be removed and extensive eye irrigation done with water or 0.9% saline solution (OPCW, 2016). Patients should be directed to pay special attention to areas that can retain chemicals, such as hair, skin folds, and orifices. Decontamination units vary from simple outside showers (Fig. 10.2) that people walk through to more high-tech units divided into separate areas, with privacy screens and signs or audio directing people what to do at each stage of the process (Fig. 10.3). Ideally, the process provides clear direction to those undergoing decontamination, one-direction flow through with clear entry and exit points and a limited need for other personnel and hospital staff to be present.

In the Tokyo subway attacks there was no field decontamination, which meant that all patients who arrived at hospital were still contaminated (Okumura et al., 1996). On arrival to St. Luke's Hospital, patients were not decontaminated until after it became evident that there had been a

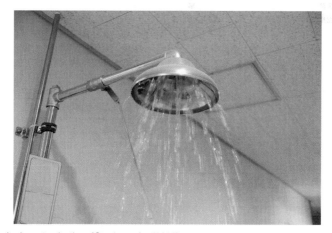

Fig. 10.2 Simple decontamination. (iStock.com\cgj0212)

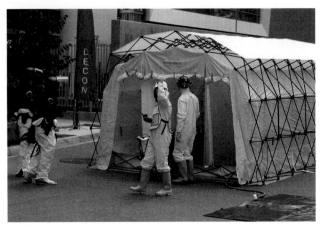

Fig. 10.3   Decontamination tent. (iStock.com\Njari)

nerve gas exposure. When it was suspected, patients were washed in their beds, and contaminated clothes were put in bags and kept on wards (Okumura et al., 1998). In addition, hospital staff were not wearing PPE, and it was reported that 23% of staff experienced secondary exposure, with nurses and nurse assistants being the highest proportion of staff affected (Okumura et al., 1998, 2005). This highlights the importance of decontamination facilities available at a safe distance from the entry points of the health care facility so that people presenting for treatment can be decontaminated as soon as possible after exposure and prevented from entering the hospital until decontamination occurs.

If "wet" decontamination is not available prior to entry into a health care facility, people affected by the exposure should be directed to do a "dry" decontamination by removing all of their clothing and accessories and then physically removing the chemical from their bodies. Methods to do this include scraping the substance off; using an absorbent material such as towels, baking soda, or flour; and vacuuming or using special preparations such as Reactive Skin Decontamination Lotion (RSDL) to remove the chemical. It is useful then to wipe down with a wet towel or bottled water. Some oily substances that are difficult to remove, such as blister agents, might require a mixture of wet and dry decontamination. Those who are present in this environment need to wear chemically resistant PPE, including a respirator. Health care facilities should have the capacity to decontaminate large numbers of people with consideration of privacy, segregation of genders, segregation of children and adults, different triage categories, and segregation of the contaminated population from the general population. This was identified as a key lesson in Japan, where complete decontamination was not possible because hospitals did not have the capacity for a large number of people to remove their clothing and shower (Okumura et al., 1996). The inability to completely decontaminate led to another problem whereby inadequate ventilation once inside the hospital led to secondary contamination of staff (Okumura et al., 1996, 1998). Although personal belongings are highly contaminated, they remain the property of the patients and should be bagged, labeled, and returned at a later stage. They also may have forensic value in case of a deliberate event.

LIFE-SAVING TREATMENT AND TRIAGE

Life-saving treatment such as giving antidotes or managing airway, breathing, and circulation can be done prior to decontamination if personnel wearing appropriate chemical-resistant PPE are available. Stockpiles of antidotes may be available at a national level, but this requires good cross-sector coordination at local and national levels. Other life-saving treatments that should be performed as soon as possible and with consideration of staff safety and resources include opening the airway, suctioning secretions, and placing casualties in a lateral position. The triage process might be performed initially at the scene of the incident by emergency responders. During the Tokyo subway attacks, 541 of the 640 patients that St. Luke's Hospital received that day bypassed emergency services, arriving on foot or via taxis or private vehicles (Okumura et al., 1996). In 1 hour, St. Luke's received 500 patients (Okumura et al., 1998), highlighting the importance of having a triage process in place to accept patients on arrival to hospital. Triage during a chemical disaster differs slightly to triage during other disaster events, as it requires consideration of the type of agent that has been used and priority for decontamination and medical treatment (Firouzkouhi et al., 2017; OPCW, 2016). Standard hospital triage scales may be altered to factor in the signs and symptoms of the agent. For example, during the Tokyo subway attacks patients were categorized into three groups—mild, moderate, and severe—whereas during the Iran-Iraq war a four-scale approach was used (Firouzkouhi et al., 2017; Okumura et al., 1998). According to the OPCW (2016), the four-scale approach outlined in Table 10.2 is one of the most commonly used chemical triage scales.

IDENTIFYING THE CHEMICAL

Identifying the chemical that caused an exposure is extremely important in determining what treatment to provide. In past events where knowledge is limited, clinicians have provided treatment by matching the signs and symptoms of casualties with a likely agent (Firouzkouhi et al., 2017; Okumura et al., 1998). It is important that nurses are aware of the effects of different chemical agents and maintain a high index of suspicion as to which one may have caused the exposure.

Two useful acronyms to help recognize nerve agent exposure are SLUDGEMM and SLOBBERED (US Department of Health and Human Services, 2020).

Salivation	**S**alivation
Lacrimation	**L**acrimation
Urination	**O**btundation
Defecation	**B**ronchoconstriction or bronchorrhea
Gastrointestinal	**B**radycardia
Emesis	**E**ye findings
Miosis	**R**educed vascular tone
Mental state (altered)	**E**mesis
	Diarrhea

MEDICAL MANAGEMENT

The treatment for a chemical exposure will be determined by the chemical compound that has caused the exposure, the dose or concentration, and the duration of exposure. This might be difficult to determine when the exposure results from multiple compounds or when the chemical in question is unknown. This was the case in Bhopal, where information from the company that operated the plant regarding the exposure and treatment was misleading (Broughton, 2005; Chernov & Sornette, 2016; Mehta et al., 1990). This example highlights the importance of knowing ahead of time what the hazards are in the region. If it is not clear what toxic chemical exposure has occurred, treatment should focus on symptom management. Medical management of chemical disasters is highly specialized; Table 10.1 is limited to a brief outline of the main treatment options per chemical classification. With most chemicals, specific antidotes are the

TABLE 10.2 ■ Four-Scale Chemical Triage

Immediate	Patients requiring emergency life-saving treatment. Requires assisted breathing. Blast injuries or other trauma. Treatment should not be time consuming or require numerous highly trained personnel, and the patient should have a high chance of survival with therapy.
Delayed	The general condition of the patient permits some delay in medical treatment, although some continuing care and pain relief may be required before definitive care is given.
Minimal	This category includes patients with relatively minor signs and symptoms who can care for themselves or who can be helped by untrained personnel.
Dead or expectant	Patients in this category have a low chance of survival, including cardiac arrest, respiratory arrest, and continued seizures. The life-threatening conditions of these patients will be beyond the treatment capabilities of the available medical personnel.

Modified from Organisation for the Prohibition of Chemical Weapons. (2016). *Practical guide for medical management of chemical warfare casualties.* https://www.opcw.org/sites/default/files/documents/ICA/APB/Practical_Guide_for_Medical_Management_of_Chemical_Warfare_Casualties_-_web.pdf

key treatment, often followed by supportive therapies. Nurses should know what antidotes are available in their facility, how to access them, and how to access the latest guidelines for medical management. Some people might be experiencing other physical symptoms associated with the event, such as penetrating injuries, burns, and blast injuries, it is important to keep in mind that medical treatment will also be required for these injuries secondary to decontamination.

PSYCHOLOGICAL IMPACTS

The psychological impacts of a chemical disaster are multifaceted and wide reaching. The psychological impact and mental health needs of three distinct groups should be considered by nurses: those people affected by the event, the health care workforce, and the wider community. Nurses must be mindful that not all people who present to a health care facility after a chemical release have actually been exposed; some people may think they were exposed or may experience psychosomatic responses. This group is referred to as the "worried well." At St. Luke's Hospital during the Tokyo subway attacks, the worried well accounted for 9.5% of the patient presentations, and there is anecdotal data that in the days following the disaster the worried well presentations increased (Okumura et al., 2005). During the Iran-Iraq war it was reported that many soldiers who did not necessarily require immediate treatment crowded in front of the medical units to receive care (Firouzkouhi et al., 2017). Post-traumatic stress disorder (PTSD) and depression are the most common disorders attributable to terror attacks, with 30% to 40% of people involved in a deliberate chemical event likely to develop a clinically diagnosable disorder within 2 years of an incident (Nakamine et al., 2018). Nurses need to be astute to the mental health impacts that involvement in the response to a chemical disaster can elicit in both themselves and their colleagues. Psychological effects of disasters are covered extensively elsewhere in this text.

Recovery

Recovery activities are aimed at returning the facility to a pre-event state. Most important to any recovery phase is a review of the emergency response and seeking input from key stakeholders involved in the response. A review and update of the emergency response plan should reflect any lessons learned from the event. Another major consideration is to monitor the health workforce for absences and sick leave. Mental health impacts might be felt among staff, particularly those working in frontline roles. A mechanism to monitor and address any mental health disturbances among staff needs to be implemented. Other facility considerations include restocking material resources used during the response. The long-term health effects of a chemical event might have a significant effect on the health system. Chronic illness and delayed effects of chemicals are understood and more uncertain than acute effects (OPCW, 2016). As previously mentioned, chemical disasters have mental health implications, and the health care facility might experience an increase in mental health presentations such as anxiety, depression, loss of libido, and PTSD (OPCW, 2016). There might also be an increase in health problems directly related to the type of chemical exposure. Examples include skin lesions from blister agents, which may take up to 60 days to heal; chronic debilitating pulmonary disease in casualties of sulfur mustard exposure; and carcinogenesis, teratogenesis, and perhaps mutagenesis due to the fact that some chemicals are carcinogens (OPCW, 2016). The effects of the Bhopal disaster remain to this day. The term *Bhopal syndrome* has been used to refer to the combination of symptoms and damage to human organs that the gas leak caused (Eckerman & Børsen, 2018). Permanent disability resulting from the incident has left people with physical disability, airway dysfunction, and decreased resistance to infection, particularly of the airways (Eckerman & Børsen, 2018). Furthermore, although the pesticide plant was dismantled the year after the incident, the site itself continued to leak chemicals for many years, leading to widespread water and soil pollution in the region and ongoing health impacts for the community (Dhara & Dhara, 2002; Eckerman & Børsen, 2018). Research conducted among people involved in the Tokyo subway attacks demonstrated that they continued to experience both physical and psychological symptoms (Okumura et al., 2005).

Legal Considerations

According to the International Council of Nurses (ICN, 2019), nurses must practice within the applicable nursing and emergency-specific laws, policies, and procedures during a chemical disaster. That is, nurses must observe the same local, national, and international laws that govern their everyday practice. At St. Luke's Hospital it was reported that due to an influx of 500 patients in a 1-hour period, documentation was limited to essential information such as name, address, and physical complaints on one piece of paper (Okumura et al., 1998). Documentation such as patient records is a valuable legal document, useful in creating a timeline of events, and may be used as forensic evidence. In terms of the Bhopal disaster, legal wrangling began as early as 4 days after the event when the first lawsuit was filed (Broughton, 2005; Eckerman & Børsen, 2018). Despite all evidence against them, the plant operators have consistently denied responsibility for the incident, and as a result the people affected by the exposure, their families, and the wider Bhopal community received inadequate representation and were poorly recompensed for their ordeal. The long-term health and socioeconomic effects were also ignored in the compensatory process (Eckerman & Børsen, 2018).

Ethical Considerations

Nurses must apply institutional or national disaster ethical frameworks in the care of individuals, families, and communities in a chemical disaster as they would in their everyday practice (ICN, 2019). Different nursing organizations across the world have developed specific ethical standards relevant to nurses in their countries. From a global perspective the ICN has published a code of ethics for nurses that outlines four elements of conduct related to nurses and people, nurses and practice, nurses and the profession, and nurses and coworkers. Similarly, different disciplines also have codes of ethics that their members are expected to follow. Ethical issues that may arise in the response to a chemical disaster could include allocation of resources, altered standards of care, staff working outside their usual scope of practice, diminished safety of staff, lack of patient privacy, and triaging effectively under pressure when it is not possible to attempt life-saving interventions on all casualties. When the health care facility is overwhelmed, such as in mass casualty events, it becomes necessary to do the greatest good for the greatest number rather than to focus resources on a small number of casualties who have less chance of survival. This means difficult decisions and protocols that need to be made and communicated broadly, well in advance.

In addition, Okumura et al. (2005) point out that the public is defenseless against chemical weapons because of their lack of knowledge about their effects and how to protect themselves, making attacks with chemical weapons ethically unsound. Terrorism and the use of chemical warfare agents such as sarin are aimed at causing not only injury and illness but also psychological effects due to the horror and dread that they inspire (OPCW, 2016). From an ethical standpoint, events such as the Tokyo subway attacks breach basic human rights. In reference to the Bhopal disaster, the notable ethical issues were safety failings at the plant, failing to respond to warnings such as persistent leaks, inadequate emergency procedures, and lack of community preparedness. Perhaps one of the biggest ethical issues arising from the Bhopal incident was a decision by the local government to approve persons to live permanently around the plant, which was an area zoned for light industry and not for residential purposes (Broughton, 2005; Chernov & Sornette, 2016; Eckerman & Børsen, 2018).

Special Considerations

Nurses must remember that the process of decontamination can be fear inducing and undignified for those who are exposed to hazardous chemicals. The water used during the decontamination process is often cold, so nurses should be aware of and mitigate against any negative physiological effects of cold water and outside temperatures. Hospital staff should not be present in the pre-decontamination environment unless they are wearing the appropriate PPE and adequately trained in wearing it. Wearing high-level PPE is difficult, as heat stress and fatigue are common. For the patient, the person wearing the PPE may appear intimidating and scary, and it may be difficult to understand instructions, as speech is often muffled by a face mask. During the decontamination process in particular, nurses need to observe those who are vulnerable. Children, for example, should not be separated from parents and should not be in situations where they are physically exposed in front of adults. People from culturally and linguistically different backgrounds might have difficulty understanding directions and expectations during the decontamination process. Elderly people and people with physical or cognitive disabilities might need more time for the decontamination process. The effects of chemicals on children or on the elderly and people with comorbidities might be more exaggerated than in the general population.

Points to Remember

- **Planning:** The Bhopal and Tokyo case studies highlight the importance of having in place a mass casualty plan with relevance to chemical disasters. All hospitals should have the ability to decontaminate a surge of patients.
- **Training:** It was reported in both events that medical staff were ill prepared for chemical events and were not familiar with the medical management of chemical disasters and exposures.
- **Risk assessment:** Particularly in Bhopal, a thorough risk assessment would have identified the power plant as a potential hazard. A thorough risk assessment in Tokyo would have identified the possibility of a chemical attack, as the city had experienced a chemical attack the year before.
- **Communication:** Both case studies identified poor communication around the identification of the chemical. Hospitals should know what industries are active in the region, what chemicals are used by those industries, and what treatment is required when exposure

occurs. In both scenarios, hospital and industry leaders and emergency services should have developed clear communication channels in advance to facilitate more robust emergency responses and lower mortality rates.

Test Your Knowledge

1. The most common types of chemicals used in chemical warfare are:
   a. Nerve agents, blister agents, lung irritants, bioxins, and riot control agents
   b. Nerve agents, blister agents, lung irritants, blood agents, and incapacitants
   c. Nerve agents, lung irritants, blood agents, bioxins, and riot control agents
   d. Blister agents, lung irritants, blood agents, incapacitants, and riot control agents
2. Nerve agents:
   a. Are highly toxic in small doses
   b. Cause blisters and burns
   c. Affect the oxygen-carrying capacity of red blood cells
   d. Include phosgene, chlorine, and ammonia
3. The type of agent used in the Tokyo subway attacks was:
   a. Arsenic
   b. Sarin
   c. Tabun
   d. Ricin
4. A key planning failure from the Bhopal disaster that could have been mitigated in the preparedness phase was:
   a. Limited knowledge about chemical agents among hospital staff
   b. Lack of hospital emergency response plans
   c. Poor communication between the Union Carbide plant and the hospital
   d. All of the above
5. If unable to identify the specific chemical exposure, the best treatment is:
   a. Oxygen
   b. Symptom management
   c. Atropine
   d. Diazepam
6. What is the most common triage scale used for chemical disaster?
   a. ATS
   b. CTS
   c. Three scale
   d. Four scale
7. Indicators that a chemical release has occurred include:
   a. An unusual odor, color, or mist
   b. A cluster of people with similar signs, symptoms, and stories
   c. The presence of dead or injured animals in the area
   d. All of the above
8. When managing patients who have been exposed to a chemical release, you must protect yourself by:
   a. Wearing chemical-resistant personal protective equipment with a respirator at all times
   b. Using standard precautions at all times
   c. Wearing chemical-resistant personal protective equipment with a respirator prior to decontamination and using standard precautions thereafter
   d. Wearing nitrile glove, surgical mask, and fluid-resistant gown at all times

9. The antidote for nerve agents is:
    a. BAL
    b. Atropine and oximes
    c. Naloxone
    d. Sodium thiosulfate
10. Which of the following is true of decontamination?
    a. Personnel working in the decontamination area must wear standard PPE.
    b. No one from the scene of a chemical release should be allowed to enter a health care facility without being decontaminated first.
    c. Wet decontamination is best for blister agent exposure.
    d. All of the above.

References

Broughton. E. (2005). The Bhopal disaster and its aftermath: A review. *Environmental Health, 4*(1), 6.

Chernov, D., & Sornette, D. (2016). *Man-made catastrophes and risk information concealment.* Switzerland: Springer.

Dhara, V. R., & Dhara, R. (2002). The Union Carbide disaster in Bhopal: A review of health effects. *Archives of Environmental Health: An International Journal, 57*(5), 391–404.

Eckerman, I., & Børsen, T. (2018). Corporate and governmental responsibilities for preventing chemical disasters: Lessons from Bhopal. *HYLE: International Journal for Philosophy of Chemistry, 24*

Firouzkouhi, M., Zargham-Boroujeni, A., Kako, M., & Abdollahimohammad, A. (2017). Experiences of civilian nurses in triage during the Iran-Iraq war: An oral history. *Chinese Journal of Traumatology, 20*(5), 288–292.

Hammad, K. (2017). The lived experience of nursing in the emergency department during a disaster [Unpublished thesis]. Flinders University, School of Nursing & Midwifery.

International Council of Nurses. (2019). *Core competencies in disaster nursing, version 2.0.*

Mehta, P. S., Mehta, A. S., Mehta, S. J., & Makhijani, A. B. (1990). Bhopal tragedy's health effects: A review of methyl isocyanate toxicity. *JAMA, 264*(21), 2781–2787.

Nakamine, S., Kobayashi, M., Fujita, H., Takahashi, S., & Matsui, Y. (2018). Posttraumatic stress symptoms in victims of the Tokyo subway sarin attack: Twenty years later. *Journal of Social and Clinical Psychology, 37*(10), 794–811.

Okumura, T., Hisaoka, T., Yamada, A., Naito, T., Isonuma, H., Okumura, S., et al. (2005). The Tokyo subway sarin attack—Lessons learned. *Toxicology and Applied Pharmacology, 207*(2), 471–476.

Okumura, T., Suzuki, K., Fukuda, A., Kohama, A., Takasu, N., Ishimatsu, S., et al. (1998). The Tokyo subway sarin attack: Disaster management, part 2: Hospital response. *Academic Emergency Medicine, 5*(6), 618–624.

Okumura, T., Takasu, N., Ishimatsu, S., Miyanoki, S., Mitsuhashi, A., Kumada, K., et al. (1996). Report on 640 victims of the Tokyo subway sarin attack. *Annals of Emergency Medicine, 28*(2), 129–135.

Organisation for the Prohibition of Chemical Weapons. (2016). *Practical guide for medical management of chemical warfare casualties.* https://www.opcw.org/sites/default/files/documents/ICA/APB/Practical_Guide_for_Medical_Management_of_Chemical_Warfare_Casualties_-_web.pdf

Organisation for the Prohibition of Chemical Weapons. (2020). *What is a chemical weapon?* https://www.opcw.org/our-work/what-chemical-weapon

Taki, K., Suzuki, K., & Satoh, T. (2009). The Tokyo subway sarin attack: Toxicological whole truth. In R. C. Gupta (Ed.), *Handbook of toxicology of chemical warfare agents* (pp. 25–32). Academic Press.

US Department of Health and Human Services. (2020). *Chemical hazards emergency medical management.* https://chemm.nlm.nih.gov/index.html.

World Health Organization. (2020). *Deliberate events.* https://www.who.int/environmental_health_emergencies/deliberate_events/en/

CHAPTER 11

Biological or Infectious Disease Outbreaks

Samah Hawsawi, MSN, RN, PhD student

CHAPTER OUTLINE

Introduction	**212**	Middle East Respiratory Syndrome (MERS)	214
Natural and Unnatural Biological or		Coronavirus Disease 2019 (COVID-19)	214
Infectious Disease Outbreaks	**212**	Infectious Disease Spread	214
Natural Infectious or Biological Diseases	212	**Case in Point**	**219**
Unnatural Infectious or Biological Diseases	213	Actual Disaster and Public Health	
Deliberate	213	Emergency: Covid-19	219
Accidental	213	Description	219
Emerging Biological or Infectious		Lessons Learned	220
Disease Outbreaks	214	Questions for Discussion	220
Zika Virus	214	**Points to Remember**	**220**
Ebola Virus Disease (EVD)	214	**Test Your Knowledge**	**221**
Severe Acute Respiratory Syndrome		**References**	**222**
(SARS)	214		

OBJECTIVES

After reading and studying this chapter, you should be able to:
- Understand biological or infectious disease outbreaks.
- Distinguish natural from unnatural biological or infectious disease outbreaks.
- Identify intentional disease outbreaks using key features.
- Explain how infectious disease spreads globally.
- Discuss emerging biological or infectious diseases.

KEY TERMS

biological weapon: An intentionally released pathogen.

bioterrorism: A type of terrorism that involves the intentional release or threat to release or disseminate biological agents such as bacteria, viruses, insects, fungi, or toxins.

deliberate: The action of doing something consciously and intentionally.

infectious agents: Organisms such as bacteria, viruses, fungi, protozoa, helminths, and prions that can cause infectious disease.

outbreak: An unexpected increase in the incidence of a disease or numbers of a harmful organism.

pandemic: The global spread of infectious disease; worldwide epidemic.

pathogen: The agent that produces infectious disease.

viral hemorrhagic fever (VHF): A common term that describes a severe illness caused by various groups of viruses. These viruses are characterized by damaging multiple systems in the body, including the vascular system, hence causing hemorrhage.

virulent: The capability of pathogens or microbes to infect or destroy a host.

Introduction

A biological or infectious disease outbreak is a disaster that increases the risk of transmittable disease spread during and after its occurrence. The incidence of infectious disease outbreaks has been increasing globally since 1980 (Smith et al., 2014). The world has witnessed several infectious disease outbreaks, including severe acute respiratory syndrome (SARS), Middle East Respiratory Syndrome (MERS; Centers for Disease Control and Prevention [CDC], 2019b), Ebola (Centers for Disease Control and Prevention, 2019a), Zika virus (Centers for Disease Control and Prevention, 2019c), and COVID-19 (Centers for Disease Control and Prevention, 2020a, 2020b), all of which threatened human health and safety worldwide. The seriousness of infectious disease outbreaks is overwhelming because disease agents are unseen and consequences are unpredictable. Compare this to other disasters, such as a chemical disaster, where by the agent can be seen when it is spilled or released. In this chapter, we discuss the types of biological or infectious disease outbreaks, including emerging outbreaks, and infectious disease spread, A table describing each disease process is included. A case study is presented to highlight an international nurse's reflection on a global pandemic.

Natural and Unnatural Biological or Infectious Disease Outbreaks

Infectious or biological diseases are illnesses caused by microorganisms that can be cellular (bacteria and fungi) or acellular (viruses and prions) and are capable of causing disease outbreaks that risk human lives and health security. When speaking about biological disease risk, we must consider a wide range of potential factors from natural exposure to the microorganism responsible for an infection to the possibility of deliberate release of nonnatural agents (caused by bioterrorism) that lead to epidemics (Mancon, Mileto, & Gismondo, 2018). Some types of pathogens occur naturally but are considered unnatural when they re-emerge due to an accident in a research laboratory. Regardless of the type of infectious disease, these diseases often spread nationally or internationally with little to no warning.

NATURAL INFECTIOUS OR BIOLOGICAL DISEASES

All infectious diseases of humans that emerge and re-emerge and lead to outbreaks occurring cyclically over time are considered naturally occurring infectious diseases unless bioterrorism features are noticed in the process of prevention and containment of the outbreaks (Mancon et al., 2018). These neutral infectious diseases can also normally appear in society as acute or chronic pathogens, or they can emerge unexpectedly, leading to new or rare syndromes.

UNNATURAL INFECTIOUS OR BIOLOGICAL DISEASES

Unnatural infectious diseases are caused by microorganisms altered or created to increase the harm they inflict. The emergence of unnatural biological or infectious diseases can be deliberate or accidental and can lead to a national or global disaster (Vallat & Chaisemartin, 2017).

Deliberate

Intentional infectious or biological diseases in the form of microorganisms such as viruses, bacteria, or other contagions are one type of biological weapon created and released to cause disease and death in humans (Mancon et al., 2018). According to Dhaked (2014), to identify intentional infectious diseases, researchers in the Center of Civilian Biodefense in the United States created the following list of critical features of viral hemorrhagic fever (VHF) biological infectious agents:

- Increased morbidity and death rate
- Human-to-human transmission
- Highly infectious potential of aerosol dissemination, which can cause large outbreaks
- Unavailability of proper vaccine
- Availability of agent
- Quickness of production
- Environmental durability
- Previous research and creation of an infectious agent to be used as a biological weapon and to be a source of tension among health care providers and the public

According to Dhaked (2014), various VHF infectious agents, such as Ebola, that displayed these features were identified as biological weapons. This is in line with the Centers for Disease Control and Prevention (2018) categorization of Ebola as a bioterrorism infectious agent.

Accidental

Accidental infectious disease outbreaks are human-made pandemics caused by experimentation and diagnostic research (Fig. 11.1). Negligence or lack of biosafety standards in research laboratories could lead to the accidental release of pathogens, thereby causing infectious disease outbreaks (Mancon et al., 2018). The threat of human-made infectious diseases running rampant due to accidental release is real, as it can result in transmitting highly contagious pathogens beyond laboratory personnel.

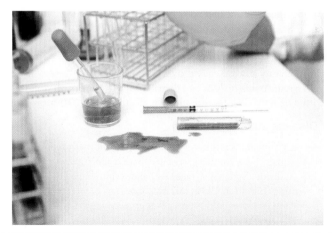

Fig. 11.1   An accidental spill of infected blood in a medical laboratory during the process of vaccine development. (iStock.com\Skarie20)

Infected people may not know they are infected and can transmit the disease to others. The historical record includes an accidental laboratory-escaped outbreak of SARS after the SARS pandemic, when researchers were analyzing SARS pathogens to prevent its outbreak (Klotz & Sylvester, 2014).

EMERGING BIOLOGICAL OR INFECTIOUS DISEASE OUTBREAKS

The terms *infection* and *disease* are not synonymous. Infection refers to the process of a microorganism attacking and progressing inside a host. Disease refers to the consequence of infection. Some infectious agents are contagious and easily transmitted, but they are not virulent enough to cause serious damage, as seen with the poliovirus. However, some infectious diseases are contagious, exhibit high virulence, and can emerge and re-emerge, leading to disease outbreaks (National Institutes of Health, 2007). Emerging infectious diseases are infections that occur in humans and have increased in the past 2 decades, threaten to increase in the near future, increase rapidly, or are new to a population or geographical region (Zumla & Hui, 2019). Examples of emerging or re-emerging infectious diseases that spread nationally and internationally include the Zika virus, Ebola virus, SARS, and MERS, as well as the more recent COVID-19 (Baylor College of Medicine, 2020; Table 11.1).

Zika Virus

Zika virus is a flavivirus initially recognized in Uganda in 1947 in monkeys and spread by the bite of an infected *Aedes* mosquito (Fig. 11.2). Zika virus is one of the most dangerous infections during pregnancy because it passes from the mother to her fetus and can lead to microcephaly, miscarriage, stillbirth, and other birth defects (Fig. 11.3; CDC, 2019c).

Ebola Virus Disease (EVD)

EVD is a rare and life-threatening disease caused by a virus originally identified in sub-Saharan Africa in 1996 that affects people and nonhuman primates, causing severe bleeding, organ failure, and death. Researchers revealed that survivors of EVD hold antibodies that can be found in the blood up to 10 years after recovery (CDC, 2019a).

Severe Acute Respiratory Syndrome (SARS)

SARS is a contagious respiratory illness caused by a coronavirus (SARS-CoV) that was initially reported in Asia in 2003, then spread to other countries, including those in North America, South America, and Europe. The virus infected 8098 people worldwide, with 774 deaths; excluding statistics for the United States, there were only 8 stable cases (CDC, 2017).

Middle East Respiratory Syndrome (MERS)

MERS is a viral respiratory disease caused by a coronavirus (MERS-CoV). MERS-CoV was initially reported in Saudi Arabia in 2012 and then spread to several other countries, including the United States, with 4 in 10 MERS cases resulting in death (CDC, 2019b).

Coronavirus Disease 2019 (COVID-19)

COVID-19 is a serious contagious respiratory illness that was initially reported in China in 2019. COVID-19 virus is caused by a coronavirus called SARS-CoV-2 and led to a pandemic that infected 12.9 million individuals globally (Fig. 11.4) and resulted in 571,000 deaths worldwide as of the date of this writing (Fig. 11.5; CDC, 2020a, 2020b).

INFECTIOUS DISEASE SPREAD

Infectious diseases present a notable threat to human and animal health due to their fast and continuous spread. Some infectious disease pathogens transmit directly from infected to uninfected

TABLE 11.1 ■ Common Emerging Biological or Infectious Diseases

Source	Disease	Transmission	Signs and Symptoms	Treatment	Duration	Vaccine
CDC, 2019c	Zika	Mosquito bites (vector-borne) Mother to fetus Sexual	Fever Rash Headache Joint pain Red eyes Muscle pain	Symptoms management	Several days to 1 week	No vaccine
CDC, 2019a	Ebola	Direct contact with infected animal, infected or dead person Blood or body fluids Semen	Fever Body aches Headache Gastrointestinal distress Unexplained bleeding Late Stage Red eyes Skin rash Hiccups	Symptoms management	2–21 days	Ervebo
CDC, 2017	SARS	Respiratory droplets Direct contact	Fever >100.4 °F Headache Discomfort Body aches Mild respiratory distress Dry cough Pneumonia	Pneumonia medication	2–10 days	Under investigation
CDC, 2019b	MERS	Direct contact Respiratory droplets	Fever Cough Shortness of breath Respiratory distress Diarrhea and nausea/vomiting Pneumonia and kidney failure	Symptoms management	2–14 days	No vaccine

(continued)

TABLE 11.1 ■ Common Emerging Biological or Infectious Diseases—cont'd

Source	Disease	Transmission	Signs and Symptoms	Treatment	Duration	Vaccine
CDC, 2020a, 2020b, 2021	COVID-19	Respiratory droplets	Fever Respiratory distress Fatigue Muscle or body aches Headache Loss of taste or smell Sore throat Congestion Gastrointestinal distress Severe Symptoms Trouble breathing Persistent chest pain Confusion Inability to wake Bluish lips or face	Symptoms management	2–14 days	Pfizer-BioNTech Moderna Johnson & Johnson's/Janssen

CDC, Centers for Disease Control and Prevention; MERS, Middle East Repiratory Syndrome; SARS, severe acute respiratory syndrome.

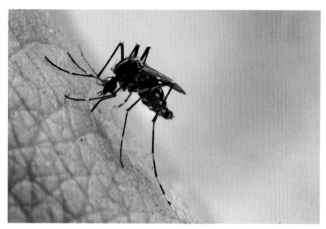

Fig. 11.2 The *Aedes aegypti* mosquito that is responsible for the spread of the Zika virus. (iStock.com\frank600)

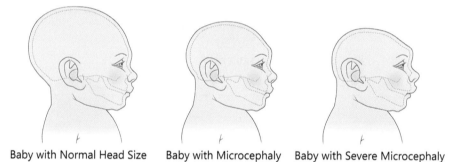

Baby with Normal Head Size   Baby with Microcephaly   Baby with Severe Microcephaly

Fig. 11.3 A comparison of a newborn child's head and skull with a normal cranium to the head and skull of a newborn child with microcephaly caused by the Zika virus. (iStock.com\juliawhite)

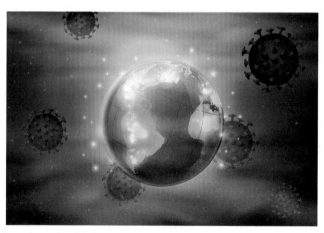

Fig. 11.4 This photo shows the global outbreak of the COVID-19 virus. (iStock.com\Egor Shabanov)

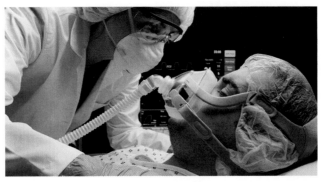

Fig. 11.5 A female patient connected to a ventilator with life-threatening disease due to the COVID-19 virus. (iStock.com\Juanmonino)

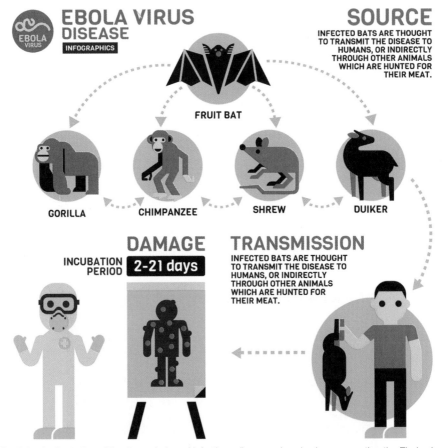

Fig. 11.6 An illustration of the transmission of infectious diseases via animals, representing the Ebola virus. (iStock.com\monkik)

individuals. Other pathogens, such as the Ebola virus, spread via multiple hosts, including animals (Fig. 11.6). There are two modes of pathogen transmission: vertical and horizontal (Fig. 11.7). Both modes promote the expansion of the infecting bacterium, fungi, or viruses. Horizontal transmission passes microorganisms via direct contact between infected individuals and uninfected

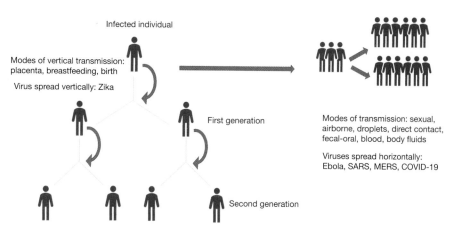

Fig. 11.7   The vertical and horizontal modes of infectious disease transmission. *MERS*, Middle East Respiratory Syndrome; *SARS*, severe acute respiratory syndrome.

individuals, which is called colonization (Kang & Castillo-Chavez, 2014). Direct contact can occur through traveling, sexual contact, sharing common areas, and more. Vertical transmission involves passing the pathogen from mother to fetus during birth, breastfeeding, or via the placenta (Kang & Castillo-Chavez, 2014). Some types of infectious viruses, such as the Zika virus, can transmit horizontally and vertically. In addition, other factors stimulate the global spread of infectious diseases, such as increasing antimicrobial resistance, connections between people (Heesterbeek et al., 2015), environmental and human behavior changes (Wong et al., 2015), and travel (Changula, Kajihara, Mweene, & Takada, 2014). All of these factors play a significant role in the spread of infectious disease locally and globally, presenting challenges for prevention and control.

Case in Point

ACTUAL DISASTER AND PUBLIC HEALTH EMERGENCY: COVID-19

A.H. is a 32-year-old Saudi female who has worked as a registered nurse (RN) in primary health care since 2010. She was interviewed by the author on July 14, 2020, for the purpose of presenting an international RN's reflection on a global pandemic (COVID-19).

Description

A.H. currently works at a hospital in Saudi Arabia. She was assigned to care for patients and conduct active screenings for COVID-19 cases beginning on May 16, 2020. She described her experience as exhausting, overwhelming, and educational. A.H. stated that, based on what she observed, approximately 70% of cases had the same signs and symptoms, including fever, shortness of breath, fatigue, dizziness, and gastrointestinal distress.

A.H. stated that, fortunately, several infectious disease outbreak preparedness initiatives were started in Saudi Arabia in 2018. She stated that the Ministry of Health (MOH) of Saudi Arabia launched a new protocol requiring all RNs to attend a licensing program called Basic Infection Control Skills License (BICSL). The program includes several teaching strategies for infectious disease management, such as lectures and workshops. She also stated that nurses were required to have meningitis and influenza vaccinations and to undergo a fit test to verify the proper fitting of the N95 respirator. The program also involves practicing hand hygiene and the use of personal protective equipment (PPE). A.H. stated that to obtain the required license to be able to work in Saudi health care settings, each RN was obligated to get the required vaccinations and attend one-on-one training sessions with a trained instructor. She stated, "Although I was uncertain about caring or being with COVID-19 patients, the BICSL program eased my burden and prepared me for such an unexpected event." Another preparedness measure taken by the MOH was that larger hospitals were required to have an isolation unit and a disaster team to respond to any disaster event.

A.H. stated that the MOH responded to COVID-19 quickly and effectively. They provided all hospitals, including private ones, with necessary equipment such as PPE, mechanical ventilators, N95 respirators, high-efficiency particulate air (HEPA) filters, and more. They also created a COVID-19 survey system so that all people in Saudi Arabia could contact the hospital if they have symptoms or concerns. Regarding legal aspects, A.H. stated that the MOH announced that during the COVID-19 pandemic, all people in Saudi Arabia, citizens and immigrants alike, would receive necessary care paid for by the MOH, and suspected cases and stable infected people would be quarantined in paid hotels. The MOH also launched a website for nurses to request a free psychiatric clinic visit.

Regarding ethical aspects, A.H. expressed her feelings by stating, "I was not excited about being a nurse at that time, but the code of ethics necessitates that nurses should care for all patients regardless of the severity and risk of their disease." She also stated that "I told myself that I have to care for all COVID-19 patients as I provide usual care for [all] patients, which helped me learn how to deal with the situation." A.H. stated that there were some special considerations for populations with chronic diseases. The MOH launched a website for people with chronic diseases to request a free at-home doctor visit, paid medication including delivery, and free transportation to and from the hospital when needed.

Lessons Learned

1. Being prepared for disasters helps nurses to handle the unexpected. Health care providers were aware of the PPE and other equipment needed during the infectious disaster; hence they provided proper care while being extremely cautious.
2. Protecting yourself as a nurse helps you to protect other people.
3. Teaching patients about the disease is better than letting them rely on myths spread via social media.
4. All patients, regardless of their disease severity, race, gender, and nationality, need to be treated equally.

Questions for Discussion

1. When should professional nurses begin to learn and prepare for disasters, specifically infectious disease outbreaks?
2. What are some of the patient characteristics nurses should consider when given a patient assignment when an infectious disease is suspected?

Points to Remember

- Lessons learned from all previous infectious disease outbreaks nationally or internationally are aiding health care providers to respond effectively to new, unexpected disease outbreaks.
- The seriousness of infectious disease outbreaks is that they are unexpected and unseen, hence preparedness for the unexpected is always effective.

Test Your Knowledge

1. Which of the following statements are true about biological or infectious disease outbreaks? *(Choose all that apply.)*
   a. There is increased risk of transmittable disease spread.
   b. The incidence of infectious disease outbreaks has been increasing globally.
   c. There are fewer outbreaks now than there were 13 years ago.
   d. Infectious disease outbreaks are typically resolved quickly.
2. Examples of global infectious disease outbreaks include: *(Choose all that apply.)*
   a. MERS
   b. Ebola
   c. COVID-19
   d. Influenza
3. The distinguishing feature of unnatural biological infections is that they:
   a. Emerge and re-emerge cyclically
   b. Are caused by microorganisms altered or created to increase harm inflicted
   c. Normally appear in society as acute pathogens
   d. Normally appear in society as chronic pathogens
4. Which of the following features would cause health care providers to suspect an intentional biological weapon? *(Choose all that apply.)*
   a. Increased morbidity and death rate
   b. Human-to-human transmission
   c. Nonavailability of effective vaccine
   d. Highly infectious potential
5. Emerging infectious diseases have which of the following characteristics? *(Choose all that apply.)*
   a. Infections occur in humans.
   b. Infections occur in animals.
   c. Occurrence increases rapidly.
   d. They are new to a population or region.
6. Which of the following statements are true regarding the spread of infectious disease pathogens? *(Choose all that apply.)*
   a. Some pathogens transmit directly from infected to uninfected individuals.
   b. Some pathogens spread via uninfected humans and animals.
   c. Some pathogens do not spread between some cultures of people.
   d. Some pathogens can be spread without the knowledge of the host or exposed individual.
7. Which of the following statements are true about horizontal transmission? *(Choose all that apply.)*
   a. Microorganisms are passed by direct contact between infected and uninfected individuals.
   b. Horizontal transmission is also called colonization.
   c. Direct contact can occur through traveling.
   d. Direct contact can occur through sexual contact or sharing common areas.
8. Which of the following statements are true about vertical transmission? *(Choose all that apply.)*
   a. It promotes the transmission of the infecting bacteria, fungi, or viruses.
   b. The transmission can occur from mother to fetus during birth.
   c. The transmission cannot occur through a mother breastfeeding her infant.
   d. The pathogen cannot be passed from mother to fetus via the placenta.

9. Challenges to the prevention and control of the global spread of infectious diseases include: *(Choose all that apply.)*
    a. Some infectious viruses can be transmitted horizontally and vertically
    b. Increasing antimicrobial resistance related to overuse of antibiotics
    c. Increased mobility of global citizens through worldwide travel
    d. Social distancing

10. One of the strongest messages nurses can share about decreasing the spread of infectious diseases is that:
    a. Regular exercise is an effective means of staying healthy
    b. Dental health is part of maintaining overall health
    c. Regular handwashing is one of the best ways to remove germs, avoid getting sick, and prevent the spread of germs to others
    d. Visiting a health care provider once each year is sufficient for most adults

References

Baylor College of Medicine. (2020). *Emerging infectious diseases.* https://www.bcm.edu/departments/molecular-virology-and-microbiology/emerging-infections-and-biodefense/emerging-infectious-diseases.

Centers for Disease Control and Prevention. (2017). *SARS basics factsheet.* https://www.cdc.gov/sars/about/fs-sars.html.

Centers for Disease Control and Prevention. (2019a). *Ebola virus disease.* https://www.cdc.gov/vhf/ebola/index.html.

Centers for Disease Control and Prevention. (2019b). *Middle East Respiratory Syndrome (MERS).* https://www.cdc.gov/coronavirus/mers/index.html.

Centers for Disease Control and Prevention. (2019c). *Zika virus.* https://www.cdc.gov/zika/index.html.

Centers for Disease Control and Prevention. (2018). *Ebola viral hemorrhagic fever.* https://emergency.cdc.gov/agent/vhf/index.asp.

Centers for Disease Control and Prevention. (2020a). *Coronavirus disease 2019 (COVID-19).* https://www.cdc.gov/coronavirus/2019-ncov/index.html.

Centers for Disease Control and Prevention. (2020b). *Coronavirus disease 2019 (COVID-19).* https://www.cdc.gov/coronavirus/2019-ncov/symptoms-testing/symptoms.html.

Centers for Disease Control and Prevention. (2021). *Approved and authorized COVID-19 vaccines.* https://www.cdc.gov/coronavirus/2019-ncov/vaccines/different-vaccines.html.

Changula, K., Kajihara, M., Mweene, A. S., & Takada, A. (2014). Ebola and Marburg virus diseases in Africa: Increased risk of outbreaks in previously unaffected areas? *Microbiology and Immunology, 58*(9), 483–491. https://doi.org/10.1111/1348-0421.12181.

Dhaked. R. K. (2014). Re-emergence of Zaire Ebola virus disease: Lessons to be learnt. *Journal of Bioterrorism & Biodefense, 5*(1). https://doi.org/10.4127/2157-2526.1000e116.

Heesterbeek, H., Anderson, R. M., Andreasen, V., Bansal, S., De Angelis, D., Dye, C., & Viboud, C. (2015). Modeling infectious disease dynamics in the complex landscape of global health. *Science, 347*(6227). https://doi.org/10.1126/science.aaa4339.

Kang, Y., & Castillo-Chavez, C. (2014). Dynamics of SI models with both horizontal and vertical transmissions as well as Allee effects. *Mathematical Biosciences, 248*, 97–116. https://doi.org/10.1016/j.mbs.2013.12.006.

Klotz, L. C., & Sylvester, E. J. (2014). The consequences of a lab escape of a potential pandemic pathogen. *Frontiers in Public Health, 2.* https://doi.org/10.3389/fpubh.2014.00116.

Mancon, A., Mileto, D., & Gismondo, M.R. (2018). The global threats from naturally occurring infectious diseases. In V. Radosavljevic, I. Banjari, & G. Belojevic (Eds.), *Defence against bioterrorism. NATO science for peace and security series A: Chemistry and biology* (pp. 13–24). Springer. 13-24. https://doi.org/10.1007/978-94-024-1263-5-3.

National Institutes of Health. (2007). *Understanding emerging and re-emerging infectious diseases.* https://www.ncbi.nlm.nih.gov/books/NBK20370/.

Smith, K. F., Goldberg, M., Rosenthal, S., Carlson, L., Chen, J., Chen, C., & Ramachandran, S. (2014). Global rise in human infectious disease outbreaks. *Journal of the Royal Society Interface, 11*(101). https://doi.org/10.1098/rsif.2014.0950.

Vallat, B., & Chaisemartin, D. (2017). The importance of intergovernmental standards in reducing biological threats associated with accidental, natural or deliberate acts. *Revue Scientifique et Technique-Office International des Epizooties, 36*(2), 615–620. https://pdfs.semanticscholar.org/354b/2edc0aec27f7c135f77 2d07eebb1d6d158cd.pdf.

Wong, G., Liu, W., Liu, Y., Zhou, B., Bi, Y., & Gao, G. F. (2015). MERS, SARS, and Ebola: The role of super-spreaders in infectious disease. *Cell Host & Microbe, 18*(4), 398–401. https://doi.org/10.1016/j.chom.2015.09.013.

Zumla, A., & Hui, D.S. (2019). Emerging and re-emerging infectious diseases: An issue of infectious disease. Elsevier Health Sciences.

CHAPTER 12

Human-Made Disasters

Joanne C. Langan, PhD, RN, CNE ▪ Jeff F. Evans, RN, BNurs, MSc, SFHEA

CHAPTER OUTLINE

Introduction	**225**	Nonconventional Terrorist Weapons	230
Human-Made Disasters Versus		**Points to Remember**	**234**
Natural Disasters	**226**	**Test Your Knowledge**	**234**
Accidental or Deliberate Acts	226		
Terrorism	228	**References**	**235**
Conventional Terrorist Weapons	230		

OBJECTIVES

After reading and studying this chapter, you should be able to:
- Differentiate natural disasters from human-made disasters and their aftermath.
- Discuss the differences in motive between intentional and accidental disasters.
- Express the value of all nurses having a working knowledge of disaster preparedness and response.
- Analyze past terrorist events and the factors that affected the degree of each event's damage.

KEY TERMS

anthropogenic disasters: Disasters caused by humans; human-made disasters.

biological terrorism or bioterrorism: The use and dissemination of various kinds of microbes or toxins with the intent to intimidate or coerce a government or civilian population to further political or social objectives. Humans, animals, and plants are often targets.

chemical terrorism: Attacks meant to cause mass devastation in which terrorist organizations release toxins; chemical attacks meant primarily to terrorize, blackmail, or cause economic damage; a specific attack in a particular product, particularly a food product.

chemical warfare agents: Highly toxic chemicals that can be disseminated as vapors, gases, liquids, or aerosols or adsorbed to dust particles.

conventional weapons: More frequently used weapons of terrorism such as bombs and guns.

dirty bomb: See *radiological dispersion bomb*.

disaster: An occurrence, either natural or human-made, that causes large-scale human suffering and creates human needs and social dysfunction that victims cannot alleviate without assistance.

domestic terrorism: Terrorist acts by individuals or groups within a given country without foreign direction or involvement.

hazardous materials: Substances that, because of their chemical, biological, or physical nature, pose a potential risk to life, health, or property if released.

international terrorism: Terrorist acts directed by foreign groups that transcend national boundaries, affecting people in several countries.

ionizing radiation: Causes the long-term destructive force of the dirty bomb. Ionizing radiation may lead to unnatural chemical reactions inside the cells and break DNA chains, causing either DNA strand death or DNA mutation; unlikely ill effects in very small doses.

mass casualty incident: A situation with a number or severity of casualties that significantly overwhelms available emergency medical services, facilities, and resources.

nonconventional weapons: Less frequently used weapons of terrorism such as chemical, nuclear, and biological weapons.

nuclear terrorist attack: An incident in which a terrorist organization uses a nuclear device to cause mass murder and devastation. Includes the use or threat of the use of fissionable radioactive materials in an attack or an assault on a nuclear power plant for the purpose of causing extensive or irreversible environmental damage.

post-traumatic stress disorder (PTSD): An anxiety disorder that can develop after exposure to a terrifying event or ordeal in which grave physical harm occurs or is threatened and that causes prolonged meaningful interference in daily life.

post-traumatic stress symptoms: Normal psychological, cognitive, and emotional responses to direct or indirect exposure to terrifying events or ordeals, including exposure through media reports and personal accounts.

radiation sickness: One of the results of DNA mutation inside cells exposed to ionizing radiation; can be deadly, but survivable with bone marrow transplantation.

radiological dispersion bomb: The most accessible nuclear device to be used by a terrorist, it consists of a conventional explosive such an trinitrotoluene (TNT) packed with radioactive waste byproducts from nuclear reactors and discharges deadly radioactive particles into the environment; also called a dirty bomb.

terrorism: The systematic use of terror; the deliberate creation and exploitation of fear for bringing about political change.

trauma: Physical injury caused by violent or disruptive action, by the introduction into the body of a toxic substance, or by a psychic injury resulting from a severe emotional shock.

Introduction

A number of human-made disasters have commanded the attention of the global humanitarian community. Some of these disasters include conflicts between the forces of the government and opposition forces in South Sudan, the Central African Republic, and throughout the Middle East. These events, although tragic, taught government leaders powerful lessons in disaster preparedness and how to react and respond to large-scale disasters (Centers for Disease Control and Prevention, 2018). This chapter discusses basic concepts in human-made disasters and provides examples so that "lessons learned" may be a means to improve disaster response and recovery on a global level.

Human-Made Disasters Versus Natural Disasters

Whereas natural disasters occur due to forces beyond human control, human-made or anthropogenic disasters are human generated. Anthropogenic disasters are generally caused by human action or inaction. The broad categories of anthropogenic disasters are biological and biochemical terrorism, chemical spills, radiological (nuclear) events, fire, explosions, transportation accidents, group violence such as riots, food or water contamination, deforestation and building collapses, armed conflicts, and acts of war. Injuries caused by acts of war are blunt, blast, and penetrating traumas. The majority of terrorist and criminal acts against humanity use conventional weapons such as firearms and explosives (Powers, Monson, Zimmerman, Einov, & Dries, 2019). Whereas terrorist acts are classified as deliberate, some human-made disasters are accidental. These differences and the impact on human life are discussed further.

ACCIDENTAL OR DELIBERATE ACTS

Regardless of the category of the event, accidental or deliberate, disasters that involve large numbers of victims or even a smaller number that overwhelms available emergency medical services, facilities, and resources are called mass casualty incidents. Disasters of this magnitude require the assistance of neighboring community resources, such as equipment and personnel, as described in previous chapters.

A wrecked tanker truck or railroad car carrying dangerous chemicals that overturns due to a collision is a human-made disaster and considered accidental. Terrorist bombings, the release of sarin gas into the Tokyo subway system, and the deliberate crashing of planes into the World Trade Center and the Pentagon are deliberate acts, not accidental. (See Table 12.1 for real-world examples of deliberate acts.)

Hazardous materials are substances that, because of their chemical, biological, or physical nature, pose a potential risk to life, health, or property if they are released in an uncontrolled environment (Fig. 12.1). Potential hazards can occur during any stage of use from production and storage to transportation to disposal. Production and storage of hazardous materials commonly occur in chemical plants, gas stations, hospitals, and a wide range of industrial sites and businesses. Hazardous materials accidents can range from a chemical spill on a highway to groundwater contamination by naturally occurring methane gas to a household hazardous materials accident. Household chemicals such as nail polish and remover, cleaning supplies, pesticides, and motor oil are considered hazardous and may lead to residential accidents. Radiological accidents involving specific hazardous materials, such as at nuclear power plants, during transport of radiological materials, and during disposal of radioactive waste, are also a concern to the public's health.

In the United States, two major disastrous events occurred at Three Mile Island (TMI) power station in Pennsylvania and at the Love Canal landfill in New York. In the TMI power station, radioactive gas was released 2 days after a cooling malfunction caused part of the core to melt in reactor number 2. Deficient control room instrumentation and inadequate emergency response training were believed to be the root causes of the accident. Further review concluded that personnel error, design deficiencies, and component failure were additional causal factors. As a result, major changes occurred in the nuclear industry and the United States Nuclear Regulatory Commission (NRC, 2018), including enhanced oversight. In New York, chemical odors from toxic waste filled the basements of homes bordering the Love Canal landfill. A chemical company had used the Love Canal as an industrial dump. The area was later covered with soil and many homes were built nearby. Heavy rains caused the contents of the rotting containment drums to percolate up through the soil and into the backyards and basements of the nearby homes. The indiscriminate disposal of toxic materials caused the relocation of 235 families and the expense of public monies and efforts to contain the disaster and restore a degree of normalcy to the lives of

TABLE 12.1 ■ Shootings, Bombings, and Terrorism Events

Event, Location, and Date*	Number Injured/Deaths	Weapons or Attack Types	Motive or Other
École Polytechnique massacre Montreal, Canada, 1989	14/15	Ruger Mini-14, hunting knife	Antifeminism
Columbine High School massacre Colorado, USA, 1999	24/15	Hi-Point Carbine, explosive, knife	Murder-suicide, arson, shootout
Virginia Tech shooting Virginia, USA, 2007	23/33	GLOCK 19 pistol, Walther P22 pistol	Mass murder, murder-suicide
Sandy Hook Elementary School shooting Connecticut, USA, 2012	2/28	Bushmaster XM 15-E2S rifle, GLOCK 20 SF handgun	Deaths included 20 children between the ages of 6 and 7 years
Pulse nightclub shooting Florida, USA, 2016	58/50	Semiautomatic rifle, semiautomatic pistol	Mass shooting
Las Vegas shooting Nevada, USA, 2017	869/59	24 firearms	Mass shooting
Christchurch mosque shootings New Zealand, 2019	49/51	Semiautomatic rifles, shotguns	Far Right politics, white supremacy
Oklahoma City bombing Oklahoma, USA, 1995	680+/168	Domestic terrorist truck bombing	Ruby Ridge, Waco siege
Centennial Olympic Park bombing Georgia, USA, 1996	111/2	Domestic terrorist pipe bomb	Anticommunism
Madrid train bombings Spain, 2004	2000/193	Goma-2, backpack bomb	Islamic extremism, opposition to Spanish participation in Iraq War
Boston Marathon bombings Massachusetts, USA, 2013	264/3	2 homemade pressure cooker bombs	Retribution for US military action in Afghanistan and Iraq
September 11 attacks USA, 2001	25,000/2996	4 coordinated terrorist attacks, aircraft hijacking	Islamic terrorist group al-Qaeda against the United States
Khobar massacre Saudi Arabia, 2004	25/22	Guns, bombs	Hostages, mass murder, terrorism

*Refer to reference list for websites relating to these events.

those affected. According to the US Environmental Protection Agency (EPA, 2016), this event is one of the worst environmental tragedies in United States history.

Using the term *accidental* can make it seem like "accidents just happen," as if by magic. However, as the "accidents" at TMI and Love Canal illustrate, human negligence, ignorance, or reckless stupidity often lie behind so-called accidents. This point is important to remember, as human factors such as negligence and stupidity have a direct impact on the mental well-being of victims and

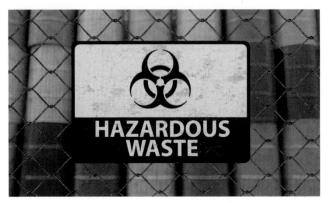

Fig. 12.1 A hazardous waste sign with oil barrels in the background. (iStock.com\vchal)

survivors. Accidents associated with human failings can lead to powerful feelings of anger directed at those considered responsible. True accidents, events that are unforeseen and not attributable to negligence and human failings, also present psychological difficulties to survivors. In true accidents, survivors may struggle to answer the fundamental questions of "Why me?" "Why my family?" "Why my neighborhood?" These questions can begin to unravel a survivor's worldview, ideas of justice and just deserts can be undermined, and confidence in religious beliefs may be challenged. Survivors may also carry feelings of guilt at having survived devastating but seemingly random acts (see BOX 12.1).

TERRORISM

Terrorism is the systematic use of terror. To terrorize is to fill with terror, to scare, or to coerce by threat or violence. The Federal Bureau of Investigation (FBI, 2020) defines domestic terrorism as "violent criminal acts committed by individuals or groups to further ideological goals for political, religious, social, racial, or environmental causes." Some incidents of domestic terrorism (described in this section) have included acts against ethnic or religious groups (Fig. 12.2). International terrorism is defined as "violent criminal acts committed by persons who are inspired by or associated with foreign terrorist organizations" (FBI, 2020). All terrorist acts have one key element in common—violence or the threat of violence. The goal of terrorism is to create lasting psychological effects that reach a much wider audience than the immediate victims or object of the attack. Through their use of dramatic, bloody, and destructive acts of violence, terrorist groups choose to frighten and intimidate large populations such as rival ethnic or religious groups, a country and its political leadership, or the international community. The following high-profile acts draw attention to the terrorists and their cause.

Terrorist acts include murder, kidnapping, bombing, and arson. These acts have been defined in both national and international law as crimes. Most countries around the world regard terrorism as a serious crime and have legal statutes in place to prosecute terrorists.

It is important to remember the underlying purpose of terrorism, that is, to terrorize. As a result, psychological morbidity can far outstrip the number of dead, injured, and wounded. All devastating events are linked to post-traumatic stress symptoms. However, terrorist events have the potential to create much stronger and more widespread post-traumatic symptoms than other events, such as a bus crash. In addition, terrorist events have the potential to drastically alter how everyday life is lived. Security operations, such as closure of access routes, grounding of flights, and checking personal baggage at stores and shopping malls, not only improve safety but also affect everyday life and can heighten feelings of danger and vulnerability. Post-traumatic

---

BOX 12.1 ■ Survival After a Human-Made Accidental Disaster

They had taken the cruise and the special small aircraft excursion several times before this fateful day. Although the cruise line was familiar, this small aircraft company was new to them. They relied on the cruise line to assure the quality and safety of the vendor and assumed it was safe. The only way to observe some of the spectacular views of the vast lands of Alaska is by air. Several family members and friends embarked on this sightseeing journey and were on their way back to land when tragedy struck. A midair collision with another small sightseeing aircraft occurred. The aircraft plunged into the frigid waters of only 8°F to 10°F. Survivors could not remove their seatbelts without help, as they had broken bones, other injuries, and varying degrees of consciousness. They were barely able to simply float on their backs, weighted down by heavy jackets and boots. Luckily, a fisherman in a Zodiac was able to get to the passengers and direct them to hold on to straps outside his inflatable boat. He was able to get some passengers to shore while a tour boat and the Coast Guard were able to rescue the others. A small 17-bed hospital stabilized the wounds and prepared the survivors for transport to a larger city and hospital. There, at least one of the survivors spent nearly 1 month having multiple surgeries and procedures and recovering. All surviving passengers are in varying states of recovery with physical therapy, occupational therapy, and sessions with a psychologist who is helping them to assimilate the trauma of their experiences.

Several lessons were learned from this disaster.

1. Do homework or research on vendors for excursions. Ask about their safety record as well as licenses and certifications.
2. Pay attention to safety instructions of all kinds when they are provided. If they are not provided, ask for them. If they still are not provided, remove yourself from the event.
3. Survivors appreciate the calm, professional, competent demeanor of rescuers and all health care providers. Honesty about the injuries and what the patient might anticipate in the short term and long term is an essential element of excellent care.
4. Patients are very perceptive as to how health care providers and ancillary workers treat each other; mutual respect gives the patient a feeling of confidence that all are working as a team and know what they are doing.

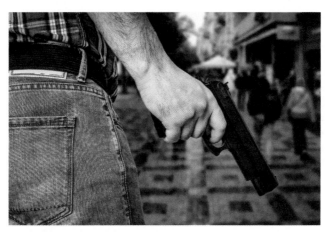

Fig. 12.2 A killer with a pistol amid a crowd of people. (iStock.com\andriano_cz)

stress disorder (PTSD) is characterized by the development of a persistent anxiety response following a traumatic event. The individual experiences or witnesses a traumatic event and develops feelings of helplessness, intense fear or horror. Symptoms are grouped into three categories: 1) re-experiencing the traumatic event with intrusive thoughts, nightmares, or flashbacks; 2) avoidance as indicated by marked efforts to stay away from activities related to the trauma; and 3) hyperarousal, as indicated by difficulty concentrating, insomnia, and exaggerated startle reactions. Symptoms may last more than one month and are severe enough to impair functioning (Torres, 2020).

Conventional Terrorist Weapons

Terrorists use more easily accessible conventional weapons such as homemade bombs and commercially purchased guns more frequently than they use nonconventional terrorist weapons such as chemical, nuclear, and biological weapons. Car and truck bombs are especially common in suicide attacks. The Oklahoma City bombing of 1995 is a prime example of a car bomb causing a major disaster. Terrorists use both explosive bombs such as letter and parcel bombs and incendiary bombs such as Molotov cocktails. Other weapons, such as handguns, rifles, semiautomatic weapons, and grenades have been used in assassinations, armed attacks, and massacres. A variety of grenades may be used, ranging from hand grenades to rocket-propelled devices. A few terrorist groups are known to possess surface-to-air, shoulder-fired missiles that can bring down aircraft. Specific organizations are designed to help combat the use of these weapons for acts of terrorism. The United Nations Office on Drugs and Crime (UNODC, 2020) is committed to seeking health, security, and justice for all through global programs and an extensive network of field offices. This international body monitors drug activity, organized crime, corruption, and terrorism (UNODC, 2020).

Improvised explosive devices are all explosive devices that are not manufactured by arms companies. They may consist of commercially produced explosive materials such as plastic explosives or TNT. Alternatively, they may make use of homemade explosives that are created from commercially available materials. Although the sale and transfer of manufactured arms and explosives are highly regulated, the purchase and shipment of commercially available components that are only dangerous in combination are less regulated. Being less regulated, homemade explosives present a greater challenge to domestic and international law enforcement agencies.

Nonconventional Terrorist Weapons

Nonconventional terrorist weapons include those in chemical, biological, and nuclear categories. Each of these categories is explained.

Chemical Terrorism. Chemical terrorism is grouped into two main types:

1. Attacks meant to cause mass devastation, in which the terrorist organization releases a toxin in congested population centers, bodies of water, or unventilated areas to create as many victims as possible.
2. Chemical attacks meant primarily to terrorize, blackmail, or cause economic damage (as in tainted food supply and loss of business); a specific attack in a particular product—particularly a food product—mainly by introducing a toxic chemical substance into the product itself.

Chemical weapons can be dispersed in gas, liquid, and solid forms (Williams & Sizemore, 2020) and can be spread through the air, water supply, and food supply.

Chemical warfare agents are highly toxic chemicals that can be disseminated as vapors, gases, liquids or aerosols or adsorbed to dust particles. Chemical weapons are categorized by the major organ system affected. These categories include blister agents or vesicants, such as mustard that affects the skin and lungs; chemicals that affect the blood such as arsine, hydrogen chloride, and hydrogen cyanide; and agents such as chlorine gas, nitrogen oxide, sulfur trioxide-chlorosulfonic acid, and zinc oxide that affect the respiratory system. Other categories of chemical agents include those that cause mental incapacitation, those that affect the central and peripheral nervous systems, and those that are used for riot control such as tear gas, and those that induce vomiting. When these materials are found, the Centers for Disease Control and Prevention (CDC) is notified and the Department of Defense uses mobile equipment to dispose of them to mitigate risks to the public's health (CDC, 2014).

Biological Terrorism. Biological terrorism (or bioterrorism) is the use and dissemination of biological weapons (bacteria, fungi, toxins, or viruses) in population centers by various means in order to cause morbidity and numerous casualties in humans, animals, and plants. These weapons may be naturally occurring or modified by humans in a laboratory; for example, to increase their ability to be spread into the environment or to increase their resistance to antibiotics (Williams & Sizemore, 2020). Unlike chemical weapons, biological weapons are not designed and ordinarily cannot be used for specific, circumscribed attacks; their principal purpose is mass devastation, which is often political in nature. The results of a biological attack may not be immediate and may become apparent only several hours or days later. Biological weapons are not as common, accessible, or available as chemical weapons.

Radiological and Nuclear Terrorism. A nuclear terrorist attack is an incident in which a terrorist organization uses a nuclear device to cause mass murder and devastation. This type of terrorism also includes the use or threat of the use of fissionable radioactive materials in an attack or an assault on a nuclear power plant with the intent to cause extensive or irreversible environmental damage. In the nuclear power plant example, a terrorist organization does not need to develop, acquire, or gain control of a nuclear bomb to cause extensive damage. Instead, it can cause great damage and havoc by using conventional weapons against a nuclear reactor. This type of action would seriously damage the reactor and release radioactive matter into the atmosphere, potentially endangering large population centers. Terrorist organizations consider the use of nuclear weapons a major advantage because they can inflict wide-scale damage and command worldwide media attention. Although it is possible for terrorist organizations to acquire nuclear weapons, it is unlikely, and currently no evidence exists for a terrorist group successfully obtaining the amounts of material required to make a nuclear weapon (Williams & Sizemore, 2020).

Radiological Dispersion Bomb Use in War. Another name for the radiological dispersion bomb is *dirty bomb*. It contains organotropic isotopes or explosives such as TNT packed with radioactive waste byproducts from nuclear reactors. Upon detonation, a dirty bomb discharges deadly radioactive particles into the environment. The dirty bomb uses the gas expansion as a means of propelling radioactive material over a wide area. The long-term destructive force of the dirty bomb is caused by the ionizing radiation from the radioactive material. In a person's body, an ion's electrical charge may lead to unnatural chemical reactions inside the cells. If the DNA mutates, a cell may become cancerous or cells may malfunction. This may result in a wide variety of symptoms collectively referred to as radiation sickness. Radiation sickness can be deadly but people can survive it, especialy if they receive a bone marrow transplant (Harris, n.d.). Radioactive waste is found throughout the world as byproducts of nuclear processing, as in industries such as nuclear medicine and research and nuclear power manufacturing (Fig. 12.3).

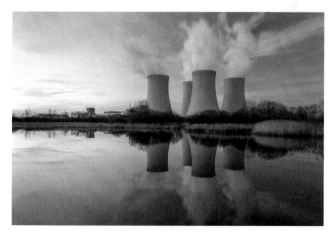

Fig. 12.3 A nuclear power plant. (iStock.com\vlastas)

In battlefields, the use of nonconventional weapons were found in the conflicts of two Gulf Wars and warfare in Iraq, Afghanistan, and the Balkans. These wars introduced radioactive weapons to modern war zones (Durakovic, 2017). (see Box 12.2).

BOX 12.2 ■ Afghanistan—Victims of War: A Trauma Nurse Responds

Kabul, Spring 2006

In the spring/summer of 2006 I deployed to Kabul, Afghanistan, with an international nongovernmental organization (NGO) for 3 months. This NGO already had an established presence in Afghanistan. They had operated in the country during the civil war in the mid-1990s after the withdrawal of Soviet forces, the eruption of violence between multiple warring factions, and the eventual installation of a Taliban-led government.

In 2006 the NGO operated three surgical hospitals across southern Afghanistan, numerous First Aid Posts in rural communities across several provinces, and a prison health service for the main civilian prison in Kabul. At that time, the hospitals run by the NGO were the only ones outside of the government and military spheres that could offer trauma care that included computerized tomography (CT), vascular surgery and neurosurgery, and intensive care including ventilation.

Because the NGO had remained in Afghanistan for more than 10 years through civil war and the Taliban, it had achieved a position of legitimacy among the Afghan populace. Rather than being seen to cut and run, the NGO was viewed as a steadfast friend of the Afghan people, a friend that had weathered the same storms as they had and stood by them in solidarity. The perception of being a true and steadfast friend of the Afghan people and the upholding of the humanitarian principle of neutrality were the cornerstones of operational security and our humanitarian legitimacy. The biggest threat to this perception, and paradoxically to our security, was when we worked closely with the International Security Assistance Force (ISAF).

We were a receiving hospital for civilians brought to us from across Afghanistan by ISAF. This always led to an interesting standoff outside the main gate. All of our facilities were weapons-free; everyone entering was searched and all knives and guns had to be left at the security checkpoints. Because ISAF troops were never separated from their weapons, it was definitely a case of an immovable object meeting an irresistible force. This led to lengthy handovers of patients outside the main gate. Having ISAF troops and vehicles parked at the front gate drew fire and also undermined the NGO's assertion that it was not associated with ISAF.

A workaround was developed whereby we would send a 4×4 SUV to the ISAF base at the airport to affect patient recovery. This 4×4 was by no means an ambulance. The vehicle usually was staffed by myself and an anesthetist with little equipment beyond a sphygmomanometer, some intravenous (IV) fluids, a bag valve mask (Ambu bag), and a cylinder of oxygen. The patient was laid in the back of the truck on a foam mattress and slowly transported back to hospital through numerous security checkpoints, crowded marketplaces, and congested traffic. We traveled unarmed and unescorted.

Even this short account might give some insight into what it is like to work within a conflict setting. In terms of personal preparation, I had very little. I am a civilian intensive care nurse but with experience working in austere prehospital settings as a volunteer medic with a local mountain rescue team. My decision to deploy to Kabul was part of my professional development as a senior lecturer in disaster health care. While deployed I had the good fortune to be placed on paid leave from my home university. Personally, it was definitely a question of "ignorance is bliss" or maybe "fools rush in where angels fear to tread." Before leaving I received a number of immunizations and wrote a will, then I set out on a week-long trip via the NGO headquarters for a briefing and to collect equipment to take out on resupply, a day's layover in the United Arab Emirates, and a final flight on a United Nations (UN) charter to Kabul. In 2006 the airport still looked like a battle zone, with craters and wrecked military equipment scattered around the periphery of the airport.

Needless to say, the clinical case load was significantly different. Although I worked in a surgical center for war victims, a large proportion of our day-to-day work involved motor vehicle accidents and assaults leading to blunt force trauma, penetrating injuries, lacerations, and gunshot wounds. We also had a regular influx of blast injuries from bombings, handling unexploded ordnance such as shells and detonators, and landmines, as well as "failed" bomb makers who would appear with very little left of their hands.

Our "emergency department" consisted of a smallish concrete room with two metal trolleys, a large oxygen cylinder, manual sphygmomanometers, stethoscopes, a range of cervical spine collars, a lot of IV fluids, and a tray of drugs for rapid sequence intubation; that was it. Our blood bank was limited to around six or eight units of whatever blood had been donated. However, we did have a fantastic surgical team of European and Afghan vascular, orthopedic, and neuro surgeons. We also had (at that time) the only free-to-use CT scan outside of military and government hospitals. We had a six-bed intensive care unit (ICU) that allowed us to ventilate patients, again the only such unit open to the general public in Afghanistan at that time. However, resupply was a constant problem. We ended up reusing "single patient use" devices, especially ventilator circuits, after cleaning and resterilizing them, again working within "altered standards of care."

We had a limited formulary of drugs. Pain relief was with pentazocine (Talwin), and our IV antibiotics included benzylpenicillin, Amoxiclav, chloramphenicol, and gentamicin. However, we had no way of measuring gentamicin levels and only a rough snapshot of renal function through urea, sodium, potassium, and creatinine levels. We did our best but always ran the risk of not achieving therapeutic ranges, leading to antibiotic resistance, or leaving the patient hearing impaired through ototoxicity. We relied on adrenaline and dopamine as our inotropes to support cardiovascular function. Both of these are first-generation drugs that have been superseded for good reason, being associated with numerous drawbacks and unwanted side effects. We had no volumetric syringe driver pumps for inotrope infusions, but we did have IV fluid rate minders. The senior anesthetist created a formula for the dilution of adrenaline or dopamine into 500 mL IV bags in such a way that the hourly infusion rate in milliliters was equivalent to the μg/min/kg infusion rate usually managed through a volumetric syringe driver pump. It was an ingenious approach but one fraught with risk, especially when the inotropes had sat on the apron at the airport in 80 °F heat for 2 days awaiting customs clearance.

Working in Kabul at that time also raised unique and unexpected ethical problems to work through. As Afghanistan began to emerge from the wreckage of civil war and the Taliban government, there was no social security system, no community primary health care system, and no rehabilitation services, and poverty was rife. To borrow a phrase from Thomas Hobbes, life was "nasty, brutish and short." This led us as clinicians to question to what end we were pursuing life-saving interventions. We had to question what quality of life would be achieved and what enduring burdens would be created for any survivor and their family. The question of futility was common. We knew that in Europe many of our most seriously injured casualties had the hope of a decent quality of life supported by extensive health care and social services. However, we knew that there was no support outside of the family for any severely physically or neurologically disabled patients we saved to the point of discharge. On several occasions we had to decide that enough was enough. Sometimes these decisions were based on the realization that death was the inevitable outcome, either sooner or later in hospital or within a matter of days after discharge. Sometimes mixed with this was the contemplation of a form of bodily survival with intolerable suffering where the only escape was into death. These are tough calls to make when you know the person is a victim of the circumstances of time and place as much as a bombing or shooting.

Personally, the most difficult cases to deal with emotionally were the deliberate, well-thought-through targeted attacks on individuals. Women run through with swords where the only explanation was that "they fell"; babies falling 30 feet onto concrete, again a stony-faced "they fell" as the only explanation; explosive devices set overnight outside the threshold of homes in the knowledge that the first people to step out of the compound would be children heading to school. Two things went through my heart in such cases: first, the calculated destructive inhumanity of one person toward another, and second, the knowledge that we would be sending the patient back to that place where their safety from attack was anything but guaranteed.

In terms of lessons learned, I can pick out three take-home messages:

1. It is surprising how little physical equipment you need to provide emergency care; skills of rapid assessment are skills we carry with us everywhere, and management of hemorrhage, airway, and breathing can be achieved with gravity, IV cannula, IV fluids, and good use of positioning.
2. People do terrible things to other people.
3. Nurses are in a unique position to bring humanity to the darkest of human experiences. We recognize the unique value of each person as valuable without any qualification. Through our nursing practice, we can rescue and rebuild the dignity of those who have been the victims of the worst of humankind's endeavours.

Points to Remember

- All nations of the world have become acutely aware of the varying degrees of vulnerability to terrorist attacks.
- Nurses have a unique opportunity to learn about disasters of all types and take an active role in preparedness and response in places of employment and in the community, including neighborhoods and private residences.
- Many issues must be well thought out when considering the major topic of disasters, such as the devastating effects of trauma and human physical and mental healing.

Test Your Knowledge

1. The production and storage of hazardous materials occur in: *(Choose all that apply.)*
   a. Chemical plants
   b. Gas stations
   c. Hospitals
   d. Industrial cleaning supply companies
2. The exodus of families from the Love Canal area was the result of:
   a. A nuclear power plant accident
   b. The indiscriminate disposal of toxic materials
   c. A biological experiment gone awry
   d. The community plan to build a shopping center at that site
3. An example of an accidental disaster is:
   a. A car loaded with bombs that steers into a bus loaded with passengers
   b. A fuel tanker that runs aground due to poor visibility in a storm
   c. Anthrax spores that are disseminated to a large population through the mail
   d. A toxic agent that is discovered in a jar of baby food
4. Conventional terrorist weapons: *(Choose all that apply.)*
   a. Include car and truck bombs
   b. Include bacteria, fungi, and toxins
   c. Are often used in suicide attacks
   d. Include handguns, rifles, and semiautomatic weapons
5. Which of the following events is most likely to be linked to negligence?
   a. A bus crash in icy weather
   b. A mass shooting of students on a college campus
   c. Release of nuclear material from a nuclear plant after an earthquake
   d. Collapse of a poorly maintained highway overpass
6. A lone gunman livestreams an attack on a mosque over the internet. He kills more than 50 worshippers. Which of the following statements is true?
   a. Those with gunshot wounds will make up the majority of survivors.
   b. Women will make up the majority of survivors.
   c. The psychologically traumatized will make up the majority of survivors.
   d. There will be no survivors.
7. In 1984 salad bars in numerous food outlets in Oregon were deliberately contaminated with *Salmonella enterica* bacteria by a local political group, causing more than 400 cases of food poisoning. Which terms best characterize this event? *(Choose all that apply.)*
   a. Domestic terrorism
   b. International terrorism
   c. Bioterrorism
   d. Mass murder

8. Which of the following phrases is true?
   a. Improvised explosive devices can be readily manufactured from commercially available components.
   b. Improvised explosive devices always contain homemade explosives.
   c. Improvised explosive devices are produced by regulated arms manufacturers.
   d. Improvised explosive devices are used only in conflict zones.
9. Which of the following are indicators of PTSD? *(Choose all that apply.)*
   a. Having persistent nightmares
   b. Avoiding usual activities
   c. Re-engagement in religious practices
   d. Extreme physical reactions to reminders of an event such as a nausea, sweating, or a pounding heart
10. Chemical terrorism can include: *(Choose all that apply.)*
    a. Poisonous gas sprayed from aircrafts
    b. Liquid cyanide added to bodies of water
    c. Infecting populations with a virus
    d. Deliberate contamination of food

References

Centers for Disease Control and Prevention. (2014). History of U.S. chemical weapons elimination. https://www.cdc.gov/nceh/demil/history.htm

Boston Marathon Bombing. (n.d.) Retrieved from https://www.google.com/search?sa=X&rlz=1C1VFKB_enUS639US706&q=Boston+Marathon+bombing&stick=H4sIAAAAAAAAAONgFuLSz9U3KDA2ySnJUAKzS0yqsvMqtaSzk630U8tS80r0UzKLE4tLUousijNTUssTK4sXsYo75ReX5Ocp-CYWJZZkABlJ-blJmXnpO1gZAZT0kiVUAAAA&ved=2ahUKEwjD0_aAwLjoAhXFWM0KHRVSCPUQ-BYwMHoECBUQNg&biw=1366&bih=625

Centennial Olympic Park Bombing. (n.d.) Retrieved from https://www.google.com/search?rlz=1C1VFKB_enUS639US706&biw=1366&bih=625&ei=gNF8Xt_7BZOStAaRp6TgCQ&q=atlanta+olympics+bombing&oq=Atlanta+O&gs_l=psy-ab.1.1.0j0i131j0l7j0i131.23310.29276..34668...0.0..0.152.2369.24j4......0....1..gws-wiz.....6..0i67j0i7i30j0i362i308i154i357j0i131i67j0i273.aZYxdIYP4Qs

Centers for Disease Control and Prevention. (2018). *Natural and human-made disasters.* https://www.cdc.gov/eis/field-epi-manual/chapters/Natural-Human-Disasters.html

Christchurch Mosque Shootings. (n.d.) Retrieved from https://www.google.com/search?sa=X&rlz=1C1VFKB_enUS639US706&q=Christchurch+mosque+shootings&stick=H4sIAAAAAAAAAONgFuLVT9c3NEwzNDIyNCrOVoJysy1SUnKNK7QEXDKLE4tLUouCM1NSyxMrixexyjpnFGUWlyRnlBYlZyjk5hcXlqYqFGFk55dk5qUX72BlBAAwQYNmVQQAAAA&ved=2ahUKEwiuk9Gbv7joAhVQQ80KHbmxCNwQ-BYwOHoECBUQSw&biw=1366&bih=625

Columbine High School Massacre. (n.d.) Retrieved from https://www.google.com/search?sa=X&rlz=1C1VFKB_enUS639US706&q=Columbine+High+School+massacre&stick=H4sIAAAAAAAAAONgFuLVT9c3NEwzNDIyNCrOVuLQz9U3SDdPqtIScMksTiwuSS0KzkxJLU-sLF7EKuecn1Oam5SZl6rgkZmeoRCcnJGfn6OQm1hcnJhclLqDlREAwmc8ylEAAAA&ved=2ahUKEwjNqbLsvrjoAhWaaM0KHVEICpgQ-BYwMXoECBUQPA&biw=1366&bih=625

Durakovic. A. (2017). Medical effects of a transuranic "dirty bomb. *Military Medicine, 182*(3–4), e1591–e1595. https://academic.oup.com/milmed/article/182/3-4/e1591/4099766.

E'cole Polytechnic Massacre. (n.d.) Retrieved from https://www.google.com/search?rlz=1C1VFKB_enUS639US706&biw=1366&bih=625&ei=XdJ8Xu2GO8a_tQb04LWgBg&q=university+of+montreal+mass acre&oq=University+&gs_l=psy-ab.1.3.0i273j0i67l5j0l2j0i67j0.30855.35103..43991...0.2..3.164.1622.13j5......0....1..gws-wiz.....6..0i71j0i362i308i154i357j0i131j0i131i67.OgQacNv91yw

Federal Bureau of Investigation. (2020). *Terrorism.* https://www.fbi.gov/investigate/terrorism

Harris, T. (n.d.) How dirty bombs work. https://science.howstuffworks.com/dirty-bomb.htm

Khobar Massacre. (n.d.) Retrieved from https://www.google.com/search?sa=X&rlz=1C1VFKB_enUS639US706&q=2004+Khobar+massacre&stick=H4sIAAAAAAAAAONgFuLUz9U3MKwyLqpQAj

ONjZNzs7QEXDKLE4tLUouCM1NSyxMrixexihgZGJgoeGfkJyUWKeQmFhcnJhel7mBlBACMEvB
rRAAAAA&ved=2ahUKEwj7-rXQwbjoAhWSbc0KHUMSBW4QxA0wFHoECBMQCw&biw=136
6&bih=625

Las Vegas Shooting. (n.d.) Retrieved from https://www.google.com/search?rlz=1C1VFKB_enUS639US706
&biw=1366&bih=625&ei=EdJ8Xo-fBIeQtAbN5J-oCA&q=las+vegas+massacre&oq=Las&gs_l=psy-
ab.1.0.0i67l2j0l2j0i131j0l3j0i131j0.67881.71681..75308...0.0..1.147.1425.9j6......0....1..gws-wiz.....6..0i8i
30j0i22i30j0i362i308i154i357j0i273._W2dYw0W72Y

Madrid Train Bombings.(n.d.) Retrieved from https://www.google.com/search?rlz=1C1VFKB_enUS639US7
06&biw=1366&bih=625&ei=gNF8Xt_7BZOStAaRp6TgCQ&q=atlanta+olympics+bombing&oq=A
tlanta+O&gs_l=psy-ab.1.1.0j0i131j0l7j0i131.23310.29276..34668...0.0..0.152.2369.24j4......0....1..gws-
wiz.....6..0i67j0i7i30j0i362i308i154i357j0i131i67j0i273.aZYxdIYP4Qs

Oklahoma City Bombing. (n.d.) Retrieved from https://www.google.com/search?sa=X&rlz=1C1VFKB_
enUS639US706&q=Oklahoma+City+bombing&stick=H4sIAAAAAAAAAONgFuLSz9U3KDGpys6
rVOIAsU1z08q1BFwyixOLS1KLgjNTUssTK4sXsYr6Z-ckZuTnJio4Z5ZUKiTl5yZl5qXvYGUEALsY
BapFAAAA&ved=2ahUKEwimiPiDwLjoAhXPHM0KHdR0AfUQxA0wHHoECBMQCQ&biw=13
66&bih=625

Powers, M., Monson, M. J. E., Zimmerman, F. S., Einov, S., & Dries, D. J. (2019). Anthropogenic disasters.
Critical Care Clinics, 35(4), 647–658. https://www.ncbi.nlm.nih.gov/pubmed/31445611.

Torres, F. (2020).What is posttraumatic stress disorder? https://www.psychchiatry.org/patients-families/ptsd/
what-is-ptsd

Pulse Nightclub Shooting. (n.d.) Retrieved from https://www.google.com/search?sa=X&rlz=1C1VFKB_
enUS639US706&q=Orlando+nightclub+shooting&stick=H4sIAAAAAAAAAONgFuLVT9c3N
EwzNDIyNCrOVoJwk6qKstOrUky0BFwyixOLS1KLgjNTUssTK4sXsUr5F-Uk5qXkK-RlpmeUJ
OeUJikUZ-Tnl2Tmpe9gZQQQARhbrrlIAAAA&ved=2ahUKEwja0d7BvrjoAhVPV80KHRbqD
cEQ-BYwLXoECBYQKg&biw=1366&bih=625

Sandy Hook Elementary School Shooting. (n.d.) Retrieved from https://www.google.com/search?rlz=
1C1VFKB_enUS639US706&q=Sandy+Hook+Elementary+School+shooting&stick=H4sIAAA
AAAAAAONgFuLVT9c3NEwzNDIyNCrOVuLSz9U3KDA2ySnJ0BJwySxOLC5JLQrOTEk
tT6wsXsSqGpyYl1Kp4JGfn63gmpOam5pXklhUqRCcnJGfn6NQDCRLMvPSd7AyAgBmFy8-WgAA
AA&sa=X&ved=2ahUKEwicmoGGvrjoAhUcIDQIHWT9CkwQxA0wF3oECBQQBQ&biw=1366&
bih=625

September 11 Attacks. (n.d.) Retrieved from https://www.google.com/search?sa=X&rlz=1C1VFKB_
enUS639US706&q=September+11+attacks&stick=H4sIAAAAAAAAAONgFuLUz9U3MMquKEx
RAjNTDMoKjLWks5Ot9FPLUvNK9FMyixOLS1KLrIozU1LLEyuLF7GKBKcWlKTmJqqUWKRga
KiSWlCQmZxfvYGUEAIkfOeZPAAAA&ved=2ahUKEwi5irnywLjoAhUEa80KHerQCS0Q-BYwH
XoECBUQIw&biw=1366&bih=625

United Nations Office on Drugs and Crime. (2020). *About the United Nations Office on Drugs and Crime.*
https://www.unodc.org/unodc/en/about-unodc/index.html

US Environmental Protection Agency. (2016). *The Love Canal tragedy.* https://archive.epa.gov/epa/aboutepa/
love-canal-tragedy.html

US Nuclear Regulatory Commission. (2018). *Backgrounder on the Three Mile Island accident.* https://www.nrc.
gov/reading-rm/doc-collections/fact-sheets/3mile-isle.html

Virginia Tech Shooting. (n.d.) Retrieved from https://www.google.com/search?rlz=1C1VFKB_enUS63
9US706&q=Virginia+Tech+shooting&stick=H4sIAAAAAAAAAONgecRYyC3w8sc9YamMSWt
OXmNM4uIKzsgvd80rySpFNLgYoOy5Lj4pLj0c_UNjApziw2TNBikeLiQ-EpaRjK7Lk07xyYmyA
AE2xxCHZQ4ORnA4IG9FoMDY9O-FYfYWDgYBRh4FrGKhWUWpWfmZSYqhKQmZygUZ
Tnl2TmpQMAz5_W5o8AAAA&sa=X&ved=2ahUKEwi71e6Tw7joAhWGXc0KHZcSC4gQ6RMwF
XoECA0QBA&biw=1366&bih=625

Williams, M., Armstrong, L., & Sizemore, D. C. (2020). Biologic, chemical and radiation terrorism review.
StatPearls [Internet] https://www.ncbi.nlm.nih.gov/books/NBK493217/.

Anticipating the Future:
Brainstorming Exercises

Anticipating the Future: Hazard Vulnerability Analysis and Resource Assessment

Joanne C. Langan, PhD, RN, CNE

CHAPTER OUTLINE

Introduction 239

Disasters: Global Events 239

Nurses Recognized for Honesty and Ethics 240

Obligation To The Public 240

Participating in Disaster Planning and Preparedness Activities 240

Hazard Vulnerabilty Analysis 241

Facility Assessment 241

Tools For Measuring Vulnerability To Hazards 242

Brainstorming in Anticipation of Future Disaster Events 243

Sustainability Lists Of Resources And Assets 243

US Example of Strategic National Stockpile 244

Case in Point 244

Applying a Hazard Vulnerability Assessment Tool 244

Questions for Discussion 244

Possible Responses 245

Points to Remember 245

Test Your Knowledge 245

References 246

OBJECTIVES

After reading and studying this chapter, you should be able to:

- Identify existing hazards to human health in your community.
- Apply the point scoring schematic to determine the hazards that are most threatening to your community.
- Describe how hazard vulnerability analysis informs disaster and emergency planning efforts.
- Evaluate the membership of the disaster preparedness team at your agency to determine the inclusiveness of the health care team's representation.

capability inventory: Assesses a community's resources and its ability to respond to the consequences of disasters.

hazard vulnerability chart: Tool used in planning for disasters that addresses types of emergencies, the probability of each emergency's occurrence, human impact, property impact, business impact, and internal and external resources. High scores indicate that the agency should develop additional contingency plans.

vulnerability analysis: Assesses the potential consequences of disasters that are likely to occur within the community.

Introduction

Although we cannot anticipate all disasters that will occur on a local, state, country, or global level, there are tools to assist in preparing for and mitigating the effects of disasters. This chapter discusses the importance of nurse and other health care professionals' involvement in disaster planning and preparedness. A key tool in the planning and preparedness process is the use of the hazard vulnerability analysis. The tool and essential elements in its proper use are presented.

Disasters: Global Events

Unfortunately, multiple tragedies and disasters are reported on a daily basis around the globe. Natural disasters, terrorist attacks, disease outbreaks, cyber-attacks, and war are among those events that occur all too frequently around the world. Although it is impossible to predict all of the events that will occur, it is prudent to anticipate some of those most likely to occur and what will be needed to be prepared for them, to mitigate their effects, and to build resilience to recover from them (Fig. 13.1). Mass media coverage of recent disaster events and public health emergencies suggests that most individuals are aware of the threats of disasters to themselves and their families. However, a recent survey in the United States indicated that more than half (51%) of the adult citizens polled do not have an emergency plan in place (Healthcare Ready, 2019). Many people across the globe rely on their governments to support them during an emergency. An emergency management person stated after Hurricane Katrina that "emergency management

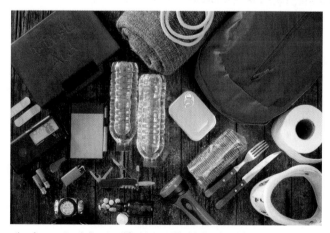

Fig. 13.1   Preparation for a natural disaster. (iStock.com/GulcinRagiboglu)

personnel are experiencing the same disaster and its effects as the citizens the agencies are charged to protect." These government agencies often become overwhelmed as the result of the disaster event and "the agency assets (equipment and personnel) are often damaged or incapacitated and unable to offer assistance" (C. Butler, personal communication, June 1, 2009).

Robert Glasser is the former representative of the Secretary General for Disaster Risk Reduction and head of the United Nations International Strategy for Disaster Reduction (UNISDR). To emphasize the importance of disaster planning, in 2016 Glasser stated:

If you see that we're already spending huge amounts of money and are unable to meet the humanitarian need—and then you overlay that with not just population growth…[but] you put climate change on top of that, where we're seeing an increase in the frequency and severity of natural disasters, and the knock-on effects with respect to food security and conflict and new viruses like the Zika virus…you realise that the only way we're going to be able to deal with these trends is by getting out ahead of them and focusing on reducing disaster risk. (*The Guardian*, 2016, para. 4)

All disaster response begins on the local level. Therefore, preparedness efforts must begin on the local level and consider the vulnerabilities of each community in planning efforts to reduce the disaster risk. Hospitals and other health care organizations; community groups; and the state, local, and territorial governments should convene standing disaster and public health emergency planning committees. These committees have broad representation across disciplines and often include emergency managers; local politicians; health care providers; and representatives from the government, tribal agencies, or ministries of health. Nurses can bring an important perspective to disaster preparedness and should be encouraged to participate as important members of these planning teams. As advocates for organizational and community disaster preparedness, nurses can bring their knowledge of health care systems and clinical care to the forefront of planning efforts.

Nurses Recognized for Honesty and Ethics

A 2019 Gallup poll asked adults in the United States to rate the degree of honesty and ethical standards of people in different professional fields. Nurses were rated highest for the 18th year in a row. In this poll, 85% of Americans indicated nurses' honesty and ethical standards as "very high" or "high." The same poll indicated that medical doctors, pharmacists, and dentists have high levels of these qualities as well (Reinhart, 2020).

OBLIGATION TO THE PUBLIC

With health care professionals being held in such high esteem, it follows that these professionals should uphold the sense of obligation to the public to be well informed about potential disasters and knowledgeable of the correct actions to take and to advise others (Fig. 13.2). The general public will seek the advice of health care professionals to direct their actions in a variety of circumstances, not the least of which are biological, radiological, or chemical terrorist threats. Communities across the globe will want to know if they should be taking medications prophylactically or in response to an exposure. They will need to know if the medications are available to them, the cost, age-appropriate dosage, length of time to take the medications, and risks versus benefits of not taking the medications.

PARTICIPATING IN DISASTER PLANNING AND PREPAREDNESS ACTIVITIES

Nurses are an integral part of the health care team in disaster response and recovery and should also be "at the table" during disaster preparedness activities. A key activity during the preparedness phase of the disaster cycle is assessment of vulnerabilities for each community or potential

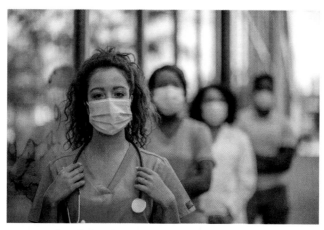

Fig. 13.2 A diverse group of medical professionals outside a hospital wear protective face masks. (iStock. com/FatCamera)

consequences of disasters that are likely to occur within the community and its ability to cope with these consequences. These functions are called vulnerability analysis and capability inventory. How well a community is able to adapt or respond to a disaster is largely dependent on the inventory of its resources that will be needed in a response. A hazard vulnerability analysis (HVA) is a useful tool in the assessment of the potential risks and consequences of disasters that are likely to occur within the community. The US Department of Health and Human Services' (2020) HVA definition refers to the process of "identifying risks that are most likely to have an impact on a healthcare facility and the surrounding community." The goal of the risk assessment is to inform organizations, such as hospitals and emergency management entities, of the greatest risks they face and areas of vulnerability in the event of natural disasters or other civil hazards. A thorough HVA should guide organizations toward the areas of greatest risk so that they can focus attention and resources on risk mitigation efforts. The community disaster planning committee maps the locations of nuclear power or chemical plants, rivers, dams, bridges, and other potential hazards to human health. The planning also takes note of hospitals, schools, nursing homes, and emergency facilities to identify those who are most vulnerable. Health care agencies assess what is needed and predict what additional resources will be needed in the event of a disaster in order to meet patient needs and maintain utilities such as communication, water, power, and other basic functions. The inventory of resources will suggest how well a community is able to adapt or respond to a disaster. A hazard vulnerability chart is a useful tool to complete the vulnerability assessment. (see Appendices A and B.)

Hazard Vulnerabilty Analysis

FACILITY ASSESSMENT

To prepare for a massive disaster with large numbers of casualties, hospitals and other health care facilities need to assess their ability to meet patient needs and to maintain basic operational functions well in advance of the event occurring (Fig. 13.3). The organizational disaster plans that are developed should include processes for the rapid discharge or evacuation of patients and some prediction of the organization's capacity for a sudden surge in demand for health care and the admission of disaster victims. It is possible that the health care facility may be unable to operate due to internal damage sustained from the event. A seminal tool, the *Mass Casualty*

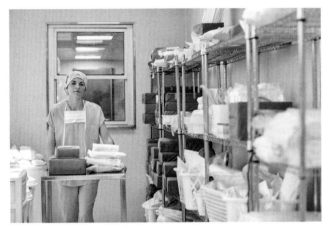

Fig. 13.3   A doctor with medical supplies in a storage room. (iStock.com/MorsalImages)

Disaster Plan Checklist: A Template for Healthcare Facilities (World Health Organization [WHO], 2001), is very effective in assessing the agency's ability to respond to major disasters or public health emergencies. This tool was originally written by the security team for the 2000 Olympics in Sydney, Australia, to assess its readiness for disasters. The original document was modified by the Association for Professionals in Infection Control and Epidemiology's Bioterrorism Task Force and the Institute for Biosecurity at Saint Louis University. It is important that assessments also include a plan to obtain background data for both victims and rescue personnel. Public health departments will collect this data, including medical needs, lodging, water, sanitation, and feeding arrangements. An excellent assessment tool, the *Hospital Disaster Preparedness Self-Assessment Tool*, is published by the American College of Emergency Physicians (2013). A more recent disaster and emergency preparedness tool, the *Hospital Emergency Response Checklist*, is published by the WHO (2011). An additional preparedness tool kit is published by Ready.gov (2019).

TOOLS FOR MEASURING VULNERABILITY TO HAZARDS

Tools to measure a health care organization's hazards and vulnerabilities and instructions for completion and sample worksheets are found in this chapter (see Appendix A, Kaiser Permanente Medical Center [2014], and Appendix B, Federal Emergency Management Agency [2014]). The instruction sheets guide users through the analysis of considering potential hazards and the impact each event might have on the daily operations of each agency. A number of elements are considered in this type of analysis.

Types of emergency—identifies types of emergencies that have a historical, geographical, technological, or other likelihood of occurrence in a specific area

Probability—rates the likelihood of each emergency's occurrence

Preparedness—status of current plans and training, insurance, availability of backup systems and community resources

Response—time to assemble an on-scene response, capability of response and historical data related to response success

Human impact—analyzes the potential human impact of each emergency, the potential for death or injury

Property impact—considers the potential property losses and damages, considering cost to replace, cost to set up temporary replacements, and cost to repair

Business impact—considers the potential impact on the agency's ability to provide services to patients, assesses the impact of employees' inability to report to work, patients' inability to reach the facility, interruption of critical supplies, ability to reach patients or transport them, and the impact on utility services supplying the agency

Internal and external resources—examines each type of emergency from beginning to end by asking: "Do we have the needed resources and capabilities to respond?" and "Will external resources be able to respond to us in this emergency as quickly as we may need them to or will they have other priority areas to serve?"

High scores indicate that the agency should develop additional contingency plans (Kaiser Permanente Medical Center, 2014).

Brainstorming in Anticipation of Future Disaster Events

Having completed the HVA, health care facilities and community planners need collaborative efforts in brainstorming about required resources and assets to maintain life and function. Critical functional categories include communications, managing resources and assets, safety and security, staffing, utilities, and clinical activities. A comprehensive list of resources and assets should be identified and included in each critical category and any potential points of systems failure also should be identified. These points of failure could include a power failure or loss of water, ventilation, or air conditioning. Next, based on the HVA and the assessment of available resources, a determination should be made as to the realistic amount of time that the organization can be expected to sustain its own operations. Most entities will need to be self-sufficient for at least 96 hours before additional support or assets can arrive to assist in the disaster relief effort.

SUSTAINABILITY LISTS OF RESOURCES AND ASSETS

Some of the key resources and assets needed to be self-sufficient for at least 96 hours are listed. This list should not be considered exhaustive, and ultimately the needed resources will vary across organizations and communities. Thus, this list should be considered carefully and customized to meet the needs of each health care entity.

Redundant communications—landline and cellular phone service, computer function, overhead paging, batteries, satellite phone service, and any other emergency communications strategies

Supply logistics—linen supplies, cleaning cloths and wipes, hand sanitizer, enzymatic cleaner, bleach, sterile processing department (SPD) materials, food (perishable and nonperishable), paper products (patient and general), medical waste containers, hazardous waste containers, personal protective equipment (PPE), N-95 respirators, disposable gowns, gloves, foot covers, powered air-purifying respirators (PAPRs), Level C chemical suits, nitrile gloves, protective boots, patient decontamination kits, disposable stethoscopes

Safety and security—fire alarm systems, barricades, security officer equipment (vests, batons), TASERs, fixed decontamination showers, tent decontamination showers, visitor labels or tags, security door-locking systems with badge-only access or alarms for elopement

Staffing—physicians, registered nurses (RNs), licensed practical nurses (LPNs), medical technologists, pharmacists, pharmacy technologists, surgical teams, security, human resources (HR), environmental services, plant operations, employee health, sterile processing, health technology management (HTM), information technology (IT), interactive health technology (IHT), laboratory, blood bank, administration

Utilities—emergency backup generator, domestic hot water, steam pressure, building heat, natural gas, propane, potable (domestic cold) water, nonpotable water or process water, chiller system, boiler system, elevators, bulk oxygen, medical air, medical vacuum, nitrogen

Clinical activities—medications, intravenous (IV) fluids, medical supplies, bandages, isopropyl alcohol (IPA) wipes, surgical supplies, blood, blood products, surgical packs, sutures

US Example of Strategic National Stockpile

In the event that local, state, tribal, or territorial responders need federal assistance to augment their response efforts, they may request supplies from the Strategic National Stockpile (SNS). The SNS is the United States' largest supply of pharmaceuticals and medical supplies. It is used for public health emergencies where local entities cannot meet demand. This supply is prepositioned in select communities across the United States, and additional stores can be delivered simultaneously to multiple large-scale emergency events or a variety of public health threats (US Department of Health and Human Services, 2019). The SNS ensures the availability and rapid deployment of necessary pharmaceuticals, antidotes, medical supplies, and equipment to respond to events involving nerve agents, biological pathogens, and chemical agents. The packages are stored in strategic locations, which enables rapid deliver if the need arises. The stockpiles are designed to bolster the area's response. For example, if evidence shows that there has been an overt release of an agent that negatively affects public health, the state requests deployment of supplies. The appropriate medications and supplies are determined based on the identification of the hazardous substance or agent.

Obvious recurring themes throughout this text follow the nursing process closely—assessment, planning, intervention, and evaluation as a continuous cycle. Those who are engaged in disaster preparedness, response, and recovery know this continuous cycle well and have learned to apply lessons learned to save lives and property. All who support these efforts are to be commended.

Case in Point
APPLYING A HAZARD VULNERABILITY ASSESSMENT TOOL

The People's Hospital is located on an island in the South Pacific. A new director of nursing has been hired to lead the nurses in the hospital and specialized personnel. She has experience with disaster preparedness from her previous hospital, but that hospital was in the United States and the disaster threats were very different. She plans to lead a discussion with hospital department heads regarding the organization's hazards and vulnerabilities so that she can be prepared in her new role and to assist the other leaders in preparedness activities. In this way, they will enhance their collaborative relationship and select response and recovery strategies for possible future disaster events that affect their hospital's community and its people.

Use the hazard vulnerability assessment tools in Appendices A and B to assess the risk of each natural hazard for this area.

Questions for Discussion

1. What are the three most likely natural disasters that could affect this region?
2. Are mitigation efforts in effect for each of these three most likely natural disasters?
3. What would you advise this hospital regarding preparedness efforts based on the findings of this assessment?

Possible Responses

The scoring of the hazard vulnerability assessment tool (Kaiser Permanente Medical Center [2014] or Appendix B tools) may vary based on the participant's perception of threats and vulnerability. The most likely natural disasters that could affect this region are directly related to the island's location—rain, flooding, fires, tsunamis, hurricanes, storm surge, earthquakes, and possibly volcanoes. Mitigation efforts will be determined by the participant's perception and indication of the level of mitigation efforts. Advising the hospital should include an assessment of structural integrity, contingency plans for staffing, alternate care sites, evacuation of the hospital and possibly of the island, and memoranda of agreement with other health care facilities or providers on the island.

Points to Remember

- The hazard vulnerability analysis provides data to inform disaster and emergency planning efforts.
- Mitigation involves the efforts taken to reduce risk from those identified hazards that are most likely to affect a community.
- Nurses and other health care providers are essential members of the disaster preparedness team.

Test Your Knowledge

1. It is important for nurses to be knowledgeable about disaster planning and response because: *(Choose all that apply.)*
   a. Nurses will be tested on such knowledge during annual competency exams
   b. Nurses traditionally have been sought out by neighbors, friends, and communities for health care information and advice
   c. Nurses have a responsibility to teach Emergency Medical Services workers
   d. Professional nurses historically have responded to the needs of society, including in times of disaster
2. A key to effective disaster management is:
   a. Having enough managers on the planning team
   b. Anticipating the probable disasters and planning for them
   c. Postdisaster mitigation
   d. Postdisaster reconstruction teams
3. An effective risk assessment informs proposed actions by focusing attention and resources on the greatest risks. Some of the basic components of a risk assessment are: *(Choose all that apply.)*
   a. Hazard identification
   b. Profiling of personnel skills
   c. Inventory of assets
   d. Estimation of potential human and economic losses
4. A hazard identification and risk assessment provides:
   a. Reassurance to the community that certain hazards will not occur
   b. A factual basis for activities proposed in hazard mitigation
   c. Leaders with a plan for preparedness and response
   d. A strategy for hiring disaster preparedness personnel
5. Nurses should be involved in disaster preparedness, response, and recovery efforts because: *(Choose all that apply.)*

    a. The general public trust nurses

    b. Nurses have the knowledge to provide input in disaster planning

    c. Nurses have an obligation to the public to be well informed

    d. The general public will seek the advice of nurses to direct them in appropriate actions to take

6. In the United States Midwest, a small community hospital is located in a low-lying area within a mile of a river. The hospital's disaster preparedness committee likely will score which hazard as "high" on the vulnerability scale?

    a. Flooding

    b. Tsunami

    c. Tidal wave

    d. Hurricane

7. After a disaster or public health emergency in a community, it is advisable to have supplies and backup resources for at least 96 hours because:

    a. Most hospitals cannot stock more than 96 hours' worth of supplies

    b. It may take as long as 96 hours for outside relief to arrive to help the community

    c. Most communities do not want "outsiders" within their agencies in the first 96 hours

    d. The Federal Emergency Management Agency (FEMA) will organize the local response for the first 96 hours

8. The Strategic National Stockpile:

    a. Contains personal protective equipment (PPE) specifically for radiological events

    b. Contains medicines and supplies for those who need them most during an emergency

    c. Contains enough supplies for one major event every 6 months

    d. Contains equipment and plans to create temporary hospitals in disaster-prone areas

9. Which of the following are considered essential items in the category of clinical activities when selecting 96-hour sustainability resources and assets? *(Choose all that apply.)*

    a. Medications

    b. IV fluids

    c. Blood and blood products

    d. Clean uniforms for staff

10. The hazard vulnerability analysis informs disaster and emergency planning efforts. If the HVA indicates a high risk of flooding, reasonable mitigation efforts would include: *(Choose all that apply.)*

    a. Relocate high-value items to higher floors

    b. Relocate portable electronic equipment to safe areas

    c. Place external heating, ventilation, and air conditioning (HVAC) systems on the roof when designing the new building tower

    d. Shut off the air intake vents until heavy rains have stopped

References

American College of Emergency Physicians. (2013). *Hospital disaster preparedness self-assessment tool*. California Hospital Association. https://www.calhospitalprepare.org/post/hospital-disaster-preparedness-self-assessment-tool.

Federal Emergency Management Agency. (2014). *Risk assessment table*. https://www.fema.gov/media-library-data/1389015304392-877968832e918982635147890260624d/Business_RiskAssessmentTable_2014.pdf

Guardian, The. (2016, April 24). *World heading for catastrophe over natural disasters, risk expert warns*. https://www.theguardian.com/global-development/2016/apr/24/world-heading-for-catastrophe-over-natural-disasters-risk-expert-warns

Healthcare Ready. (2019, May 29). *USA: Poll reveals lack of preparedness in the face of increasingly frequent disasters*. PreventionWeb. https://www.preventionweb.net/news/view/66591

Kaiser Permanente Medical Center. (2014). *Hazard and vulnerability analysis.* California Hospital Association. https://www.calhospitalprepare.org/post/hazard-vulnerability-analysis-tool.

Ready.Gov. (2019). *Community preparedness toolkit.* https://www.ready.gov/community-preparedness-toolkit

Reinhart, R. J. (2020). *Nurses continue to rate highest in honesty, ethics.* Gallup. https://news.gallup.com/poll/274673/nurses-continue-rate-highest-honesty-ethics.aspx?version=prin.

US Department of Health and Human Services. (2019). *Strategic National Stockpile.* https://www.phe.gov/about/sns/Pages/default.aspx

US Department of Health and Human Services. (2020). Hazard vulnerability/risk assessment. https://asprtracie.hhs.gov/technical-resources/3/hazard-vulnerability-risk-assessment/1

World Health Organization. (2001). *Mass casualty disaster plan checklist: A template for healthcare facilities.* https://www.who.int/hac/techguidance/tools/5.8%20Mass%20Casualty%20disasterplan.pdf

World Health Organization. (2011). *Hospital emergency response checklist.* http://www.euro.who.int/en/health-topics/emergencies/disaster-preparedness-and-response/publications/2011/hospital-emergency-response-checklist-2011

CHAPTER 14

Exercises and Drills

Lavonne M. Adams, PhD, RN, CCRN-K

CHAPTER OUTLINE

Introduction   249
Types of Exercises   249
Exercise Design   250
Simulation   254
Exercise Evaluation   257
Planning Resources   257
Case in Point   258

Putting a Preparedness Plan to the
  Test: Taking a Plan from Paper to
  Implementation   258
  Questions for Discussion   259
Points to Remember   259
Test Your Knowledge   259
References   260

OBJECTIVES

After reading and studying this chapter, you should be able to:
- Describe the purpose of disaster exercises.
- Describe two main categories of disaster exercises.
- Compare and contrast common types of disaster exercises.
- Describe key elements of exercise planning, implementation, and evaluation.

KEY TERMS

after-action report: A review of previously undertaken actions as part of role performance evaluation and process improvement. It is used to make recommendations to improve standard procedures and an agency's ability to respond to future disasters.

discussion-based exercises: Activities in which participants from a single organization talk through disaster plans, policies, and procedures.

drill: An operations-based exercise focused on a specific capability, designed to validate a specific capability within a single organization; may also be used to support training on new equipment or maintenance of current skills.

fidelity: The degree to which an activity replicates reality and encompasses the physical, psychological, and environmental dimensions of a real-world event.

full-scale exercise: An operations-based exercise in a realistic real-time scenario often involving multiple agencies or jurisdictions in real-time activity and resource mobilization and in operationalizing cooperative systems such as the incident command system

(ICS) or Unified Command. Often described as the most complex and resource-intensive of the disaster exercise types.

functional exercise: An operations-based exercise in a realistic, real-time scenario that may involve either a single agency or multiple agencies. Resources typically are not fully mobilized. Designed to test and evaluate capabilities and multiple functions in a simulated high-stress environment.

operations-based exercises: Full-scale live exercises in which multiple entities deploy resources in real-time response to a simulated event.

simulation: An educational strategy in which a particular set of conditions is created or replicated to resemble authentic situations that are possible in real life.

tabletop exercise: A discussion-based exercise using a hypothetical scenario in a low-stress setting, designed to improve understanding of and assess emergency preparedness plans, policies, and procedures; also used to identify areas of strength and the need for improvement.

Introduction

To meet a community's health needs effectively after a disaster, first responders, health care professionals, and volunteers must work together within a strong and interconnected infrastructure and systems, implementing plans that address all phases of the disaster cycle. Plans and procedures must be tested and validated, and health care professionals must practice their assigned roles prior to an actual disaster or public health emergency. Activities ranging from discussion-based to full-scale live exercises offer opportunities to test and train in a low-risk environment. Exercises play a crucial role in preparedness and should be used to promote continuous improvement and enhance capabilities across the disaster cycle.

Emergency preparedness exercises are activities designed to train, monitor, or evaluate the capabilities of participants through response to a simulated event (World Health Organization [WHO], 2017). They are key elements in validating and testing plans, identifying gaps in plans so that improvements can be made, familiarizing participants with their roles, and fostering relationships with stakeholders (McCormick et al., 2014; Vasa et al., 2019). Well-designed exercises allow participants the opportunity to perform disaster roles and simulate plan implementation realistically yet with minimal risk (McCormick et al., 2014; Vasa et al., 2019). They are often divided into two main categories: discussion-based exercises and operations-based exercises. They range from activities in which participants from a single organization talk through disaster plans, policies, and procedures to full-scale live exercises in which multiple entities deploy resources in real-time response to a simulated event (Australian Institute for Disaster Resilience [AIDR], 2012; WHO, 2017).

Types of Exercises

Discussion-based exercises provide a means to develop new plans and procedures or to evaluate and improve existing plans and procedures. During these exercises, participants respond to events that potentially would arise during a disaster-related scenario. Their responses serve as the basis for evaluation of outcomes and critique of disaster-related communication, coordination, and partnership agreements. Lessons learned during these exercises can be documented and used to adapt and improve existing plans, policies, and procedures or to develop new ones if necessary. Examples include seminars, workshops, tabletop exercises (TTXs), and games (Federal Emergency Management Agency [FEMA], 2020; Pan American Health Organization [PAHO], 2011).

As with discussion-based exercises, operations-based exercises involve the use of a disaster-related scenario to evaluate outcomes of existing disaster plans; determine effective performance

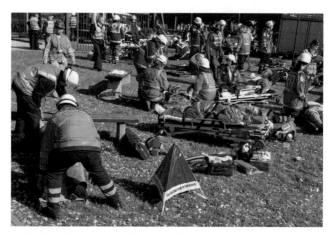

Fig. 14.1 Example of a full-scale exercise. In Wiesbaden, Germany, members of German rescue services take care of many seriously injured persons at a casualty collection point during a large antiterrorism and disaster management exercise with German and US Special Forces and emergency services. Approximately 75 actors portray wounded or injured people after being prepared by a special team of makeup artists. (iStock.com\ollo)

of disaster-related roles, communication, and partnership agreements; and use results of the exercises to improve existing plans and procedures. Operations-based exercises include drills, functional exercises, and full-scale exercises. The disaster scenarios include replication of disaster situations and require real-time communication and deployment of personnel and physical resources (Fig. 14.1). Thus, operations-based scenarios allow for greater understanding of organizational and individual capacity for disaster response through identification of response barriers and resource gaps and through clarification of disaster-related roles and responsibilities (FEMA, 2020; PAHO, 2011).

Tabletop exercises and games are among the most commonly used discussion-based exercises and drills, functional exercises, and full-scale exercises are examples of operations-based exercises. Table 14.1 provides a comparison of some of the most commonly used exercise approaches, including description, format, advantages, and disadvantages of each.

Exercise Design

No matter what type, size, or approach used, each exercise will involve common principles for planning, implementation, and evaluation. Elements essential to exercise design include needs assessment; establishing exercise purpose, scope, objectives, and evaluation parameters; scenario creation, and developing a plan for documentation, outcome evaluation, and performance improvement (AIDR, 2012; FEMA, 2020; WHO, 2017). Other items crucial to consider include organizational commitment, time and resources available for the exercise, and media or public affairs involvement (FEMA, 2020; WHO, 2017).

Needs assessment is crucial to clarify understanding of the local community's priority risks and hazards, articulate reasons to conduct the exercise, and determine the specific function to be tested. Ideally, the needs assessment will build on existing systems, plans, or capabilities and should consider analysis of after-action reports from previous exercises (FEMA, 2020; WHO, 2017). An after-action report is a review of previously undertaken actions as part of a process of performance evaluation and improvement. It is used to make recommendations to improve standard procedures and an agency's ability to respond to future disasters (US Department of Homeland Security, 2018). A thorough needs assessment will serve to inform design of the most appropriate scenario to meet exercise purpose and objectives.

TABLE 14.1 ■ Commonly-Used Discussion-Based and Operations-Based Exercises

	Tabletop Exercise (TTX)	Game	Drill	Functional Exercise	Full-Scale Exercise
Description and Purpose	Discussion-based exercise using a hypothetical scenario in a low-stress setting. Designed to improve understanding of and assess emergency preparedness plans, policies, and procedures; also used to identify areas of strength and need for improvement.	Discussion-based exercise applying structured play to a simulated scenario, also referred to as "serious games." Designed to simulate and analyze the consequences of problem solving, decisions, and actions; reinforce team training; enhance team building; and promote the improvement of capabilities.	Operations-based exercise focused on a specific capability. Designed to validate a specific capability within a single organization (such as a hospital performing a fire drill). May also be used to support training on new equipment or maintenance of current skills	Operations-based exercise in a realistic, real-time scenario that may involve either a single agency or multiple agencies; resources are typically not fully mobilized. Designed to test and evaluate capabilities and multiple functions in a simulated high-stress environment	Operations-based exercise in a realistic, real-time scenario often involving multiple agencies or jurisdictions in real-time activity and resource mobilization, operationalizing cooperative systems such as the incident command system (ICS) or Unified Command. Often described as the most complex and resource intensive of the exercise types. • Often builds on previous discussion-based or smaller operations-based exercises. Designed to implement and analyze plans, policies, and procedures in a high-stress environment. • Allows participants to demonstrate roles and responsibilities outlined in plans and procedures. • Analyzes coordination between multiple entities.

Continued

TABLE 14.1 ■ Commonly-Used Discussion-Based and Operations-Based Exercises—Cont'd

	Tabletop Exercise (TTX)	Game	Drill	Functional Exercise	Full-Scale Exercise
Format	A scenario describing a simulated event is presented by a facilitator, typically in the form of a case study that includes a list of problems. Participants apply knowledge and skills to problem solve through group discussion. Actions do not occur in real-time. Resolution is documented for later analysis.	The game is designed to portray a simulated event and scenario data, rules, and procedures are introduced to individual players or teams. Activities and decision making may be pre-scripted or allow for dynamic adjustment. Speed, stress level, and consequences of decision making will vary based on the exercise's design and objectives.	Requires existence of clearly defined plans and procedures May be conducted singly or in a series	A realistic exercise scenario that typically uses a scripted event series with updates that require rapid problem solving Typically involves a controller to manage the scenario and evaluators to observe behaviors and compare them against established plans, policies, procedures, and standard practices	A realistic exercise scenario that typically uses a scripted event series with complex updates that require rapid problem solving. Typically involves a controller to manage the scenario and evaluators to observe behaviors and compare them against established plans, policies, procedures, and standard practices.
Advantages	Generally low-stress. Particularly useful to validate plans and explore procedural weaknesses. Provides an opportunity for in-depth problem solving and discussion. Relatively inexpensive with the exception of participant time.	Does not require expenditure of physical disaster resources. Allows a safe environment in which players can: • Evaluate and critique existing plans using a "what if" approach. • Identify critical decision-making points and analyze consequences of decisions and actions. • Identify and try out potential strategies.	Allows for immediate feedback Allows for a specific narrow focus in a realistic environment Results can be measured against established benchmarks	Offers a realistic environment for testing of plans, procedures, and capabilities. Experiential learning offers participants the opportunity to gain confidence by testing their skills and applying their training in a realistic event. Provides the opportunity to strengthen cooperative relationships	Offers a realistic environment for testing of plans, procedures, and capabilities. Experiential learning offers participants the opportunity to gain confidence by testing their skills and applying their training in a realistic event. Provides the opportunity to strengthen cooperative relationships. Allows the most realistic evaluation of resources needed for the plan and identification of gaps in the plan.

TABLE 14.1 ■ **Commonly-Used Discussion-Based and Operations-Based Exercises—Cont'd**

	Tabletop Exercise (TTX)	Game	Drill	Functional Exercise	Full-Scale Exercise
Disadvantages	An experienced facilitator is needed to ensure that all participants contribute actively to discussion and problem solving. Careful planning is required.	Has specific hardware, software, and bandwidth requirements	Tests only one entity and/or one capability in isolation rather than in coordination with others.	Resource intensive, particularly human resources (controller and evaluators) and time (time-consuming to build scenario, prepare for and set up event).	Typically requires a greater level of support than needed for other types of exercises Resource-intensive due to the mobilization of staff and resources. Often requires a large space to accommodate activities. Site logistics must be closely monitored for safety.

Data from Federal Emergency Management Agency. (2020). *Homeland Security Exercise and Evaluation Program (HSEEP)*. https://www.fema.gov/media-library-data/1580929080128-43a6a087f3956a7e51ae506514598053/Homeland-Security-Exercise-and-Evaluation-Program-Doctrine2020Revision.pdf; Kerins, D., Barishansky, R.M., & Cortacans, H.P. (2012, June). *How to conduct EMS exercises and drills*. *EMS World*, 33–38; and World Health Organization. (2017). *WHO simulation exercise manual*. https://www.who.int/ihr/publications/WHO-WHE-CPI-2017.10/en/

The purpose of the exercise arises from the needs assessment and should provide a clear rationale for the activity. Factors to consider in determining the purpose include awareness of local threats or hazards, understanding of existing plans, and findings noted in previous after-action reports (FEMA, 2020). The purpose is the basis for specific objectives that will serve as the exercise's foundation and help determine its scope and scale. Clearly defined objectives support the development of specific, measurable outcomes that lead to evaluation and process improvement. The use of "SMART" criteria can be useful for both writing effective objectives and developing clear outcome criteria for evaluation (FEMA, 2020). These criteria are included by the International Nursing Association for Clinical Simulation and Learning (INACSL, 2016a) as part of its best practices for simulation. SMART criteria include the need to be:

- **S**pecific, addressing who, what, when, where, and why for each objective and including a clear time frame.
- **M**easurable, defining an outcome through various methods, including quantity, quality, cost, and change.
- **A**chievable, asking if participants can reasonably complete the objective in the proposed time frame with available resources and support.
- **R**elevant, clearly linked to the desired goal or outcome.
- **T**ime bound, identifying when each objective should be accomplished (FEMA, 2020).

Once objectives and outcome criteria have been articulated, scope can be determined. Major elements of scope include type of emergency, type of exercise, duration, location, participants and their level of participation, and functions to be practiced (FEMA, 2020; WHO, 2017). Additional key considerations include availability of resources (including human, financial, and time), impact on daily operations, stakeholder commitment, and organizational commitment. Time and money can be significant considerations. For example, a TTX takes minimal time to plan and is relatively inexpensive (although planners must consider costs related to salaries, printing, copying, and refreshments), whereas a full-scale exercise can take up to 1 year to plan and can be expensive, depending on costs associated with salaries; shift differential; overtime pay; and expenditures on fuel, food, supplies, and simulation aids (Kerins et al., 2012). Human resources involve more than salary considerations; the scope and scale of the exercise also will determine the number of people required to plan and conduct it. Large, complex exercises likely will require a team, including at least one subject-matter expert. In contrast, a small, uncomplicated exercise may require only one person (AIDR, 2012). The impact of the exercise on standard operations also must be considered; the benefits of a full-scale live exercise must be weighed against potential disruption to ongoing patient care (Wexler & Flamm, 2017). Exercise scope should be sufficient to meet the objectives of the exercise while remaining within resource capabilities.

Exercises must be seen as useful to the organization or community as well as realistic and manageable. "Dual-purpose" activities that clearly meet a community health or organizational need as well as an emergency preparedness goal may garner more commitment from participants. Nurses can play a key role in promoting interprofessional and interagency training and exercises. Nurses are essential in engaging those who can assist with such activities, including nurses who are either retired or not employed full time, students, and volunteers (Association of Public Health Nurses [APHN] Public Health Preparedness Committee, 2014; Jakeway et al., 2008). Regardless of desired outcomes, resource availability and buy-in from stakeholders ultimately may determine the type, scale, and scope of an exercise (WHO, 2017). It may be more feasible to develop an ongoing program of exercises and related activities to meet the purpose and objectives incrementally rather than to attempt a single large-scale exercise that tries to accomplish all objectives simultaneously (AIDR, 2012).

Simulation

An integral part of exercises is the use of simulation, which INACSL describes as "an educational strategy in which a particular set of conditions are created or replicated to resemble authentic situations that are possible in real life" (INACSL, 2016b, p. S44). Exercises are designed to simulate reality to varying degrees based on their stated objectives. The degree to which an activity replicates reality is fidelity, and although fidelity is often described in terms of technology use, it also encompasses physical, psychological, and environmental dimensions of a real-world event (Lioce et al., 2020). The more realism that participants perceive in the exercise, the more their psychological processes such as emotions, beliefs, and self-awareness will mimic the processes produced by a real-world event. Physical and environmental fidelity are major factors in promoting realism, and examples of items that contribute to increased fidelity include realistic room or location design, use of functional equipment, application of moulage with either complex high-fidelity manikins or simulated patients, and sensory props (Figs. 14.2, 14.3, and 14.4). Multiple simulation modalities are available and may be combined within the same scenario to enhance realism; examples include unfolding case studies, manikin-based simulation, computer- and Web-based formats, virtual reality, augmented reality, and standardized patients (Farra & Smith, 2015). The specific modalities selected will depend on exercise objectives; desired level of realism for environment, equipment, and psychological involvement of participants; and level of available simulation technology.

Medium- and high-fidelity activities often include opportunities to develop and demonstrate critical thinking, decision making, and higher skill levels such as triage and assessment through the use of standardized patients, virtual reality, augmented reality, or complex high-fidelity manikins (Farra & Smith, 2015). However, simulation success does not depend on the level of technological fidelity. For example, if exercise objectives focus on information sharing and consensus attainment for policies, plans, and procedures, low-fidelity discussion-based exercises would be both feasible and appropriate. Likewise, to meet objectives that require task-related competency checks for medication administration or dressing application, the use of a low-fidelity task trainer would be highly effective.

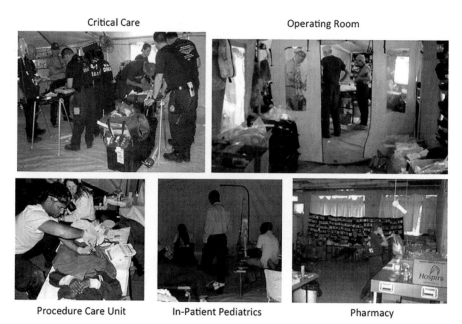

Fig. 14.2 Realism in an austere environment. (Weiner, D. L., & Rosman, S. L. [2019]. Just-in-time training for disaster response in the austere environment. *Clinical Pediatric Emergency Medicine, 20*[2], 95–110.)

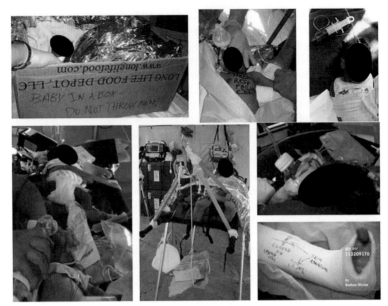

Fig. 14.3 Realistic equipment in an austere environment. (Weiner, D. L., & Rosman, S. L. [2019]. Just-in-time training for disaster response in the austere environment. *Clinical Pediatric Emergency Medicine, 20*[2], 95–110.)

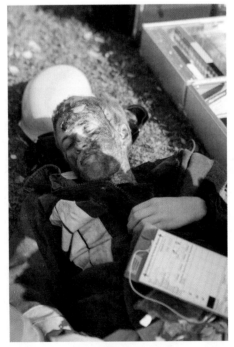

Fig. 14.4 A simulated patient. In Wiesbaden, Germany, a simulated seriously injured person with burn wounds on his face lies on a stretcher at a casualty collection point during a large antiterrorism and disaster management exercise with German and US Special Forces and rescue services. On his chest is a triage card for categorization of his injuries. (iStock.com\ollo)

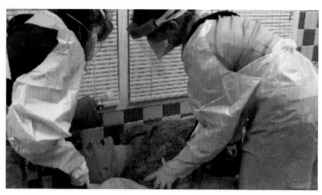

Fig.14.5   A simulation for competency attainment. (Scott, L. A., Ross, T., Davis, C. A., Tueber, J., & Seymore, A. [2013]. Competencies during chaos: Life-saving performance of patient care providers using a multi-actor, competency-based emergency preparedness curriculum. *Annals of Emergency Medicine, 62*[4], S160–S160.)

Simulation has become a key method of training for disaster response roles and assessing role performance in low-frequency, high-risk events during which it would be impractical to evaluate competency directly (Fig. 14.5). When selecting a simulation modality for training purposes, alternative media such as digital story format (Walkner et al., 2014), computer adaptive scenarios (Uden-Holman et al., 2014), and virtual reality (Farra et al., 2019) offer promise as strategies that can serve as effective training tools for individuals and groups. Such modalities have the potential to be more accessible and financially feasible than full-scale exercises. They have an added benefit of being asynchronous, which allows an individual user to review, practice, and reinforce learning.

Exercise Evaluation

Disaster preparedness depends on organizations and community stakeholders having the opportunity to operationalize disaster plans through the use of exercises, evaluate their effectiveness and pursue continuous improvement. Evaluation of exercises allows participants to identify strengths and areas for improvement and recommend corrective actions using an after-action report and improvement plan, thus serving as a vital means to enhance response capability and promote continuous improvement (AIDR, 2012; FEMA, 2020). Because it is crucial to identify operational gaps, weaknesses, and needed improvements prior to an actual event rather than during an event, participants should be encouraged to "drill to failure" rather than to focus only on "passing" to maximize the effectiveness of exercises.

Planning Resources

Guidelines, frameworks, and templates can be valuable tools to help organizations and exercise designers systematically approach the process of exercise development. Multiple resources exist; Table 14.2 provides a list of some readily available resources. Some elements of the various resources can be used in multiple countries or regions, whereas others will either be specific to a country or region or require adaptation for use. Nurses, particularly those involved with exercise design and planning processes, will find it valuable to be aware of guidelines that are setting- or location-specific as well as generic resources that can be applied to a variety of settings or locations.

TABLE 14.2 ■ Exercise Planning Resources

Source	Reference
Australian Institute for Disaster Resilience (AIDR)	Australian Institute for Disaster Resilience. (2012). *Australian disaster resilience handbook 3: Managing exercises* (2nd ed.). https://knowledge.aidr.org.au/resources/handbook-3-managing-exercises/
Centers for Disease Control and Prevention (CDC)	Centers for Disease Control and Prevention. (2018). Writing SMART objectives. *Evaluation Briefs* (3b). https://www.cdc.gov/healthyyouth/evaluation/pdf/brief3b.pdf
Federal Emergency Management Agency (FEMA)	Federal Emergency Management Agency. (2020). *Homeland Security Exercise and Evaluation Program (HSEEP)*. https://www.fema.gov/hseep, https://www.fema.gov/media-library-data/1580929080128-43a6a087f3956a7e51ae506514598053/Homeland-Security-Exercise-and-Evaluation-Program-Doctrine2020Revision.pdf
International Nursing Association for Clinical Simulation and Learning (INACSL)	INACSL Standards Committee. (2016, December). INACSL standards of best practice: Simulation^SM: Simulation design. *Clinical Simulation in Nursing, 12*(S), S5–S12. https://doi.org/10.1016/j.ecns.2016.09.005
Pan American Health Organization (PAHO)	Pan American Health Organization. (2011). *Guidelines for developing emergency simulations and drills*. https://www.paho.org/disasters/index.php?option=com_content&view=article&id=1637:guidelines-for-developing-emergency-simulations-and-drills&Itemid=807&lang=en
United Kingdom Central Government Emergency Response Training (CGERT)	United Kingdom. (2014). *United Kingdom CGERT guidance*. https://www.gov.uk/guidance/emergency-planning-and-preparedness-exercises-and-training
University of Oklahoma Health Sciences Center	Wendelboe, A. M., Miller, A., Drevets, D., Salinas, L., Miller, E. J., Jackson, D., Chou, A., & Raines, J. (2020). Tabletop exercise to prepare institutions of higher education for an outbreak of COVID-19. *Journal of Emergency Management, 18*(2), S1–S20. doi:10.5055/jem.2020.0464
World Health Organization (WHO)	World Health Organization. (2017). *WHO simulation exercise manual*. https://www.who.int/ihr/publications/WHO-WHE-CPI-2017.10/en/

Case in Point

PUTTING A PREPAREDNESS PLAN TO THE TEST: TAKING A PLAN FROM PAPER TO IMPLEMENTATION

Faculty members of a senior-level nursing course designed an emergency preparedness exercise that used an annual mass immunization clinic as the basis for a simulated response to an infectious disease outbreak. During the project, students were given a scenario in which the local public health department (PHD) has requested the College of Nursing to open a points of dispensing (POD) clinic. Students had to plan POD logistics, social marketing, and community education to meet the goal; implement the plan; and complete an after-action report.

In response to an outbreak of Type A influenza at a local university, the local PHD recommended that the university prevent spread into the larger community by beginning vaccinations for its students, faculty, and staff as soon as possible. Health center staff at the university and nursing faculty collaborated on an immediate POD clinic targeted toward the campus population at greatest risk for exposure and spread of influenza.

The POD operation used the plan for the university's annual mass immunization clinic as its basis ("systems"), and senior nursing majors in a public health nursing (PHN) course served as the primary workforce ("staff") under faculty supervision. The vaccine ("supplies") was requested from the Centers for Disease Control and Prevention (CDC) for immediate shipment, and an appropriate location was selected for the clinic ("structure").

The POD clinic was offered over several days, and more than 900 doses were administered. At the conclusion of the POD clinic, the PHN students immediately resumed planning for the annual vaccination clinic, incorporating lessons learned during the after-action debriefing.

Continued tracking of influenza incidence revealed that the majority of positive influenza cases occurred prior to the POD clinic being established, during its operation, or during the period needed for antibody formation, suggesting that the POD operation—combined with social isolation for those testing positive for influenza—successfully limited further spread. After-action analysis suggested that continued practice and improvement of this emergency preparedness activity allowed it to be successful when put to the test by an actual outbreak.

Note: Further details of this case are described by Adams et al. (2019).

Questions for Discussion

1. How did the exercise address the surge capacity element of staff?
2. How did the exercise address surge capacity elements of supplies and structure?
3. How did the exercise address surge capacity elements of system(s)?

Points to Remember

- Both discussion-based exercises and operations-based exercises allow participants to test plans and perform disaster roles with little risk by responding to a simulated event.
- Exercises should not be designed to focus on strengths with a goal to "pass"; rather, successful exercises should emphasize "drilling to failure" in order to identify operational gaps, weaknesses, and areas for improvement prior to an actual event.
- Exercise design should include:
  - Needs assessment
  - Establishment of purpose, scope, objectives, and evaluation parameters
  - Creation of a scenario
  - Plans for documentation, outcome evaluation, and performance improvement

Test Your Knowledge

1. What type of exercise does the Case in Point illustrate?
   a. Full-scale exercise
   b. Game
   c. Tabletop exercise
   d. Functional exercise
2. What elements of surge capacity are necessary for a POD operation to be successful? *(Choose all that apply.)*
   a. Staff
   b. Supplies
   c. Structure
   d. Systems
3. Based on the information in the Case in Point, what populations would be at greatest risk for exposure and spread of influenza? *(Choose all that apply.)*
   a. Students, faculty, and staff of the College of Nursing
   b. Students, faculty, and staff from a department housed in the same building as the College of Nursing

   c. Student athletes and students who frequent the University Recreation Center
   d. Faculty, staff, and administrators in other colleges across the campus
4. How do operations-based exercises differ from discussion-based exercises? *(Choose all that apply.)*
   a. Allow testing of decision making in a low-risk environment
   b. May involve mobilization of resources in real time
   c. Allow the most realistic evaluation of necessary resources
   d. Promote problem solving and allow identification of gaps in the plan
5. What are important elements of planning the exercise design?
   a. Needs assessment and establishing exercise scope
   b. Identification of areas for improvement in an existing plan
   c. Evaluating participants' performance of their disaster roles
   d. Identification of gaps in a disaster plan and scenario creation
6. Which disaster exercise will allow participants to apply knowledge and problem solve through group discussion?
   a. Tabletop exercise
   b. Drill
   c. Functional exercise
   d. Full-scale exercise
7. When planning for a full-scale exercise, important considerations should include awareness that a full-scale exercise will:
   a. Focus on a single capability within one organization
   b. Require specific computer software and hardware
   c. Include real-time activity and resource mobilization
   d. Use structured play to enhance team building
8. When planning an operations-based exercise to support maintenance of a specific skill within a single organization, it would be most appropriate to design a:
   a. Tabletop exercise
   b. Game
   c. Drill
   d. Functional exercise
   e. Full-scale exercise
9. How can realism be promoted in exercises? *(Choose all that apply.)*
   a. Use of functional equipment
   b. Application of moulage to simulated patients
   c. Combining multiple simulation modalities
   d. Only through the use of full-scale exercises
10. What is the purpose of an after-action report? *(Choose all that apply.)*
    a. Evaluates participants' performance of their disaster roles
    b. Serves as a foundation to plan evaluation and process improvement
    c. Establishes measurable and achievable objectives
    d. Defines outcomes, including quantity, quality, cost, and change

References

Adams, L. M., Canclini, S. B., & Tillman, K. (2019). "This is not a drill": Activation of a student-led influenza vaccination point of distribution. *Journal of American College Health, 67*(2), 88–91. https://doi.org/10.1080/07448481.2018.1463228.

Association of Public Health Nurses Public Health Preparedness Committee. (2014). *The role of the public health nursing in disaster preparedness, response, and recovery: A position paper.* http://www.quadcouncilphn.org/wp-content/uploads/2016/03/2014_APHN-Role-of-PHN-in-Disaster-PRR-Ref-updated-2015.pdf.

Australian Institute for Disaster Resilience. (2012). *Australian disaster resilience handbook 3: Managing exercises* (2nd ed.). https://knowledge.aidr.org.au/resources/handbook-3-managing-exercises/.

Farra, S., Hodgson, E., Miller, E. T., Timm, N., Brady, W., Gneuhs, M., ... & Bottomley, M. (2019). Effects of virtual reality simulation on worker emergency evacuation of neonates. *Disaster Medicine and Public Health Preparedness*, *13*(2). 301–308. doi: 10.1017dmp.2018.58.

Farra, S. L., & Smith, S. J. (2015). Simulation in disaster education. In S. A. R. Stanley & T. A. Benecoff Wolanski (Eds.), *Designing and integrating a disaster preparedness curriculum: Readying nurses for the worst.* Sigma Theta Tau International. (2015).

Federal Emergency Management Agency. (2020). *Homeland Security Exercise and Evaluation Program (HSEEP).* https://www.fema.gov/hseep https://www.fema.gov/media-library-data/1580929080128-43a6a087f3956a7e51ae506514598053/Homeland-Security-Exercise-and-Evaluation-Program-Doctrine2020Revision.pdf.

International Nursing Association for Clinical Simulation and Learning Standards Committee. (2016a). INACSL standards of best practice: Simulation[SM]: Simulation design. *Clinical Simulation in Nursing*, *12*(S), S5–S12. http://doi.org/10.1016/j.ecns.2016.09.005.

International Nursing Association for Clinical Simulation and Learning Standards Committee. (2016b). INACSL standards of best practice: Simulation[SM]: Simulation glossary. *Clinical Simulation in Nursing*, *12*(S), S39–S47. http://doi.org/10.1016/j.ecns.2016.09.012.

Jakeway, C. C., LaRosa, G., Cary, A., & Schoenfisch, S. (2008). The role of public health nurses in emergency preparedness and response: A position paper of the Association of State and Territorial Directors of Nursing. *Public Health Nursing*, *25*(4), 353–361.

Kerins, D., Barishanksky, R. M., & Cortacans, H. P. (2012, June). How to conduct EMS exercises and drills. *EMS World*, 33–38.

Lioce, L. (Ed.); Downing, D., Chang, T. P., Robertson, J. M., Anderson, M., Diaz, D. A., & Spain, A. E. (Assoc. Eds.); & Terminology and Concepts Working Group. (2020). *Healthcare simulation dictionary* (2nd ed.). Agency for Healthcare Research and Quality. AHRQ Publication No. 20-0019. doi: https://doi.org/10.23970/simulationv2.

McCormick, L. C., Hites, L., Wakelee, J. F., Rucks, A. C., & Ginter, P. M. (2014). Planning and executing complex large-scale exercises. *Journal of Public Health Management Practice*, *20*(5). S37–S43. doi: 10.1097/PHH.000000000000068.

Pan American Health Organization. (2011). *Guidelines for developing emergency simulations and drills.* https://www.paho.org/disasters/index.php?option=com_content&view=article&id=1637:guidelines-for-developing-emergency-simulations-and-drills&Itemid=807&lang=en.

Uden-Holman, T., Bedet, J., Walkner, L., & Abd-Hamid, N. H. (2014). Adaptive scenarios: A training model for today's public health workforce. *Journal of Public Health Management Practice*, *20*(5). S44–S48. doi: 10.1097PHH.0000000000000067.

US Department of Homeland Security. (2018). *Hurricane after-action report: The full story.* https://www.fema.gov/news-release/2018/07/14/2017-hurricane-after-action-report-full-story.

Vasa, A., Madad, S., Larson, L., Kraft, C. S., Vanairsdale, S., Grein, J. D., ... & Kratochvil, C. J. (2019). A novel approach to infectious disease preparedness: Incorporating investigational therapeutics and research objectives into full-scale exercises. *Health Security*, *1*(1), 54–61. https://doi.org/10.1089/hs.2018.0100.

Walkner, L., Fife, D., Bedet, J., & DeMartino, M. (2014). Using a digital story format: A contemporary approach to meeting the workforce needs of public health laboratories. *Journal of Public Health Management Practice*, *20*(5). S49–S51. doi: 10.1097PHH.0000000000000095.

Wexler, B., & Flamm, A. (2017). Lessons learned from an active shooter full-scale functional exercise in a newly constructed emergency department. *Disaster Medicine and Public Health Preparedness*, *11*(5), 522–525. https://doi.org/10.1017/dmp.2016.181.

World Health Organization. (2017). *WHO simulation exercise manual.* https://www.who.int/ihr/publications/WHO-WHE-CPI-2017.10/en/.

Core Competencies in Disaster Nursing, Version 2.0

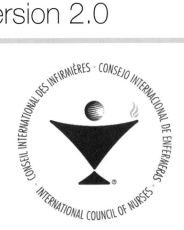

International Council of Nurses
Version 2.0 is organized into eight domains.

Domain 1	**Preparation and Planning**	(actions taken apart from any specific emergency to increase readiness and confidence in actions to be taken during an event)
Domain 2	**Communication**	(approaches to conveying essential information within one's place of work or emergency assignment and documenting decisions made)
Domain 3	**Incident Management**	(the structure of disaster/emergency response required by countries/organizations/institutions and actions to make them effective)
Domain 4	**Safety and Security**	(assuring that nurses, their colleagues and patients do not add to the burden of response by unsafe practices)
Domain 5	**Assessment**	(gathering data about assigned patients/families/communities on which to base subsequent nursing actions)
Domain 6	**Intervention**	(clinical or other actions taken in response to assessment of patients/families/communities within the incident management of the disaster event)
Domain 7	**Recovery**	(any steps taken to facilitate resumption of pre-event individual/family/community/organization functioning or moving it to a higher level)
Domain 8	**Law and Ethics**	(the legal and ethical framework for disaster/emergency nursing)

Effective nursing practice during any disaster requires clinical competency and the application of utilitarian principles (doing the greatest good for the greatest number with the least amount of harm). At Level I, the basic or generalist nurse is not expected to be an expert in response to any one kind of emergency or to be working apart from others. It is possible that outside of the working day, a nurse as a member of the community might be on the site of an emerging disaster or event, in which case the nurse should use basic first aid and professional skills until additional responders arrive and a team structure is organized. While every nurse develops greater proficiency in any competencies used in everyday practice; the acute care nurse makes little use of community-focused competencies and the public health nurse makes little use of cardiac resuscitation competencies. The altogether too frequent occurrence of cyclones, earthquakes, volcanic eruptions, transportation crashes, epidemics, chemical spills, radiation leaks, and human-initiated violence means that every nurse should take these disaster competencies seriously and use refresher training and participation in drills and exercises to maintain at least a basic level of proficiency.

ICN Core Competencies in Disaster Nursing Version 2.0

General Professional Nurse	Advanced or Specialized Nurse[1]
Level I: any nurse who has completed a program of basic, generalized nursing education and is authorized to practice by the regulatory agency of his/her country. Examples of Level I include staff nurses in hospitals, clinics, public health centers; all nurse educators.	**Level II:** any nurse who has achieved the Level I competencies and is or aspires to be a designated disaster responder within an institution, organization, or system. Examples of Level II include supervising or head nurses; a nurses designated for leadership within an organization's emergency plan; a nurses representing the profession on an institution or agency emergency planning committee, preparedness/response nurse educators.
Domain 1: Preparation and Planning	
I.1.1 Maintains a general personal, family, and professional preparedness plan	II.1.1 Participates with other disciplines in planning emergency drills/exercises at the institution or community level at least annually
I.1.2 Participates with other disciplines in drills/exercises in the workplace[2]	II.1.2 Plans nursing improvement actions based on results of drill/exercise evaluation
I.1.3 Maintains up-to-date knowledge of available emergency resources, plans, policies and procedures	II.1.3 Communicates roles and responsibilities of nurses to others involved in planning, preparation, response and recovery
I.1.4 Describes approaches to accommodate vulnerable populations during an emergency or disaster response	II.1.4 Includes actions relevant to needs of vulnerable populations in emergency plans
	II.1.5 Incorporates Level I core competencies in Disaster Nursing in any basic nursing education program or refresher course
Domain 2: Communication	
I.2.1 Uses disaster terminology correctly in communication with all responders and receivers	II.2.1 Plans for adaptable emergency/disaster communications systems
I.2.2 Communicates disaster-related priority information promptly to designated individuals	II.2.2 Includes emergency communication expectations in all orientation of nurses to a workplace
I.2.3 Demonstrates basic crisis communication skills during emergency/ disaster events	II.2.3 Collaborates with disaster leadership team(s) to develop event-specific media messages
I.2.4 Uses available multilingual resources[3] to provide clear communication with disaster-effected populations	II.2.4 Develops guidance on critical documentation to be maintained during disaster or emergency
I.2.5 Adapts documentation of essential assessment and intervention information to the resources and scale of emergency	
Domain 3: Incident Management	
I.3.1 Describes the national structure for response to an emergency or disaster	II.3.1 Participates in development of organizational incident plan consistent with national standards
I.3.2 Uses the specific disaster plan including chain of command for his/her place of education or employment in an event, exercise, or drill	II.3.2 Participates with others in post-event (actual or exercise) evaluation
	II.3.3 Develops action plans for improvement in nursing practice based on event assessment

General Professional Nurse

I.3.3 Contributes observations and experiences to postevent evaluation
I.3.4 Maintains professional practice within licensed scope of practice when assigned to an interprofessional team or an unfamiliar location

Domain 4: Safety and Security

I.4.1 Maintains safety for self and others throughout disaster/emergency event in both usual or austere environment(s)
I.4.2 Adapts basic infection control practices to the available resources
I.4.3 Applies regular assessment of self and colleagues during disaster event to identify need for physical or psychological support
I.4.4 Uses PPE[2] as directed through the chain of command in a disaster/emergency event
I.4.5 Reports possible risks to personal or others' safety and security

Domain 5: Assessment

I.5.1 Reports symptoms or events that might indicate the onset of an emergency in assigned patients/families/communities
I.5.2 Performs rapid physical and mental health assessment of each assigned patient/family/community based on principles of triage and type of emergency/disaster event
I.5.3 Maintains ongoing assessment of assigned patient/family/community for needed changes in care in response to the evolving disaster event

Domain 6: Intervention

I.6.1 Implements basic first aid as needed by individuals in immediate vicinity
I.6.2 Isolates individuals/families/clusters at risk of spreading communicable condition(s) to others
I.6.3 Participates in contamination assessment or decontamination of individuals when directed through the chain of command
I.6.4 Engages patients, their family members or assigned volunteers within their abilities, to extend resources during events
I.6.5 Provides patient care based on priority needs and available resources
I.6.6 Participates in surge capacity activities as assigned (e.g., mass immunization)
I.6.7 Adheres to protocol for management of large numbers of deceased in respectful manner

Advanced or Specialized Nurse[1]

II.3.4 Includes emergency planning guidance when reassigning staff or including unfamiliar colleagues or volunteers

II.4.1 Implements materials that support nursing decision making that maintains safety during disaster/emergency events
II.4.2 Provides timely alternative infection control practices applicable within limited resources
II.4.3 Collaborates with others to facilitate nurses' access to medical and/or mental health treatment, and other support services as needed
II.4.4 Explains the levels/difference in PPE and indications for use to nurses and others
II.4.5 Creates an action plan to address and correct/eliminate risks to personal or others' safety and security

II.5.1 Assures that all nurses have up-to-date information on potential emergency events and the process for reporting them if observed
II.5.2 Develops event-specific guidance on rapid physical and mental health assessment of individual patients/families/communities based on available information
II.5.3 Includes principles of disaster/emergency triage in all assessment courses taught in basic and continuing education programs
II.5.4 Identifies event-specific vulnerable population(s) and actions needed to protect them

II.6.1 Assures that emergency plans and institutional policy include the expectation that basic first aid can be administered by all nurses
II.6.2 Includes organizationally specific guidance on implementation of isolation in an emergency
II.6.3 Describes the range of CBRNE[5] exposures and the exposure-related decontamination methods to be used
II.6.4 Plans for expanded patient, patient's family, or volunteer participation in extending resources in emergency/disaster plan
II.6.5 Guides implementation of nursing reassignments within an organization's emergency plan
II.6.6 Guides nursing participation in surge activities when required by event

General Professional Nurse	Advanced or Specialized Nurse[1]
Domain 7: Recovery	
I.7.1 Assists an organization to maintain or resume functioning during and postevent	II.7.1 Communicates nursing roles, responsibilities and needs to leadership throughout the recovery phase
I.7.2 Assists assigned patients/families/communities to maintain or resume functioning during and postevent	II.7.2 Maintains up-to-date referral resource lists and adds event-specific modifications as needed
I.7.3 Makes referrals for ongoing physical and mental health needs as patients are discharged from care	
I.7.4 Participates in transition debriefing to identify personal needs for ongoing assistance	
Domain 8: Law and Ethics	
I.8.1 Practices within the applicable nursing and emergency-specific laws, policies, and procedures	II.8.1 Participates in development of emergency-specific policy and procedure guidance for nurses within the organization/institution
I.8.2 Applies institutional or national disaster ethical framework in care of individuals/families/communities	II.8.2 Participates in the development of disaster/emergency frameworks for allocation of resources (e.g., staff, supplies, medications)
I.8.3 Demonstrates understanding of ethical practice during disaster response that is based on utilitarian principles[6]	II.8.3 Develops guidance for nurses expected to apply utilitarian principles in practice during emergency and disaster response

[1]Level II, Disaster-specific advanced nurse

[2]Some drills/exercises done in a basic educational setting may not involve other disciplines

[3]Resources include such things as interpreters, signs, or pictures

[4]Personal Protective Equipment

[5]Chemical, biological, radiation, nuclear, explosive

[6]Utilitarian principles place highest value on actions that lead to the greatest good for the greatest possible number of persons, rather than actions that are prioritized based on the needs of any

Sample List: Readiness Resources and Toolkits

AARP: The New Go Bag: What You Need in Your Emergency Escape Kit
  https://www.aarp.org/home-family/friends-family/info-2020/emergency-go-bag.html
American Red Cross: Emergency Preparedness for Older Adults
  https://www.redcross.org/get-help/how-to-prepare-for-emergencies/older-adults.html
California Department of Aging: Disaster Preparedness (tip sheets for seniors on flood, hot weather, winter, pets, earthquake, power outages, and wildfire)
  https://www.aging.ca.gov/Providers_and_Partners/Area_Agencies_on_Aging/Disaster_Preparedness/Disaster_Tip_Sheets/
Centers for Disease Control and Prevention (CDC): Caring for Children in a Disaster
  https://www.aging.ca.gov/Providers_and_Partners/Area_Agencies_on_Aging/Disaster_Preparedness/Disaster_Tip_Sheets/
Centers for Disease Control and Prevention (CDC): Communication Resources
  https://www.cdc.gov/coronavirus/2019-ncov/communication/
Centers for Disease Control and Prevention (CDC): Coronavirus Disease (COVID-19): Considerations for Alternate Care Sites
  https://www.cdc.gov/coronavirus/2019-ncov/hcp/alternative-care-sites.html
Centers for Disease Control and Prevention (CDC): COVID-19 Risks and Vaccine Information for Older Adults
  https://www.cdc.gov/aging/covid19/covid19-older-adults.html?CDC_AA_refVal=https%3A%2F%2Fwww.cdc.gov%2Fcoronavirus%2F2019-ncov%2Fneed-extra-p
Centers for Disease Control and Prevention (CDC): Disability and Health Emergency Preparedness Tools and Resources
  https://www.cdc.gov/ncbddd/disabilityandhealth/emergency-tools.html
Centers for Disease Control and Prevention (CDC): Disaster Planning: Infant and Child Feeding
  https://www.cdc.gov/nccdphp/dnpao/features/disasters-infant-feeding/index.html
Centers for Disease Control and Prevention (CDC): Disability and Health Emergency Preparedness Tools and Resources
  https://www.cdc.gov/ncbddd/disabilityandhealth/emergency-tools.html
Centers for Disease Control and Prevention (CDC): Emergency Preparedness for Older Adults
  https://www.cdc.gov/aging/publications/features/older-adult-emergency.html
Centers for Disease Control and Prevention (CDC): Emergency Preparedness: Hurricanes, Floods and Pregnancy
  https://www.cdc.gov/ncbddd/disasters/pregnancy.html
Centers for Disease Control and Prevention (CDC): 2020–21 Health Care Professional Fight Flu Toolkit
  https://www.cdc.gov/flu/resource-center/freeresources/toolkit.htm

Centers for Disease Control and Prevention (CDC): Identifying Vulnerable Older Adults and Legal Options for Increasing Their Protection During All-Hazards Emergencies
https://www.cdc.gov/cpr/documents/aging.pdf

Centers for Disease Control and Prevention (CDC): Radiological Terrorism planning and response tool kits
https://www.cdc.gov/nceh/radiation/emergencies/toolkits.htm

Centers for Disease Control and Prevention (CDC): Reaching At-Risk Populations in an Emergency
https://emergency.cdc.gov/workbook/index.asp

Centers for Disease Control and Prevention (CDC): Reproductive Health in Emergency Preparedness and Response
https://www.cdc.gov/reproductivehealth/emergency/index.html

Centers for Medicare and Medicaid Services (CMS): Coronavirus (COVID-19) Partner Resources
https://www.cms.gov/outreach-education/partner-resources/coronavirus-covid-19-partner-toolkit

Healthy People.gov. Healthy People 2020: Older Adults
https://www.healthypeople.gov/2020/topics-objectives/topic/older-adults

Missouri Department of Health and Senior Services: Planning for Emergencies: Three Steps to be Prepared, A Family Safety Guide (See Appendix C)
https://health.mo.gov/emergencies/readyin3/pdf/familyguideenglish.pdf

Ready.gov: Basic Disaster Supplies Kit
https://www.ready.gov/kit

Ready.gov: Create Your Family Emergency Communication Plan (See Appendix D)
https://www.ready.gov/collection/family-emergency-communication-plan

Ready.gov: Individuals with Disabilities
https://www.ready.gov/disability

US Department of Health and Human Services, Office of the Assistant Secretary for Preparedness & Response (ASPR): Critical Care Load-Balancing Operational Template
https://files.asprtracie.hhs.gov/documents/critical-care-load-balancing-operational-template.pdf

HAZARD AND VULNERABILITY ASSESSMENT TOOL
EVENTS INVOLVING HAZARDOUS MATERIALS

KAISER PERMANENTE.

EVENT	PROBABILITY	SEVERITY = (MAGNITUDE - MITIGATION)						RISK
		HUMAN IMPACT	PROPERTY IMPACT	BUSINESS IMPACT	PREPARED-NESS	INTERNAL RESPONSE	EXTERNAL RESPONSE	
	Likelihood this will occur	Possibility of death or injury	Physical losses and damages	Interuption of services	Preplanning	Time, effectivness, resouces	Community/ Mutual Aid staff and supplies	Relative threat*
SCORE	0 = N/A 1 = Low 2 = Moderate 3 = High	0 = N/A 1 = Low 2 = Moderate 3 = High	0 = N/A 1 = Low 2 = Moderate 3 = High	0 = N/A 1 = Low 2 = Moderate 3 = High	0 = N/A 1 = High 2 = Moderate 3 = Low or none	0 = N/A 1 = High 2 = Moderate 3 = Low or none	0 = N/A 1 = High 2 = Moderate 3 = Low or none	0 - 100%
Mass Casualty Hazmat Incident (From historic events at your MC with >= 5 victims)								0%
Small Casualty Hazmat Incident (From historic events at your MC with < 5 victims)								0%
Chemical Exposure, External								0%
Small-Medium Sized Internal Spill								0%
Large Internal Spill								0%
Terrorism, Chemical								0%
Radiologic Exposure, Internal								0%
Radiologic Exposure, External								0%
Terrorism, Radiologic								0%
AVERAGE	0.00	0.00	0.00	0.00	0.00	0.00	0.00	0%

Threat increases with percentage.

RISK = PROBABILITY * SEVERITY

0.00	0.00	0.00

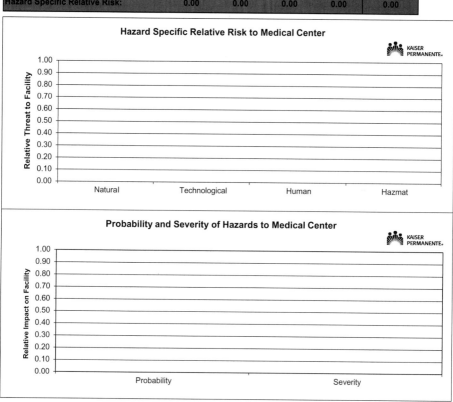

Test Answers

Chapter 1

CASE IN POINT

Ms. L. lives in a low-lying area that is less than half a mile from the river. Her house is not on stilts. She is a young single mother with an infant. She also cares for her mother, who has multiple health comorbidities, is on oxygen, and has difficulty walking. It has been raining for 7 days straight, and Ms. L. has heard that the river has breached the levee 10 miles upstream.

1. What should Ms. L.'s immediate plan include?
2. If she decides to evacuate her home, what should she consider taking with her?
3. What items should be taken for the care of the infant?
4. What items should be taken for the care of her mother?

CASE IN POINT ANSWERS

1. Ms. L. should have registered her mother with the local fire and police departments so that they are alerted to persons in the home with special needs. She needs to evacuate the home as soon as she can get essential items packed. When the rains started, she should have filled her car with gas and checked that it was road-ready to drive to a safe harbor.
2. Ms. L. needs to carry essential documents such as birth certificates, Social Security numbers, driver's license, money, credit cards, sturdy boots, rain gear, maps or a GPS system to indicate evacuation routes, first aid kit, nonperishable food, water, and a list of shelters or evacuation centers.
3. The infant will need diapers, clothes, blankets, formula or (if breastfeeding) breast pump and breast milk storage containers if refrigeration is available, baby food if old enough, medicines, and health care providers' information.
4. Her mother will need her oxygen tank and backup tank if available, O_2 tubing, medicines, assistive devices, health care providers' information, identification and health care cards, money, and credit cards.

TEST YOUR KNOWLEDGE ANSWERS

1. Which of the following is an example of an accidental disaster?
   b. A fuel tanker that runs aground due to poor visibility in a storm
2. The final stage of recovery after a disaster, which involves future-oriented activities to prevent subsequent disasters or to minimize their effects, is called:
   c. Mitigation
3. The types of activities that occur during the predisaster or pre-impact stage include: *(Choose all that apply.)*
   a. Rescue equipment is pre-staged
   b. Citizens are evacuated to safe areas
   c. Rescue and recovery teams are mobilized

       d. Public service announcements are made to instruct communities on appropriate safety actions

4. After a disaster event, which of the following actions should take place? *(Choose all that apply.)*

       a. Review actions taken that were most helpful

       b. Review actions taken that were of little use

       d. Modify the disaster plan to include lessons learned

5. Mitigation includes which of the following activities? *(Choose all that apply.)*

       a. Reinforcing existing structures

       b. Building new structures to withstand the forces of a disaster

       c. Recruiting and preparing volunteers to assist in disaster prevention, preparedness, and relief efforts

       d. Extensive education for health care providers in multiple settings about types of injuries that might occur in future disasters

6. Key activities that occur during the preparedness stage include: *(Choose all that apply.)*

       a. Plans and preparations made to save lives and help with response and rescue operations

       b. Evacuation plans that include routes, shelters, and alternate care sites

       c. Stocking food and water

7. Responding safely in an emergency includes: *(Choose all that apply.)*

       a. Actions taken to save lives and prevent further immediate damage

       b. Putting preparedness plans into action

       c. Seeking shelter

       d. Turning off gas valves in an earthquake

8. Recovery from an emergency or disaster situation takes time. Some of the activities during the recovery stage include: *(Choose all that apply.)*

       a. Actions taken to return to normal

       c. Getting financial assistance to pay for home repairs

       d. Making one's home safer than it was prior to the disaster

9. Which of the following persons would be considered vulnerable and need special consideration by nurses in a disaster situation? *(Choose all that apply.)*

       a. A near-term pregnant woman

       b. A person who is sight impaired

       c. A person who is hearing impaired

       d. A person who does not understand the primary language where the disaster is occurring

10. An example of a deliberate human-made disaster is:

       c. Multiple deaths after patrons ate anthrax-contaminated food from a restaurant salad bar

Chapter 2

CASE IN POINT

You work in a rural hospital that covers three small counties in your state (total population for the area is 30,000). The closest state health care coalition is located in a large urban county 120 minutes away from your facility. During the COVID-19 pandemic, your facility was the lead for your area's response and does not currently have a local health care coalition. There were many lessons learned from the COVID-19 response and numerous accounts of duplication of services in your area. Nationally and state-wide, there has been a 6-month decrease in COVID-19 cases. Your hospital has just appointed you to update your facility EOP and form a new health care coalition that will serve the counties your hospital covers.

1. What is the first thing you should do?
2. Who would you need to involve in your hospital to update the EOP?
3. What stakeholders would you need to seek to serve in your area health care coalition?

CASE IN POINT ANSWERS

1. Initial steps would include:
   a. Develop an internal team within your organization that will compile the lessons learned from the COVID-19 response and review the current EOP. Include a list of all health care providers who worked collaboratively during the response.
   b. Contact the emergency management agency (EMA) director for your county. The EMA at the county level is the lead agency for planning efforts for the entire response. It can help direct you to potential partnerships for planning efforts.
   c. Contact the local health department. Public health is the lead agency for Emergency Support Functions (ESF) #8, and they have assigned emergency preparedness teams that will work with you on steps to develop a local health care coalition.
   d. Contact the health care coalition located in the urban area. It will be a great resource for next steps.
2. First, determine who wrote the current EOP and when. These people will help guide you to who they included in the process along with additional people who should have been included. Departments you would need to involve include the emergency department, surgical, specialty areas, medical-surgical, laboratory, ancillary services, and finance. The more departments you include, the better your response. A key point is that everyone has a part to play in patient care. Talk with your direct care staff as well as administration. It is essential to involve the people who are delivering direct care to help guide you to making your EOP work for everyone.
3. Make sure that you review where duplication of health care services exists. Some organizations you would need to include are public health, hospitals, assisted living facilities, nursing homes, and clinics.

TEST YOUR KNOWLEDGE ANSWERS

1. The emergency planner understands that global and national frameworks are meant to:
   a. **Guide planners through the planning process Global and national frameworks guide emergency planners through the process of emergency preparedness planning (FEMA, 2019; WHO, 2017a, 2017b, 2019).**
2. Which type of approach involves assuring that the emergency response can address any type of situation that can affect society and the health of people?
   a. **All-hazards**
      An all-hazards approach means assuring that the emergency response can address any type of situation that can affect society and the health of people, including both natural (e.g., hurricanes, tornados, earthquakes) and human-made (e.g., terrorist attacks, mass shootings, cybersecurity breach) events (FEMA, 2016b, 2019; WHO, 2017a, 2017b, 2019).
3. Which of the following is the potential for an unwanted outcome resulting from an incident or caused by systemic degradation, as determined by its likelihood, associated consequences, and vulnerability to those consequences?
   a. **Risk**

FEMA defines risk as "the potential for an unwanted outcome resulting from an incident or caused by systemic degradation, as determined by its likelihood, associated consequences, and vulnerability to those consequences" (FEMA, 2016b, p. 6).

4. An emergency planner understands that which of the following reduces loss of life and property by lessening the impact of disasters?

   a. **Mitigation**

   Prevention: Avoiding, preventing, or stopping a threatened or actual act of terrorism. Within the context of national preparedness, the term *prevention* refers to dealing with imminent threats. Protection: Securing the homeland against acts of terrorism and human-caused or natural disasters. Mitigation: Reducing loss of life and property by lessening the impact of disasters. Response: Saving lives, stabilizing community lifelines, protecting property and the environment, and meeting basic human needs after an incident has occurred. Recovery: Assisting affected communities with restoration and revitalization.

5. An emergency planner understands that planning efforts should be developed to support which of the following levels?

   a. **Local**

   "The most effective disaster response and recovery efforts are locally developed and executed, state/tribal/territorially managed, and federally supported" (White House Office of Intergovernmental Affairs, 2018, p. 2), and each level of the preparedness planning and response should support the local/community level (WHO, 2017a, 2017b).

6. A hospital emergency planner is coordinating with a medical supply company when developing the EOP. The planner is doing this for all of the following reasons **except**:

   a. **Abundance of medical supplies**

   There are overlaps between health care providers using the same medical supply chains, which can lead to competition for medical supplies that can be scarce during an emergency response.

7. Which of the following statements is true?

   d. **An actual emergency response can be used to meet the exercise requirements of the CMS and TJC.**

8. What should the emergency planning team do first when developing an EOP?

   a. **Conduct a threat and risk assessment**

   The first step to emergency preparedness planning is the identification and prioritization of potential threats the community could face.

9. Communication planning is critical to response operations because it outlines the importance of: *(Choose all that apply.)*

   a. **Developing a single set of objectives**

   b. **Improving information flow and coordination**

   d. **Optimizing the combined efforts of all participants**

   Communication planning is critical to response operations because it outlines the "importance of (1) developing a single set of objectives; (2) using a collective, strategic approach; (3) improving information flow and coordination; (4) creating a common understanding of joint priorities and limitations; (5) ensuring that no agency's legal authorities are compromised or neglected; and (6) optimizing the combined efforts of all participants under a single plan" (FEMA, 2019, p. 11).

10. Which of the following statements is accurate regarding a MCI?

    c. **A MCI is any event that overwhelms the local health care system, as it exceeds the capabilities of that system.**

Mass casualty incident (MCI) is "an event that overwhelms the local health care system, with a number of casualties that vastly exceeds the local resources and capabilities in a short period of time" (Ben-Ishay et al., 2016, p. 1). An MCI would differ depending on the capacity of a health care system.

Chapter 3

CASE IN POINT

A registered nurse, who primarily works in the emergency department (ED) at a large, urban hospital, becomes aware of a newly identified illness spreading across countries around the globe. To maintain awareness of current health-related information, the nurse frequently visits expert websites created by health agencies to monitor health statistics and emerging diseases and provide expert guidance to health care providers. The nurse learns that the virus continues to spread, and many countries have high levels of infection and mortality rates. As a result, many governments are mandating quarantines and orders for people to shelter in place, particularly for those with chronic underlying conditions, as they are at greatest risk for dying from this new illness. As the nurse notes predictions that the illness will reach her country, she begins thinking of the impact it could have and what she might need to do to prepare.

The nurse is a single mother of two children, but her retired parents live close by. The nurse's oldest child has autism, and is easily upset at changes in his routine, and experiences frequent seizures. The nurse is extremely concerned that if she goes in to work in the ED, one of the patients visiting the ED might have the illness and she then would bring it home to her children. Further, she is concerned that if she visits her parents, she might infect them. However, the nurse also believes it is her duty to provide care to the sick, and this is something she is committed to doing, even in these circumstances. The nurse decides that, should the infection spread to her city, she will have her children stay with her parents to prevent her from potentially transmitting the infection to her family. She discusses this plan with her parents, who agree to provide care if it becomes necessary. In addition, she speaks to her children, who are 8 and 10 years old, about what is happening with the virus and that she wants to make sure they do not get sick. She explains in an age-appropriate manner that she will not get sick because she has the proper equipment at work, but that she doesn't want them to get sick so she will have them stay with their grandparents for a while and talk to them as often as she can. The children are very excited to spend time with their grandparents and are proud that their mother is taking care of sick people.

Over the next couple of weeks, she begins to craft her emergency preparedness plans with her children in mind and sets aside oral medications for her son with autism, as well as her son's doctor's name, address, and telephone number; a copy of the prescriptions her son needs; information on what constitutes an emergency in terms of his seizures; and information on actions her parents should take if her son has a seizure while in their care. The nurse packs clothes, personal hygiene items, books, and toys for both of her children in an emergency supply kit. She also puts together a kit for herself with enough clothes, scrubs, personal hygiene items, and other supplies so that she can sleep at the hospital if necessary. She attends JIT training conducted by her hospital to ensure that she knows what is required to take care of patients who have contracted the illness. Because the nurse has no siblings, she also thinks of her parents, as her father is 75 years old with type 2 diabetes and hypertension, and her mother is 72 years old and hearing impaired. She calls her parents to discuss their preparedness plans and determine if they have enough food, water, and medications for themselves as well as her children to last for 30 days per the most recent expert recommendations. Her parents state that they do not have enough to last for that long and remind her that they are on a fixed income and do not have enough money to buy that much food, though they could refill their medications. The nurse asks her parents to refill their medications and goes to the grocery store, gets enough food for her parents and her children to last at least 30 days, and delivers it to them to store for use in case it is needed.

The illness arrives in her city with rapidly increasing rates of infection. The schools close, but the nurse needs to continue working, especially since the number of visits to the ED has been increasing dramatically and some of her coworkers haven't reported to work in the previous days so the ED is short staffed. The nurse takes her children and all their emergency supplies as well as their schoolwork to her parents' home. The nurse double-checks her parents' supplies and makes sure there is enough for at least a month and tells them that she will see them all soon and drop off additional supplies as needed. Two days later, the government issues an order for everyone in the city to shelter in place. The nurse is considered an essential employee, so she continues to report to work every day but things are getting increasingly hectic. Shifts off become less frequent because nurses are also becoming infected and unable to work. The influx of the patients and the decreasing number of nurses able to work means that every available member of the health care team must work as much as they can, so the nurse takes her own emergency preparedness supplies to work with her to sleep there between shifts. The nurse is able to provide care for her patients and get enough rest for herself, all the while speaking with her family every day yet having decreased the chance she will transmit the virus to them.

1. What are three professional preparedness activities this nurse demonstrated prior to going to work for an extended period of time?
2. How did the nurse's activities relate to quarantine mandates for herself, her children, and family members?

CASE IN POINT ANSWERS

Responses will vary, but categories to consider include food, medicines, clothing, shelter, transportation, time for rest, quarantine, and possible isolation measures.

TEST YOUR KNOWLEDGE ANSWERS

1. What type of capacity is required when space, staff, and supplies have been adapted to provide sufficient care during a catastrophic disaster but are inconsistent with usual standards of care?
   d. **Crisis capacity**
2. Preparedness plans should include all of the following **except**:
   a. **Where local municipalities will provide food immediately after the emergency**
3. Which of the following are elements of cultural competency within disaster preparedness? *(Choose all that apply.)*
   a. **Be aware of and accept cultural differences**
   b. **Be aware of one's own cultural values**
   c. **Understand and manage the "dynamics of difference"**
   d. **Adapt activities to fit different cultural contexts**
4. Considerations for the emergency preparedness plans of independent older clients with diabetes would not include:
   b. **A caregiver**
5. A tornado and severe thunderstorm sends dozens of injured people to the emergency department of a small hospital. Driving conditions are becoming hazardous due to flooded roads, and multiple hospital personnel report having difficulty getting to work. Administrators are likely to be most concerned about which element of surge capacity?
   b. **Staff**
6. A hospital setting up a tent outside the emergency department to serve as an initial triage area is an example of which element of surge capacity?
   c. **Structures**

7. Actions that a health system can take to promote disaster preparedness and mitigate loss and harm to vulnerable populations include: *(Choose all that apply.)*
   a. Getting to know and actively engaging with community partners
   d. Routinely reviewing disaster plans, procedures, and mutual aid agreements
8. A nurse participating in the development of a disaster plan that uses principles of disaster risk reduction should expect the plan to include actions that:
   a. Strengthen community resilience
9. Which of the following might be signs that a client has low health literacy? *(Choose all that apply.)*
   c. Inability to explain the purpose of their medications
   d. Not following through on instructions
10. Which disaster education resource is designed specifically for nurses in acute care settings?
   b. ASPR-TRACIE EPIMN

Chapter 4

CASE IN POINT

It is 3:00 p.m. on a Sunday afternoon. The city's professional football team is playing, and the domed stadium is filled to capacity (55,000). The EMS personnel on-site have called to report that they have seen 12 persons exhibiting symptoms of watery eyes, coughing, shortness of breath, hypertension, fever, and prostration. Family members of the victims have begun to talk with other spectators, and people have begun to respond to the news of a possible biological agent and are hurrying from the area. EMS suspects that many of these people will be coming to the hospital. You are the charge nurse in the ED.

1. What is the first thing you should do?
2. Describe the process of activating the disaster response plan.
3. What departments and services should be notified?

CASE IN POINT ANSWERS

1. Notify key agency personnel, hospital administration, and the lab director and open the hospital incident command center.
2. Typically, the senior nurse administrator on duty will activate the disaster response plan by opening the incident command center.
3. Laboratory, security, labor pool, and human resources for additional health care providers, emergency department, infection control, and administration; then local health department, state health department, and the CDC.

TEST YOUR KNOWLEDGE ANSWERS

1. Important members or groups to include when selecting for the disaster response committee include: *(Choose all that apply.)*
   a. Nursing
   b. Medicine
   c. Infection control
   d. Safety and security
2. If a bioterrorism event is suspected, the first notification entity is:
   a. Emergency department and infection control

3. The system used for analyzing data to track a perpetrator to limit further damage to persons or property is termed the responsibility of:
   b. **The FBI**
4. Which of the following reflect basic decontamination principles? *(Choose all that apply.)*
   c. **The person who decontaminates patients also will be decontaminated.**
   d. **The person who cares for the patient in the hospital will remain in the clean area.**
5. After a mass casualty event or a drill, which of the following should take place? *(Choose all that apply.)*
   a. **A careful review of actions or inactions should occur.**
   c. **A no-blame climate should permeate the debriefing session.**
   d. **An action plan should be developed to strengthen identified areas of weakness.**
6. A method of sorting disaster victims and prioritizing their care after a mass casualty event when there are limited resources of personnel and equipment is called:
   c. **Reverse triage**
7. Which of the following blood products may be used during emergency transfusion support? *(Choose all that apply.)*
   a. **Red blood cells**
   b. **Plasma**
   c. **Platelets**
   d. **Cryoprecipitate**
8. What type of red blood cell is needed when an emergency patient is a woman of childbearing age and her blood type is unknown?
   b. **Group O, Rh-negative**
9. In hemolytic disease of the fetus and newborn (HDFN), what is the source of the potentially life-threatening antibodies?
   a. **Maternal**
10. Why is it critical that severely bleeding patients have their blood drawn prior to receiving donor blood products?
    c. **Difficulty in blood typing due to donor red blood cell interference**

Chapter 5

CASE IN POINT

This case is a composite of several survivors of the Boston Marathon bombing (Fig. 5.9).

A 19-year-old runner at the 2013 Boston Marathon was injured by flying shrapnel when a homemade pressure cooker bomb detonated near the finish line of the marathon. The bombing embedded two pieces of shrapnel in his body, one in his left leg and the other in his left arm. The survivor was taken to the hospital for treatment of his wounds. After surgery, the survivor remained in the hospital for a couple of days and then was discharged to home. Although the treatment was painful, the survivor felt very lucky to be alive and to have endured the bombing with minimal injury.

Upon discharge to home, a home health nurse was assigned to visit the survivor for wound assessment and dressing changes. During the home health visit, the parents expressed concern about their son's insomnia and frequent nightmares related to the bombing. The survivor revealed that whenever he ventures outside the house, he experiences heart palpitations, dizziness, sweating, and shortness of breath. He is hesitant to leave the house or engage in any activities. When his parents leave the house, even briefly, to run an errand or visit the neighbors, he calls them, asking them to return.

1. The stress reactions of survivors following disasters are frequently complex. How is this concept expressed in this case?
2. What stress reactions is the survivor exhibiting?
3. What nursing interventions should be implemented?

CASE IN POINT ANSWERS

1. After a disaster, survivors can experience a wide range of stress reactions. These stress reactions manifest in multiple ways: physically, emotionally, behaviorally, and cognitively. For most survivors, stress reactions are temporary. However, when stress reactions are severe, they can be quite upsetting and uncomfortable. Referral to a behavioral health profession for evaluation and treatment may prevent or reduce symptoms of acute stress disorder (ASD).
2. The survivor is presenting with ASD symptoms of intrusion (nightmares and distressing thoughts about the bombing), arousal (sleep disturbances, heart palpitations, dizziness, sweating, shortness of breath), and avoidance (refusal to leave the house or engage in outside activities).
3. Nursing interventions include (1) develop a sense of rapport and empathy, (2) acknowledge the fear and distressing feelings, (3) provide education about the autonomic nervous system's survival response and stress reactions, (4) teach abdominal breathing and stress management skills, (5) convey a sense of hope, and (6) refer the survivor to a behavioral health professional for further evaluation.

TEST YOUR KNOWLEDGE ANSWERS

1. The honeymoon phase in a disaster includes which of the following behaviors?
   d. People experience a sense of optimism and persist in doing what is necessary to meet basic needs.
2. Which of the following is a parasympathetic nervous system response?
   c. Decreased heart rate
3. Psychological first aid interventions include: *(Choose all that apply.)*
   a. Providing for psychological needs
   c. Connecting survivors with family members
4. One of the most important attributes of the nurse when interviewing a survivor is:
   c. Be a good listener
5. When assessing for suicide, the nurse should: *(Choose all that apply.)*
   a. Directly ask whether the survivor has thoughts of harming self
   b. Be supportive
   d. Ask specific questions about a suicide plan
6. Which of the following are high-risk factors for difficulty with postdisaster recovery? *(Choose all that apply.)*
   a. Exposure to gruesome or massive death
   b. History of mental illness
   c. Use of dissociation during the traumatic event
7. Which of the following behaviors are associated with unresolved grief after a disaster? *(Choose all that apply.)*
   a. Continued social isolation
   b. Maintenance of the illusion that a person is not dead
   d. Development of symptoms similar to those of the deceased

8. Crisis interventions include which of the following? *(Choose all that apply.)*
    a. **Assessing accurately the crisis event**
    b. **Exploring coping mechanisms and realistic problem solving by the survivor**
    c. **Collaborating with the survivor to form a short-term, realistic plan**
9. Which of the following symptoms are reflective of the diagnosis posttraumatic stress disorder (PTSD)? *(Choose all that apply.)*
    a. **Re-experiencing distressing thoughts, dreams, or flashbacks**
    b. **Feeling numb**
    c. **Being jumpy or easily startled**
10. Which of these interventions would assist with reducing anxiety? *(Choose all that apply.)*
    a. **Abdominal breathing**
    b. **Replacing negative thoughts with positive thoughts**
    c. **Relaxation training**

Chapter 6

CASE IN POINT

Based on weather reports of a hurricane forming in the Atlantic Ocean with movement to the Northeast, state and county emergency management began planning for possible damaging winds and flooding in the state. As more information became available, it was determined that opening shelters would be necessary for the protection of those individuals living in areas at risk for flooding or heavy wind damage. The affected county opened eight shelters. Each shelter was staffed with four to six Level I nurses to provide health services, as necessary, to the shelter population. Guidelines for minimum staffing requirements for general shelters are 4 Level I nurses per 100 clients for each 24-hour period. If a shelter has a large number of individuals with chronic conditions, additional nurses are requested.

A shelter was set up in a local school with the expectation of 350 clients. Health services initially was staffed with two Level I nurses working days and two Level I nurses working nights. A request was made for additional Level I nurses, though none were immediately available due to the number of shelters open. The nurses on-site selected a room where health services could be set up, providing easy access and privacy. The nurses also made a survey of the dormitory area where clients would be staying as well as the kitchen, bathrooms, and feeding area to assure client and staff safety. In addition, the nurses identified an area where clients with special needs who could not be housed within the general population could be supported.

When clients arrived at the shelter, they needed to go through a registration process. This was a difficult process due to the number of people trying to register and client concerns that there would not be enough room for everyone. Staff circulated among the clients to let them know that there was room for all and that they would be safe. Once registered, clients were escorted to the dormitory, where they selected a space for their family to sleep. As clients moved through the registration process, a nurse greeted them and spoke with them to determine if they had any health needs or injuries requiring immediate care. For example, the nurse asked clients if they had all their medications, if they were injured, if they had their needed medical equipment, if they had a disability that limited any of their abilities to function, and if special accommodations were required.

Any client who needed immediate assistance (e.g., due to injury, medication loss, or confusion) was taken directly to the health services room, where one of the nurses assessed them and provided care as required. A client who could not be safely managed in a general population was moved to a special needs shelter or other facility, if possible. However, it was important to remember that clients needed to be managed in the general shelter until a special needs shelter became available.

The nurse then designated an area for the client and a family member that best met the client need. If a client failed to bring their medications, it was sometimes possible to send someone back to the home to retrieve the medications. If this was not possible, health services worked to obtain the needed medications from the local pharmacy. Another common issue was clients with in-home health services. Following up with the home health agency was helpful in managing care of the clients in the shelter. Frequently, the agency continued care in the shelter once it was safe to travel. Family members were expected to provide the same support to their family members with health and mobility issues as they did at home. Nurses supported the family by providing any materials they needed to care for their family member or any needed training that helped the family better meet identified needs. One area that was particularly challenging was the need for special beds for clients who could not use the regular cots. For some, this was because of mobility issues or weight. For these clients, it was sometimes necessary to obtain a hospital bed or bariatric bed. There were also times when a client needed special equipment. The nurse worked with the family and local resources to meet the need.

Once clients were settled in the dormitory area, nurses began the process of interviewing each family to identify any access or functional needs; needs to maintain health and independence, and services, support, and transportation needs. Each family was interviewed, usually in the dormitory area where they chose to sleep. Nurses went to the clients rather than having the clients go to the nurses, as this created a more comfortable dynamic. This was the first time the nurse had the opportunity to establish a relationship with the family and identify health and wellness needs that may not have been identified earlier. For example, needs identified might include that a client did not bring all their medications, a client has dialysis treatment twice a week, a child's wheelchair is lost, a family member is autistic, or a client needs a medical treatment once a week. With this information, the nurse could begin to plan how to meet the client needs. It was important that the nurse had access to resource lists and phone numbers. It was not unusual for clients to come to the shelter without contact information for the resources they needed. The nurses worked with the family to identify the resources and arrange for the needs to be met. Most of the health services kits used by the nurses contained resource lists that helped with meeting client needs.

The health room in the shelter, staffed 24 hours a day, was designed to provide care for injured or ill clients and staff. Needs ranged from a situation requiring a Band-Aid to a serious illness or injury. The great majority of the health room visits in any shelter are for minor injuries: clients needing an aspirin for a headache or Band-Aids or clients wanting a blood pressure check. Over-the-counter (OTC) medications were stocked in the health room and managed by the nurses. A health services record was completed for every client treated. For example, a client coming in to request an aspirin would have a health services record completed. It was necessary to complete the health services record even for a single aspirin because if the client returned for aspirin multiple times, this may indicate a need for additional assessment. Since nurses changed regularly, documentation was the only way to track care, even with OTC medications.

Nurses in the shelter made periodic rounds of the client and staff areas throughout the day and night. They monitored activities such as feeding to ensure that food was not being left out for too long without proper storage. They reminded workers to wash their hands, talk with clients and staff, and listen to concerns. Nurses also monitored the health of kitchen volunteers, and others who were volunteering in the shelter. The importance of the presence of a nurse was illustrated by the following example. Client A mentioned to a nurse that she had seen client B going in and out of the bathroom multiple times that morning. The nurse was concerned and sought out client B. Client B stated that she had not been feeling well but thought it was from the worry and stress of the hurricane. The nurse walked her back to the health room, where she assessed client B, determining that the client's blood pressure was high and heart rate was irregular. The nurse immediately arranged for transport to the hospital, where client B remained for several days. Had the nurse not been interacting with clients in the dormitory, client B might have suffered a far worse outcome. Another incident within the shelter occurred with one of the kitchen volunteers who, despite having a cold, continued working as her illness got worse. It was not until several staff also got colds that the nurse realized the volunteer in the kitchen was spreading the virus.

1. Which of the competencies in the ICN *Core Competencies in Disaster Nursing, Version 2.0* are illustrated by the nurses' actions in this case study? Give specific examples.

CASE IN POINT ANSWERS

1. As part of the local health department education training program, notably within Domain 1: Preparation and Planning, the majority of health department nurses in the affected area had received Red Cross disaster health services training and followed Red Cross disaster protocol before the arrival of the hurricanes. Preparation and planning continued after the shelter was set up as the nurses determined where services within the shelter would be best located (e.g., health room area, kitchen, dormitory, bathrooms). Level I nurses were integral in the planning for each general population shelter, in staffing, and in services provided in each of the shelters for this disaster.

Once the shelter opened, the role of the nurse working in the shelter was to maintain the health and wellness of the shelter population and address the unmet disaster-related health needs of affected individuals, families, and communities. It was expected that nurses in the shelter work within their scope of practice. Common health needs in shelters include injuries, acute onset of illness, stress-related symptoms, aggravation of chronic health conditions, and loss of medications or health-related equipment. Nurses communicated regularly with shelter residents (Domain 2: Communication), working to register clients as they arrived, but also to provide calm reassurance during a difficult time. Further, they noted any injuries, medications needed, medical equipment needs, and access functional needs requiring special accommodations. Through such assessments, they determined the needs that the clients and their families had and worked through difficulties in meeting those needs. The importance of communication was exemplified in the nurse's conversations with client A and client B, preventing a potential poor health outcome. Further, Domain 5: Assessment and Domain 6: Intervention were woven throughout each encounter and each conversation the nurse on duty had with the clients in the shelter to identify needs and address them. These skills were used to determine if a client could remain in the general population shelter or if their needs required a higher level of care. They were also critical in supporting families in the provision of care, resolving issues related to medical needs, and the maintenance of health and independence.

Within Domain 4: Safety and Security, the nurse also must be cognizant of the health of staff. It is typical of staff to overwork or take on tasks that are more strenuous than they are accustomed to handling. This also may include working in the rain, cold, or heat; failing to remain hydrated; or working when not feeling well. Staff can be very insistent about wanting to keep working, despite such hardships. In this shelter, an example of this was seen in one of the kitchen volunteers who, despite having a cold, continued working as her cold got worse. It was not until several staff also got colds that the nurse realized that the volunteer in the kitchen was spreading the virus. It is important that health services volunteers monitor staff to ensure that they remain healthy and take action when a volunteer is ill. Regular interaction with clients and staff is paramount in managing the health of clients and staff during a disaster operation.

Nurses are a major part of every disaster response. They also must be part of planning for the future. They must understand how health services interacts with all other lines of service (e.g., sheltering, feeding, transportation, casework). Nurses bring extensive knowledge of emergency planning needs, including the health of the community, resources, needs of the community, and methods to maintain the health of the workforce. Often nurses see things from a different perspective than others, which can result in broader discussion of the topic, providing valuable input on lessons learned after each shelter operation. In addition, nurses must work with the health agencies in their communities, providing training for public health nurses and planning for disaster response in the community. Partnerships with hospitals, nursing homes, home health agencies, and medical supply companies are also important to ensure that there is an understanding of the disaster response process and how the agencies can better collaborate when a disaster occurs.

TEST YOUR KNOWLEDGE ANSWERS

1. What qualifications are required to be a competent Level I nurse or general professional nurse? *(Choose all that apply.)*
   a. **Completion of generalized nursing education**
   b. **Authorization to practice**
2. Which of the following is a principle of crisis and emergency risk communication?
   d. **All of the above**
3. Proficiency in using personal protective equipment is in which competency domain?
   b. **Safety and Security**
4. Knowledge of triage models is in which competency domain?
   a. **Assessment**
5. According to the ICN *Core Competencies in Disaster Nursing, Version 2.0*, what level are military nurses?
   c. **Level III**
6. Which of the following statements is true?
   d. **Many of the competencies taught in nursing education are also pertinent in disaster nursing.**
7. Nurses in long-term care facilities most frequently serve in which capacity during or after a disaster?
   a. **Supporting residents of the facility who must shelter in place during a disaster**
8. What are the three steps in the learning process for emergency medical teams?
   c. **License to practice and professional competence, adaptation to context, team performance**
9. Which of the steps in the learning process for emergency medical teams is an individual responsibility? *(Choose all that apply.)*
   a. **Step 1**
   b. **Step 2**
10. It is important to note that Level I nurses should:
    a. **Strive to become experts in a selected area of disaster nursing**
    b. **Understand that they may develop greater proficiency in one area of disaster nursing based on their area of practice**

Chapter 7

CASE IN POINT

Case Study 1

An earthquake with a magnitude of approximately 8 shook County A in the afternoon. There were several strong aftershocks. The earthquake triggered a large number of geohazards, including landslides and quake lakes. It also caused damage to buildings, roads, pipes, railways, and health facilities. Transportation to the nearest provincial capital and to hospitals about 200 kilometers (125 miles) away is not possible, as roads are blocked. Phone lines were damaged.

You are the nurse manager at the only hospital in the county. You have received notifications that thousands have been injured, in addition to several hundred fatalities. Most of the injuries involve broken limbs or arms or legs crushed by collapsed buildings and roads. There has also been some damage to the hospital building and facilities. The soon-to-arrive casualties will far exceed the usual capacity of your hospital and human resources.

1. What actions will you take in preparing for the arrival of casualties?
2. What other organizations will you seek assistance from, since there has been damage to the hospital's facilities, blocking your access to equipment?
3. How will you recruit enough nurses or health care workers, knowing that you do not have the human resources needed to help all the victims?
4. After the event is over, what will you do to prepare for any unforeseeable disasters in the future?

Case Study 2

You are a military nurse who has been deployed abroad to a clinic in an armed conflict zone. With the collapse of the infrastructure and health facilities in the village due to the conflict between an insurgent group and the government, your clinic has been providing medical services to soldiers as well as locals. Your team has been waiting for the arrival of necessary medical supplies, but it has been delayed by sporadic attacks from the insurgent troops. Your team is worried about the current lack of medical supplies. However, you have received a warning that the base may be attacked tonight.

You are the team leader responsible for triage today, and you predict that wounded soldiers will be coming in if attacks do occur. You surmise that you will need to save the medical supplies that you have on hand. In the afternoon, the insurgent group launches an air attack on the village near your station. Three severely injured local residents are quickly transported to your clinic. A man in his 60s and a woman in her 30s are bleeding severely upon arrival. They will die soon if they do not get immediate treatment and minor surgery. The third victim is a small boy of about 8 years old, who is suffering from multiple trauma injuries and burns; treating him will require the use of a large portion of your limited medical supplies.

1. How would you classify the three victims?
2. Would you treat these victims?
3. How would you balance the role of a nurse with that of a military nurse in charge?

CASE IN POINT ANSWERS

Case Study 1

Background. An earthquake is a major and frequent natural disaster that can lead to a large number of casualties and huge losses. In the period 2000–2019, 552 earthquakes were reported to have occurred around the world, which caused 72,315 deaths, caused 1,487,046 injuries, and affected 117 million people. However, in terms of the death toll, injuries, and total number of affected people, the 2008 Wenchuan earthquake in Sichuan Province, China, was the most severe of the earthquakes that occurred during that period. It caused 87,564 deaths, caused 368,412 injuries, and affected 47 million people. Here, the Wenchuan earthquake of 2008 is used to illustrate its impact on a hospital in a county, to facilitate discussion on the responses of advanced or specialized nurses.

Public Health Impact of a Large Earthquake. On May 12, 2008, a magnitude 8.0 earthquake occurred in the county of Wenchuan in Sichuan Province, China. The earthquake caused buildings to collapse and led to landslides, floods, and the creation of quake lakes. It also caused large numbers of trauma-related deaths and injuries, with cardiopulmonary arrest, severe craniocerebral injuries, incurable hemorrhagic shock, and crush syndrome being the major causes of on-site deaths. The damage to roads and health facilities was the major obstacle to providing appropriate medical care to victims. Days later, more than 100 medical teams from around the nation arrived to provide on-scene emergency medical care in Wenchuan. The governments in the earthquake-affected areas also adopted rapid and multistage assessments and interventions that prevented further complications and risks after the earthquake, such as outbreaks of infectious diseases or other public health emergencies.

As of February 5, 2009, nearly 9 months after the earthquake, 97.8% of patients had been treated and discharged. Among the 928 patients still in a hospital; 5.9% suffered from brain trauma; 17.6% from paraplegia; 28.0% from amputations; and 48.4% from severe spine, pelvis, and other fractures. The earthquake had caused a public health threat due to the large number of causalities and had a long-term impact on the area.

Tips for Your Deliberation

Actions to take in preparing for the arrival of casualties

The International Council of Nurses (2019) core competencies in disaster nursing illustrate the skills of advanced nurses in disaster management at various stages. As part of the disaster response effort, advanced or specialized nurses in a hospital should act as planners, leaders, and communicators to provide immediate incident management. They are expected to guide the nursing team with the appropriate specialties to develop an immediate action plan, provide rapid assessments, and identify the at-risk populations. In their leadership role, they also are responsible for maintaining the safety and security of nursing staff and patients and for communicating and collaborating with other professional teams and organizations in the earthquake rescue team and in the health emergency response effort.

Filling the need for enough nurses

Second, the advanced or specialized nurses should maintain referral resources and provide professional health care and mental health counselling to nurses as well as patients with regard to posttraumatic stress disorder, depression, and anxiety in the postdisaster recovery stage.

Preparing for unforeseeable disasters in the future

Third, the advanced or specialized nurses should work with community leaders to increase levels of awareness, knowledge, and skills in disaster response at the organizational and community levels. At the organizational level, the nurses should participate in evaluating and revising the emergency plans of organizations and take the lead in holding regular earthquake evaluation drills. They also should work with other professionals to increase the resilience of hospital facilities (e.g., hospital backup power, water supply, fire protection and escape, communication systems) as well as plan the human resources needed for a disaster response. At the community level, advanced or specialized nurses should initiate community health forums and offer education to the general public to increase their awareness of disaster, individual and family preparedness, and response actions upon the occurrence of an earthquake.

Case Study 2

Classification of the three victims, and decision to treat as a military nurse

All three victims would be treated as emergency cases in need of immediate care. The ethical principle of utilitarianism is to be considered to do the greatest good for the greatest number. If all three victims can be treated with available resources, they would be treated as they arrive. However, the military nurse in charge needs to reserve essential resources (equipment, supplies and skilled personnel) to treat the arrival of anticipated wounded military members who may be expected to return to service.

Military nurses have conflicting roles in the provision of nursing care during a deployment because they are nurses who see all patients as equal human beings; however, as members of the military, their priority is to care for their own service members to help them return to their missions as soon as possible. Military nurses often face a dilemma in their triage of victims because they sometimes must decide whether to treat victims in need of urgent trauma care when faced with limited help and a shortage of medical supplies.

TEST YOUR KNOWLEDGE ANSWERS

1. What is the best description of the roles of advanced or specialized nurses in disaster management?
   d. All of the above
2. Nurses who have completed a basic education program in general nursing and are authorized to practice by the regulatory agency in their country are:
   b. Equipped with Level I of the core competencies in disaster nursing
3. Nurses who are regarded as being equipped with Level III core competencies in disaster nursing are:
   b. Advanced nurses who have attained a higher level of competencies and are willing to be deployed both nationally and internationally to serve in disaster response efforts
4. What are the possible benefits to adopting a bottom-up community-based disaster reduction education program?
   d. All of the above
5. Advanced or specialized nurses in public health are community health educators. Which of the following is **not** their key responsibility?
   c. Teaching medical knowledge to the general public
6. The practice of disaster nursing during an epidemic emergency response includes:
   d. All of the above
7. A specialized disaster nurse description does **not** include:
   a. General professional nurses
8. The zoning in wards for infectious disease does **not** include:
   c. An office zone
9. Which of the following descriptions of the roles of military nurses in response to a disaster is **not** true?
   b. Military nurses are deployed to a disaster only by military command.
10. All of the following statements about the work of advanced or specialized military nurses during triage at a disaster site are true, **except**:
    b. Should exclude prisoners or detainees of war from receiving treatment

Chapter 8

CASE IN POINT

The home health nurse is visiting a 59-year-old married male client who was discharged from the hospital yesterday. The purpose of the visit is to review the care and dressing change instructions for his new central line catheter through which he will receive chemotherapy. While driving to the client's home, the nurse notices the couple's close proximity to the town's main river. They have a dock at the back of their home. It has been raining off and on for the past 3 days, and the forecast calls for several more days of heavy rainstorms.

1. What types of questions will the nurse ask this client and his wife regarding their proximity to the water?
2. What will the nurse assess regarding their preparations for emergencies?
3. What items should the couple keep with them at all times, especially if swift evacuation is required?
4. What will the nurse teach about foods and water if they should lose power to their home?
5. What other information will the nurse share to prepare them for emergencies?

Case In Point Answers

1. The nurse will ask the client and his wife if they have experienced flooding in the past at their current location. What have they done in this situation in the past? Do they have an evacuation plan? How soon must they leave to drive to a shelter before the water rises and makes major streets and thoroughfares impassable due to flooding? Do they have a boat prepared in the event of a water evacuation?

2. Some of the questions in #1 will be repeated. The nurse also will assess if they have a "go bag" prepared ahead of time to take with them if a rapid evacuation is required. Do they have an alternative site to visit for chemotherapy if the usual office is inaccessible? How far away are they from a medical facility, as they should be seen within 1 to 2 hours of spiking a fever?

3. The client should have treatment calendars with him at all times that indicate the treatment protocols and a medication log that any health care provider can review to save valuable treatment time should an emergency arise. Keep all medications together, stored where they will be able to get to in an emergency, including medications to prevent nausea, constipation, diarrhea, allergic reactions, and fevers. Have a basic "ready kit" to help keep them safe and healthy during a disaster. This includes water, nonperishable foods, battery-powered radio and weather radio, flashlight, cell phone with batteries, and cell phone charger. Important documents (such as health insurance information, cancer treatment, allergies, blood type, home care instructions, and a list of whom to contact) should be stored in a seal-tight container. Personal care items, face mask, sturdy shoes, hat, gloves, underwear, and a warm blanket are some other recommended items.

4. Do they know not to eat raw seafood or drink water that is possibly contaminated? Infection control is a major issue for immunocompromised patients. Teach patients to have bottled water ready and not to risk drinking water of questionable purity. It may be risky to eat fresh fruits and vegetables due to the risk of contamination and subsequent infection. They may consume processed or canned foods if these can be heated to the proper temperatures.

5. Make sure that anyone who can turn off the gas, water, and electricity in their home knows how to do this. Have a plan for pets. If they need life-sustaining equipment such as pumps or oxygen tanks, they should contact their utility company. If they are doing central line dressing changes, they need to have supplies readily available. The supplies need to be double bagged to keep them dry.

TEST YOUR KNOWLEDGE ANSWERS

1. Which of the following are examples of meteorological natural disasters? *(Choose all that apply.)*
   a. **Tornadoes**
   b. **Hurricanes**
2. Which of the following are examples of biological natural disasters? *(Choose all that apply.)*
   c. **COVID-19**
   d. ***Salmonella* poisoning**
3. Which of the following are examples of geological natural disasters? *(Choose all that apply.)*
   a. **Earthquakes**
   b. **Volcanoes**
4. A patient suspected of having heat stroke is brought to the emergency department. Which of the following is true?
   c. **Core body temperature of at least 41°C (106°F)**

5. A person who is diagnosed with hypothermia would likely exhibit which of the following symptoms? *(Choose all that apply.)*
   a. **Shivering**
   b. **Exhaustion**
   d. **Slurred speech**
6. Appropriate treatment for persons diagnosed with hypothermia would include: *(Choose all that apply.)*
   a. **Warm the core areas of the body**
   b. **Seek medical attention quickly**
   c. **Cardiopulmonary resuscitation**
   d. **Remove wet clothing**
7. Nurses should be aware of the immediate health needs after disasters, such as: *(Choose all that apply.)*
   a. **Clean drinking water**
   b. **Nutritious food**
   c. **Shelter**
   d. **Medical care for injuries**
8. Nurses are in a position to teach the general public about secondary health effects of disasters. Which of the following statements are true? *(Choose all that apply.)*
   b. **Those most at risk are those who handle bodies and prepare them for burial.**
   d. **Contaminated food and water may cause worsening illnesses that already exist in the affected region.**
9. The long-term duties of public health officials and others engaging in disaster relief and recovery include: *(Choose all that apply.)*
   a. **Monitoring for infectious water or disease-transmitted diseases**
   b. **Restoring primary health services, water systems, and housing**
   c. **Diverting medical supplies from nonaffected areas to meet the needs of the affected regions**
   d. **Assisting community members to recover mentally and socially when the crisis has subsided**
10. Massive heat waves such as the European heat wave of 2019 can cause which of the following effects? *(Choose all that apply.)*
    a. **An extensive number of deaths**
    b. **Wildfires that destroy land, homes, and vehicles**
    c. **Deaths and injuries among first responders, police, and firefighters**

Chapter 10

TEST YOUR KNOWLEDGE ANSWERS

1. The most common types of chemicals used in chemical warfare are:
   b. **Nerve agents, blister agents, lung irritants, blood agents, and incapacitants**
2. Nerve agents:
   a. **Are highly toxic in small doses**
3. The type of agent used in the Tokyo subway attacks was:
   b. **Sarin**
4. A key planning failure from the Bhopal disaster that could have been mitigated in the preparedness phase was:
   d. **All of the above**
5. If unable to identify the specific chemical exposure, the best treatment is:

    b. Symptom management
6. What is the most common triage scale used for chemical disaster?
    d. Four scale
7. Indicators that a chemical release has occurred include:
    d. All of the above
8. When managing patients who have been exposed to a chemical release, you must protect yourself by:
    c. Wearing chemical-resistant personal protective equipment with a respirator prior to decontamination and using standard precautions thereafter
9. The antidote for nerve agents is:
    b. Atropine and oximes
10. Which of the following is true of decontamination?
    b. No one from the scene of a chemical release should be allowed to enter a health care facility without being decontaminated first.

Chapter 11

CASE IN POINT

A.H. is a 32-year-old Saudi female who has worked as a registered nurse (RN) in primary health care since 2010. She was interviewed by the author on July 14, 2020, for the purpose of presenting an international RN's reflection on a global pandemic (COVID-19).

Description

A.H. currently works at a hospital in Saudi Arabia. She was assigned to care for patients and conduct active screenings for COVID-19 cases beginning on May 16, 2020. She described her experience as exhausting, overwhelming, and educational. A.H. stated that, based on what she observed, approximately 70% of cases had the same signs and symptoms, including fever, shortness of breath, fatigue, dizziness, and gastrointestinal distress.

    A.H. stated that, fortunately, several infectious disease outbreak preparedness initiatives were started in Saudi Arabia in 2018. She stated that the Ministry of Health (MOH) of Saudi Arabia launched a new protocol requiring all RNs to attend a licensing program called Basic Infection Control Skills License (BICSL). The program includes several teaching strategies for infectious disease management, such as lectures and workshops. She also stated that nurses were required to have meningitis and influenza vaccinations and to undergo a fit test to verify the proper fitting of the N95 respirator. The program also involves practicing hand hygiene and the use of personal protective equipment (PPE). A.H. stated that to obtain the required license to be able to work in Saudi health care settings, each RN was obligated to get the required vaccinations and attend one-on-one training sessions with a trained instructor. She stated that "although I was uncertain about caring or being with COVID-19 patients, the BICSL program eased my burden and prepared me for such an unexpected event." Another preparedness measure taken by the MOH was that larger hospitals were required to have an isolation unit and a disaster team to respond to any disaster event.

    A.H. stated that the MOH responded to COVID-19 quickly and effectively. They provided all hospitals, including private ones, with the necessary equipment such as PPE, mechanical ventilators, N95 respirators, high-efficiency particulate air (HEPA) filters, and more. They also created a COVID-19 survey system so that all people in Saudi Arabia could contact the hospital if they have symptoms or concerns. Regarding legal aspects, A.H. stated that the Saudi MOH announced that during the COVID-19 pandemic, all people in Saudi Arabia, citizens and immigrants alike, would receive necessary care, paid for by the MOH, and suspected cases and stable infected people would be quarantined in paid hotels. The MOH also launched a website for nurses to request a free psychiatric clinic visit.

Regarding ethical aspects, A.H. expressed her feelings by stating, "I was not excited about being a nurse at that time, but the code of ethics necessitates that nurses should care for all patients regardless of the severity and risk of their disease." She also stated that "I told myself that I have to care for all COVID-19 patients as I provide usual care for [all] patients, which helped me learn how to deal with the situation." A.H. stated that there were some special considerations for populations with chronic diseases. The MOH launched a website for people with chronic diseases to request a free at-home doctor visit, paid medication including delivery, and free transportation to and from the hospital when needed.

Lessons Learned

1. Being prepared for disasters helps nurses to handle the unexpected. Health care providers were aware of the PPE and other equipment needed during the infectious disaster; hence, they provided proper care while being extremely cautious.
2. Protecting yourself as a nurse helps you to protect other people.
3. Teaching patients about the disease is better than letting them rely on myths spread via social media.
4. All patients, regardless of their disease severity, race, gender, and nationality, need to be treated equally.

Questions for Discussion

1. When should professional nurses begin to learn and prepare for disasters, specifically infectious disease outbreaks?
   Professional nursing disaster preparedness programs should be initiated well in advance of a disaster event or public health emergency. Ideally, disaster education should occur as nurses are being prepared for practice in their basic nursing education programs.
2. What are some of the patient characteristics nurses should consider when given a patient assignment when an infectious disease is suspected?
   Nurses should provide optimal care for all patients equally.

TEST YOUR KNOWLEDGE ANSWERS

1. Which of the following statements are true about biological or infectious disease outbreaks? *(Choose all that apply.)*
   a. **There is increased risk of transmittable disease spread.**
   b. **The incidence of infectious disease outbreaks has been increasing globally.**
2. Examples of global infectious disease outbreaks include: *(Choose all that apply.)*
   a. **MERS**
   b. **Ebola**
   c. **COVID-19**
3. The distinguishing feature of unnatural biological infections is that they: *(Choose all that apply.)*
   b. **Are caused by microorganisms altered or created to increase harm inflicted**
4. Which of the following features would cause health care providers to suspect an intentional biological weapon? *(Choose all that apply.)*
   a. **Increased morbidity and death rate**
   b. **Human-to-human transmission**
   c. **Nonavailability of effective vaccine**
   d. **Highly infectious potential**
5. Emerging infectious diseases have which of the following characteristics? *(Choose all that apply.)*

      a. **Infections occur in humans.**
      c. **Occurrence increases rapidly.**
      d. **They are new to a population or region.**

6. Which of the following statements are true regarding the spread of infectious disease pathogens? *(Choose all that apply.)*
      a. **Some pathogens transmit directly from infected to uninfected individuals.**
      b. **Some pathogens spread via uninfected humans and animals.**
      d. **Some pathogens can be spread without the knowledge of the host or exposed individual.**

7. Which of the following statements are true about horizontal transmission? *(Choose all that apply.)*
      a. **Microorganisms are passed by direct contact between infected and uninfected individuals.**
      b. **Horizontal transmission is also called colonization.**
      c. **Direct contact can occur through traveling.**
      d. **Direct contact can occur through sexual contact or sharing common areas.**

8. Which of the following statements are true about vertical transmission? *(Choose all that apply.)*
      a. **It promotes the transmission of the infecting bacteria, fungi, or viruses.**
      b. **The transmission can occur from mother to fetus during birth.**

9. Challenges to the prevention and control of the global spread of infectious diseases include: *(Choose all that apply.)*
      a. **Some infectious viruses can be transmitted horizontally and vertically**
      b. **Increasing antimicrobial resistance related to overuse of antibiotics**
      c. **Increased mobility of global citizens through worldwide travel**

10. One of the strongest messages nurses can share about decreasing the spread of infectious diseases is that:
      c. **Regular handwashing is one of the best ways to remove germs, avoid getting sick, and prevent the spread of germs to others.**

Chapter 12

TEST YOUR KNOWLEDGE ANSWERS

1. The production and storage of hazardous materials occur in: *(Choose all that apply.)*
      a. **Chemical plants**
      b. **Gas stations**
      c. **Hospitals**
      d. **Industrial cleaning supply companies**

2. The exodus of families from the Love Canal area was the result of:
      b. **The indiscriminate disposal of toxic materials**

3. An example of an accidental disaster is:
      b. **A fuel tanker that runs aground due to poor visibility in a storm**

4. Conventional terrorist weapons: *(Choose all that apply.)*
      a. **Include car and truck bombs**
      c. **Are often used in suicide attacks**
      d. **Include handguns, rifles, and semiautomatic weapons**

5. Which of the following events is most likely to be linked to negligence?
      d. **Collapse of a poorly maintained highway overpass**

6. A lone gunman livestreams an attack on a mosque over the internet. He kills more than 50 worshippers. Which of the following statements is true?
      c. **The psychologically traumatized will make up the majority of survivors.**

7. In 1984 salad bars in numerous food outlets in Oregon were deliberately contaminated with *Salmonella enterica* bacteria by a local political group, causing more than 400 cases of food poisoning. Which terms best characterize this event? *(Choose all that apply.)*
    a. **Domestic terrorism**
    c. **Bioterrorism**
8. Which of the following phrases is true?
    a. **Improvised explosive devices can be readily manufactured from commercially available components.**
9. Which of the following are indicators of PTSD? *(Choose all that apply.)*
    d. **Extreme physical reactions to reminders of an event such as a nausea, sweating, or a pounding heart**
10. Chemical terrorism can include: *(Choose all that apply.)*
    a. **Poisonous gas sprayed from aircrafts**
    b. **Liquid cyanide added to bodies of water**
    d. **Deliberate contamination of food**

Chapter 13

CASE IN POINT

The People's Hospital is located on an island in the South Pacific. A new director of nursing has been hired to lead the nurses in the hospital and specialized personnel. She has experience with disaster preparedness from her previous hospital, but that hospital was on the US mainland and the disaster threats were very different. She plans to lead a discussion with hospital department heads regarding the organization's hazards and vulnerabilities so that she can be prepared in her new role and to assist the other leaders in preparedness activities. In this way, they will enhance their collaborative relationship and select response and recovery strategies for possible future disaster events that affect their hospital's community and its people.

Use the hazard vulnerability assessment tools in Appendix B to assess the risk of each natural hazard for this area. What are the three most likely natural disasters that could affect this region? Are the mitigation efforts in effect for each of these three most likely natural disasters? What would you advise this hospital regarding preparedness efforts based on the findings of this assessment?

Possible Responses

The scoring of the hazard vulnerability assessment tool (Kaiser Permanente Medical Center [2014] or Appendix B tools) may vary based on the participant's perception of threats and vulnerability. The most likely natural disasters that could affect this region are directly related to the island's location: rain, flooding, fires, tsunamis, hurricanes, storm surge, earthquakes, and possibly volcanoes. Mitigation efforts will be determined by the participant's perception and indication of the level of mitigation efforts. Advising the hospital should include an assessment of structural integrity, contingency plans for staffing, alternate care sites, evacuation of the hospital and possibly of the island, and memoranda of agreement with other health care facilities or providers on the island.

TEST YOUR KNOWLEDGE ANSWERS

1. It is important for nurses to be knowledgeable about disaster planning and response because: *(Choose all that apply.)*
    b. **Nurses traditionally have been sought out by neighbors, friends, and communities for health care information and advice.**

    d. Professional nurses historically have responded to the needs of society, including in times of disaster.

2. A key to effective disaster management is:

    b. Anticipating the probable disasters and planning for them

3. An effective risk assessment informs proposed actions by focusing attention and resources on the greatest risks. Some of the basic components of a risk assessment are: (*Choose all that apply.*)

    a. Hazard identification

    c. Inventory of assets

    d. Estimation of potential human and economic losses

4. A hazard identification and risk assessment provides:

    b. A factual basis for activities proposed in hazard mitigation

5. Nurses should be involved in disaster preparedness, response, and recovery efforts because: (*Choose all that apply.*)

    a. The general public trusts nurses.

    b. Nurses have the knowledge to provide input in disaster planning.

    c. Nurses have an obligation to the public to be well informed.

    d. The general public will seek the advice of nurses to direct them in appropriate actions to take.

6. In the US Midwest, a small community hospital is located in a low-lying area within a mile of a river. The hospital's disaster preparedness committee likely will score which hazard as "high" on the vulnerability scale?

    a. Flooding

7. After a disaster or public health emergency in a community, it is advisable to have supplies and backup resources for at least 96 hours because:

    b. It may take as long as 96 hours for outside relief to arrive to help the community.

8. The Strategic National Stockpile:

    b. Contains medicines and supplies for those who need them most during an emergency

9. Which of the following are considered as essential items in the category of clinical activities when selecting a 96-hour sustainability resources and assets? (*Choose all that apply.*)

    a. Medications

    b. IV fluids

    c. Blood and blood products

10. The hazard vulnerability analysis informs disaster and emergency planning efforts. If the HVA indicates a high risk of flooding, reasonable mitigation efforts would include: (*Choose all that apply.*)

    a. Relocate high-value items to higher floors

    b. Relocate portable electronic equipment to safe areas

    c. Place external heating, ventilation, and air conditioning (HVAC) systems on the roof when designing the new building tower

Chapter 14

CASE IN POINT

This case study illustrates how ICN's *Core Competencies in Disaster Nursing, Version 2.0* can be operationalized. It is a realistic example of a points of dispensing (POD) operation that evolved from an annual mass immunization clinic led by public health nursing (PHN) students. The annual clinic is a "dual-purpose" activity because it includes health promotion and disease prevention by immunizing members of the campus community as well as providing emergency preparedness training in which students are expected to respond to a scenario involving a Centers for Disease Control and Prevention (CDC) announcement of a virulent strain of influenza followed by the local public health department's request for mass immunization from various community partners.

The Case

Faculty members of a senior level nursing course designed an emergency preparedness exercise that used an annual mass immunization clinic as the basis for a simulated response to an infectious disease outbreak. During the project, students were given a scenario in which the local public health department (PHD) has requested the College of Nursing to open a points of dispensing (POD) clinic. Students had to plan POD logistics, social marketing, and community education to meet the goal; implement the plan; and complete an after-action report.

In response to an outbreak of Type A influenza at a local university, the local PHD recommended that the university prevent spread into the larger community by beginning vaccinations for its students, faculty, and staff as soon as possible. Health center staff at the university and nursing faculty collaborated on an immediate POD clinic targeted toward the campus population at greatest risk for exposure and spread of influenza.

The POD operation used the plan for the university's annual mass immunization clinic as its basis ("systems"), and senior nursing majors in a public health nursing (PHN) course served as the primary workforce ("staff") under faculty supervision. The vaccine ("supplies") was requested from the Centers for Disease Control and Prevention (CDC) for immediate shipment, and an appropriate location was selected for the clinic ("structure").

The POD clinic was offered over several days, and more than 900 doses were administered. At the conclusion of the POD clinic, the PHN students immediately resumed planning for the annual vaccination clinic, incorporating lessons learned during the after-action debriefing.

Continued tracking of influenza incidence revealed that the majority of positive influenza cases occurred prior to the POD clinic being established, during its operation, or during the period needed for antibody formation, suggesting that the POD operation—combined with social isolation for those testing positive for influenza—successfully limited further spread. After-action analysis suggested that continued practice and improvement of this emergency preparedness activity allowed it to be successful when put to the test by an actual outbreak.

Analyzing the Case

For the POD operation to be successful, all elements of surge capacity (staff, supplies, structure, and systems) had to be in place. Scalable "systems" were already in place for the POD operation because the basis for its setup was a well-established plan used for the university's annual mass immunization clinic. Potential "staff" were identified, with senior nursing majors acting as the primary workforce and faculty serving in dual roles as supervisors of the nursing students and vaccinators as needed. The vaccine ("supplies") was requested from the CDC for immediate shipment. The clinic site ("structure") was selected to ensure that it was readily accessible to the target population and large enough for all POD components to be located within it.

For more than a decade, the College of Nursing has offered a 1-day annual mass immunization clinic for more than 3000 students, staff, and faculty based on core PHN concepts and resources including *Healthy People 2020*. Senior nursing students in a PHN course play a leading role in the clinic's design and delivery; development and delivery of "just in time" (JIT) training for junior and senior nursing students; and related health education, outreach, and marketing. This larger scale event functions with as many as 21 vaccination stations, staffed by junior and senior nursing students who have completed JIT training conducted by senior nursing students. More experienced students monitor and coach incoming students who have completed JIT training, and faculty provide ongoing consultation and intervention as needed.

To allow for both POD clinic operation and ongoing class schedules, the clinic was offered over 3 days, 3 to 6 hours at a time, with 6 vaccination stations. The team of student participants was smaller, but faculty supervision needs were greater because the clinic fell so early in the semester. Unlike the annual mass immunization clinic in which faculty focus most of their attention to activities at delivery stations, faculty supervisors for the POD clinic were also dedicated to consenting, JIT training, priming of vaccinations, and monitoring for adverse reactions. Due to the time constraints, JIT training was conducted using the previous year's documentation, literature review, and educational posters, with lessons learned through debriefing after the POD operation incorporated into JIT training and planning for the annual clinic. More than 900 doses were administered, with the health center continuing to vaccinate until the annual vaccination clinic. At the conclusion of the POD clinic, the PHN students immediately resumed planning for the annual vaccination clinic scheduled for October, incorporating lessons learned during the debriefing. The annual clinic resumed its usual student-led format but took only half a day because the majority of doses had already been administered.

Continued tracking of influenza-like illness (ILI) incidence through the fall semester revealed that 86% of the positive influenza cases occurred prior to the POD clinic, during its operation, or during the period for antibody formation. The health center and PHD determined that the POD operation—combined with social isolation for those testing positive for influenza—successfully limited further spread of ILI. After-action analysis suggested that continued practice and improvement of this emergency preparedness activity allowed it to be successful when put to the test by an actual outbreak.

TEST YOUR KNOWLEDGE ANSWERS

1. What type of exercise does the CASE IN POINT illustrate?
   a. **Full-scale exercise**
2. What elements of surge capacity are necessary for a POD operation to be successful? *(Choose all that apply.)*
   a. **Staff**
   b. **Supplies**
   c. **Structure**
   d. **Systems**
3. Based on the information in the CASE IN POINT, what populations would be at greatest risk for exposure and spread of influenza? *(Choose all that apply.)*
   a. **Students, faculty, and staff of the College of Nursing**
4. How do operations-based exercises differ from discussion-based exercises? *(Choose all that apply.)*
   b. **May involve mobilization of resources in real time**
   c. **Allow the most realistic evaluation of necessary resources**
5. What are important elements of planning the exercise design?
   a. **Needs assessment and establishing exercise scope**
6. Which disaster exercise will allow participants to apply knowledge and problem solve through group discussion?
   a. **Tabletop exercise**
7. When planning for a full-scale exercise, important considerations should include awareness that a full-scale exercise will:
   c. **Include real-time activity and resource mobilization**
8. When planning an operations-based exercise to support maintenance of a specific skill within a single organization, it would be most appropriate to design a:
   c. **Drill**

9. How can realism be promoted in exercises? *(Choose all that apply.)*
   a. **Use of functional equipment**
   b. **Application of moulage to simulated patients**
   c. **Combining multiple simulation modalities**
10. What is the purpose of an after-action report? *(Choose all that apply.)*
    a. **Evaluates participants' performance of their disaster roles**
    b. **Serves as a foundation to plan evaluation and process improvement**

INDEX

Note: Page numbers followed by *f* indicate figures, *t* indicate tables, and *b* indicate boxes

A

Accidental acts, 226–228
Accidental infectious disease outbreaks, 213–214, 213*f*
Acute stress disorder (ASD), 100–101
Advanced or specialized nurses (ASNs)
 case study, 146–147, 282–283
 core competencies, 136–139, 137*t*–138*t*
  assessments, 139
  communications, 136
  incident management, 136–139
  intervention, 139
  law and ethics, 139
  preparedness and planning, 136
  recovery, 139
  safety and security, 139
 Korean Armed Forces Nurses, 143–146
 public health disaster management, 139–143
  community leaders and villagers, workshop for,
   140–141
  COVID-19 epidemic, 141–143
Aedes aegypti mosquito, 217*f*
Afghanistan-victims of war, 232*b*–233*b*
All-hazards approach, 30
American Association of Colleges of Nursing
  (AACN), 6
American Red Cross, 28–29
ASNs. *See* Advanced or specialized nurses (ASNs)
Assessment
 advanced or specialized nurses (ASNs), 139
 general professional nurse (GPN), 120
Authority during a disaster, 63–64

B

Basic Infection Control Skills License (BICSL), 219–220
Behavioral health disorders, 100–101
Be Informed, Make a Plan, Build a Kit, and Get
  Involved, 45–47
Bhopal disaster, 195, 198–199
Biological disease outbreaks
 emerging, 214
 incidence, 212
 natural, 212
 unnatural, 213–214
 vertical and horizontal transmission modes,
  214–219, 219*f*

Biological terrorism, 230–231
Body and eye shower, 70*f*
Boston Marthon bombing, 106–107, 106*f*, 277–278
Brainstorming, 243–244

C

Car and truck bombs, 230
Casualty management
 blood components, provision of, 74–76
 patient tracking, 77–78
 preparations for care, 69–71
 staff, 72–73
 triage, 73–74
CBT. *See* Cognitive behavioral therapy (CBT)
Centers for Medicare and Medicaid Services
  (CMS), 28
Chemical disasters
 Bhopal disaster, 195, 198–199
 chemical groups, 195–198
 definition, 195
 ethical considerations, 207–208
 legal considerations, 207
 preparedness
  health facilities, 200
  plans, 200
  risk assessment, 199
 recovery activities, 206–207
 response
  chemical release indicator, 201–202
  decontamination, 203–204
  identifying the chemical, 205
  life-saving treatment and triage, 204–205
  medical management, 205–206
  personal protective equipment, 202–203
  psychological impacts, 206
  special considerations, 208
 Tokyo subway attacks, 195, 199
Chemical terrorism, 230
CHEMPACK, 28
Chernobyl Nuclear Power Plant, 178
Children, 102
Climate change, 158
Clinical activities, 244
Clinic/outpatient care nurse, 125
CMS. *See* Centers for Medicare and Medicaid
  Services (CMS)

Cognitive behavioral therapy (CBT), 101–102
Communication, 32
    advanced or specialized nurses (ASNs), 136
    general professional nurse (GPN), 117–118
Communication, 68–69
Community leaders and villagers, workshop for,
        140–141
Community Preparedness Toolkit, 28–29
Conventional terrorist weapons, 230
Core Competencies in Disaster Nursing, Version 2.0, 6,
        135–136
Coronavirus Disease 2019 (COVID-19), 214, 217*f*,
        218*f*, 219–220
    advanced or specialized nurses (ASNs), 141–143
    education for disaster response, 49
    Korean military nurses (KMNs), 145
    persons with disabilities, 14
    resources and logistics, 31, 32*f*
    rural hospital health care coalition, 33
    student nurse, 124
Crisis
    assessment, 94–97
    intervention, 94–97
Culturally appropriate preparedness measures, 51

D

Decontamination, 68
    chemical disasters, 203–204
    cold weather considerations, 71*b*
    contamination zone, 69*f*
    infographic, 72*f*
Deliberate acts, 226–228
Deliberate infectious disease outbreaks, 213
Dirty bomb. *See* Radiological dispersal device
        (RDD); Radiological dispersion bomb
Disaster and public health emergency, COVID-19,
        219–220
Disaster education resources, 49*t*–50*t*
Disaster management
    cyclical sequence, 7*f*
    stages, 7–10
Disaster Nursing Version 2.0, core competencies in,
        263*t*–265*t*
Disaster preparedness
    communication, 42–43
    planning
        tools and resources, 39
        types, 40–42
    resource management, 44–45
    risk reduction and mitigation, 43–44
    schools of nursing, 45
    volunteers, 45
Disaster response committee, 65–66

Disaster risk reduction (DRR), 38, 43–44
Disaster supply kits, 48*b*
Discussion-based exercises, 245, 249, 251*t*–253*t*
Domestic terrorism, 228
Drills, 249–250. *See also* Exercise
Drought, 157–158

E

Earthquakes, 160–162
Ebola virus disease (EVD), 214–219, 218*f*
Emergency department (ED), 12
    personal preparedness, 55–56
    professional preparedness, 55–56
Emergency evaluation kit, 47, 47*f*
Emergency medical teams (EMTs), 125–126
Emergency Nurses Association (ENA), 146
Emergency operations plan (EOP). *See* Health care
        emergency preparedness
Emergency preparedness. *See also* Preparedness
    exercise. *See* Exercise
    health care. *See* Health care emergency
        preparedness
    organizations
        community/local/state level, 28–29
        global/regional level, 23–24
        national/regional level, 24–28
Emergency & Relief Nursing for Disaster, 146
Emergency System for Advance Registration of
        Volunteer Health Professionals (ESAR-VHP), 6
Emerging infectious disease outbreaks, 214
Ethical considerations
    chemical disasters, 207–208
    radiological emergencies, 187–189
Exercise
    activities, 249
    case study, 292–294
    categories, 249
    design, 250–254
    evaluation, 257
    planning resources, 257, 258*t*
    simulation, 254–257
    types, 249–250
Explosive materials, 230
Expressive art therapy, 102
Extreme heat and cold, 160

F

Family preparedness, 31–32
Fangcang Shelter (FCS) in Hanyang District,
        Wuhan, 142–143
Federal Emergency Management Agency (FEMA),
        12, 13*f*, 28–29, 64, 65*f*

Fidelity, 254–255
Five-level triage, 74
Flooding, 157
Fukushima Daiichi Nuclear Power Plant, 178–179
Full-blown chemical disasters, 195
Full-scale exercises, 249–250, 250*f*
Functional exercises, 249–250

G

Geiger-Mueller (GM) survey meter, 185*f*
General professional nurse (GPN)
 case example, 127–129, 279–281
 core competency domains, 137*t*–138*t*
  assessment, 120
  communication, 117–118
  incident management systems, 118
  intervention, 120
  law and ethics, 122
  preparation and planning, 116–117
  recovery, 120–122
  safety and security, 118–119
 global threats, 112–114
 role, 114–116
 specialty areas of practice
  clinic/outpatient care, 125
  hospital/acute care, 122–123
  institutions of higher learning, 123–124
  international emergency medical teams, 125–126
  long-term care, 125
  public health, 123
  student nurse, 124
  volunteers, 125
Geological natural disasters
 earthquakes, 160–162
 landslides, 162–163
 tsunamis, 162
 volcanoes, 163
GPN. *See* General professional nurse (GPN)
Grenades, 230

H

Hazardous waste sign, 228*f*
Hazard vulnerability analysis (HVA), 240–243
 applications, 244–245
 case study, 291
 facility assessment, 241–242
 tools to measure, 242–243
Hazard vulnerability chart, 240–241
Head nurse
 earthquake, emergency response, 146–147

Health care emergency preparedness
 all-hazards and mass casualty incidents, 30
 checklist, 29, 30*f*
 communication, 32
 exercises, 32
 operational readiness, 31
 personal and family preparedness, 31–32
 principles, 29–33
 resources and logistics, 31
 threat assessment and risk management, 29
Health center nurse, 125
HHS. *See* US Department of Health and Human Services (HHS)
Home evacuation, considerations and planning for, 15–16
Hospital/acute care nurse, 122–123
Hospital Disaster Preparedness Self-Assessment Tool, 241–242
Hospital emergency command system, 64
Human-made disasters, 4–5
 vs. natural disasters, 226–234
 survival following, 228–230, 229*b*
Hurricane Irma, 164–167
Hurricanes, 159–160

I

Incident command system (ICS), 32, 63–64
Incident management
 advanced or specialized nurses (ASNs), 136–139
 general professional nurse (GPN), 118
Infectious disease outbreaks. *See* Biological disease outbreaks
Institutions of higher learning, 123–124
Intentional infectious disease outbreaks, 213
Interagency coordination, 64–69
International Council of Nurses (ICN), 46, 135, 207–208, 262
International emergency medical teams, 125–126
International Nursing Association for Clinical Simulation and Learning (INACSL), 254–255
International terrorism, 228
Intervention, general professional nurse (GPN), 120

J

Just in time (JIT) training, 49–51

K

Korea Armed Forces Nursing Academy (KAFNA), 143–146

Korean Armed Forces Nurses
  competencies, 143–144
  education courses, 146
  operations, 144–146
Korean Disaster Relief Team for Ebola, 146
Korean military nurses (KMNs), 144–146
Korean War, 144

L

Landslides, 162–163
Law and ethics
  advanced or specialized nurses (ASNs), 139
  general professional nurse (GPN), 122
Legal considerations
  chemical disasters, 207
  persons with disabilities, 14–15
  radiological emergencies, 187
Long-term care nurse, 125

M

Major depressive disorder (MDD), 101
Management of events, 66–67
Mass Casualty Disaster Plan Checklist: A Template for Healthcare Facilities, 241–242
Mass casualty events
  blood products, 44–45
  triage tag used in, 121*f*
Mass casualty incidents (MCI), 30
Medical Reserve Corps, 28–29
Meteorological natural disasters
  climate change, 158
  drought, 157–158
  extreme heat and cold, 160
  flooding, 157
  hurricanes, 159–160
  tornadoes, 158
  tropical storms, 159–160
Methyl isocyanate (MIC), 198–199
Middle East respiratory syndrome (MERS) pandemic, 145, 214
Mobile Army Surgical Hospital (MASH), 144

N

National Incident Management System (NIMS), 32
National League for Nursing (NLN), 124
National Voluntary Organizations Active in Disaster (VOAD), 28–29
Natural disasters, 4
  case study, 285–286
  definition, 152–153
  examples, 152*b*

geological. *See* Geological natural disasters
  vs. human-made disasters, 226–234
meteorological. *See* Meteorological natural disasters
preparation for, 239–240, 239*f*
preparedness, 164–165
recovery, 166–167
response, 165–166
school building safety, 163
Needs assessment, 250
Neurobiology of stress, 83–85
Nonconventional terrorist weapons, 230–234
Nuclear power plant accidents, 175–176, 231*f*
Nuclear terrorism, 231–234
Nuclear weapons, 174–175
Nurses, 6. *See also* Advanced or specialized nurses (ASNs); General professional nurse (GPN)
  disaster preparedness activities, 240–241
  exercises, 254, 257
  obligation to the public, 240
  radiological emergencies, 185–187

O

Occupational accidents, 176
Oklahoma City bombing of 1995, 230
Older adults with cognitive impairment or disabilities, 103–104
Operational readiness, 31
Operation Desert Storm, Iraq, 144–145
Operations-based exercises, 249–250, 250*f*, 251*t*–253*t*
Over-the-counter (OTC) medications, 128

P

People of diverse cultural backgrounds, 104
People with low socioeconomic status, 104
Personal emergency preparedness, 31–32, 45–48
  case study, 55–56, 274–275
  clients, 52–55
  nurse, 51–52
Personal protective equipment (PPE), 14, 15*f*, 202–203
Persons with disabilities, 10–12
  COVID-19 pandemic, 14
PHN. *See* Public health nursing (PHN)
Physical and communication needs, 147
Points of dispensing (POD) clinic, 258–259
Population exposure model, 85–86, 86*f*
Posttraumatic distress disorder (PTSD), 8–9, 101–102, 228–230
Potassium iodide (KI), 167–168, 180–183

Preparedness
  advanced or specialized nurses (ASNs), 136
  chemical disasters
    health facilities, 200
    plans, 200
    risk assessment, 199
  general professional nurse (GPN), 116–117
  persons with disabilities, 12
  radiological emergencies, 183
Professional emergency preparedness, 45–46
  case study, 55–56, 274–275
  nurses, 49–51
Public health disaster management
  advanced or specialized nurses (ASNs), 139–143
  community leaders and villagers, workshop for, 140–141
  COVID-19 epidemic, 141–143, 219–220
Public health nursing (PHN), 123, 258–259
Public Readiness and Emergency Preparedness (PREP) Act, 187
Public service announcements (PSAs), 7

R

Radiological dispersal device (RDD), 175
Radiological dispersion bomb, 231–232
Radiological emergencies
  ethical considerations, 187–189
  instantaneous and near-immediate health concerns, 180
  legal issues, 187
  long-term health concerns, 184
  nurses, 185–187
  potassium iodide, 180–183
  preparedness, 183
  resources, 189–190
  response, 184–187
  shelter and evacuation, 183
  short-term health concerns, 183–184
Radiological exposure device (RED), 175
Radiological terrorism, 231–234
Recovery
  advanced or specialized nurses (ASNs), 139
  chemical disasters, 206–207
  general professional nurse (GPN), 120–122
  persons with disabilities, 8–10
Red Cross, 6, 28–29
Red Cross shelter, 140*f*
Redundant communications, 243
Resiliency, 28–29, 38, 89
Resources
  and logistics, 31
  management, 44–45
  radiological emergencies, 189–190

Resources and assets, sustainability lists of, 243–244
Reverse triage, 74
Risk management, 29
Rural hospital health care coalition, 33

S

Safety and security, 243
  advanced or specialized nurses (ASNs), 139
  general professional nurse (GPN), 118–119
Schools of nursing, 123–124
  disaster preparedness, 45
Self-care, 105–106
Sentinel nuclear events, 176–179
Severe acute respiratory syndrome (SARS), 214
Simple Triage and Rapid Treatment (START), 74
Simulation, exercise, 254–257
SMART criteria, 254
Staffing, 243
Strategic National Stockpile (SNS), 28, 244
Student nurse, 124
Substance use disorders, 101
Supply logistics, 243
Surveillance, 67

T

Tabletop exercises (TTXs), 250, 254
Terrorism
  biological, 230–231
  chemical, 230
  domestic, 228
  nuclear, 231–234
  purpose, 228–230
  radiological, 231–234
Terrorist acts, 228
The Joint Commission (TJC), 28
Threat assessment, 29
Three-level triage, 73–74
Three Mile Island Nuclear Generating Station, 176–178
Tokyo subway attacks, 195, 199
Tornadoes, 158
Transportation accidents, 176
Tropical storms, 159–160
Tsunamis, 162
TTXs. *See* Tabletop exercises (TTXs)

U

Uniform Emergency Volunteer Health Practitioners Act (UEVHPA), 187
Union Carbide India Limited, 198–199

United Nations International Strategy for
    Disaster Reduction (UNISDR),
    38, 240
United Nations Office on Drugs and Crime
    (UNODC), 230
US Department of Health and Human Services
    (HHS), 14–15, 27–28
US Ready Compaign, 45–46
Utilitarian principles, 122
Utilities, 244

V

Vicarious traumatization, 104–105, 105*f*
Vietnam War, 144
Volcanoes, 163
Volunteers, 125
    disaster preparedness, 45

Vulnerable populations, 10–15
    children, 102
    emergency preparedness, 52
    older adults with cognitive impairment or
        disabilities, 103–104
    people of diverse cultural backgrounds, 104
    people with low socioeconomic status, 104

W

World Health Organization (WHO), 6
    emergency medical teams, 125–126
    emergency preparedness plans, 29
    emergency preparedness principles, 29

Z

Zika virus, 214, 217*f*